# AUTOGENIC THERAPY

## WOLFGANG LUTHE, M.D., EDITOR

## Volume V

# DYNAMICS OF AUTOGENIC NEUTRALIZATION

*By* WOLFGANG LUTHE, M.D.

*Dr. med. (Hamburg), L.M.C.C. (Ottawa),*
*Scientific Director, Oskar Vogt Institute,*
*Kyushu University, Fukuoka; (visiting)*
*Professor of Psychophysiologic Therapy,*
*Medical Faculty, Kyushu University, Japan.*
*Formerly Assistant Professor of Psychophysiology,*
*University of Montreal; College of Physicians and*
*Surgeons, Province of Quebec, Montreal, Canada.*

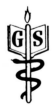

**GRUNE & STRATTON/New York and London**

## AUTOGENIC THERAPY
WOLFGANG LUTHE, M.D., *Editor*

### Vol. I. Autogenic Methods
J. H. SCHULTZ AND W. LUTHE

### Vol. II. Medical Applications
W. LUTHE AND J. H. SCHULTZ

### Vol. III. Applications in Psychotherapy
W. LUTHE AND J. H. SCHULTZ

### Vol. IV. Research and Theory
W. LUTHE

### Vol. V. Dynamics of Autogenic Neutralization
W. LUTHE

### Vol. VI. Treatment with Autogenic Neutralization
W. LUTHE

Volume IV contains the central Bibliography for all six volumes. Volume VI contains additional bibliographic information.

Grune & Stratton, Inc.
757 Third Avenue, New York, New York 10017

Library of Congress Catalog Card Number 70-76888
International Standard Book Number 0-8089-0664-X

Printed in the United States of America (G-B)

# Contents

**VOLUME V: DYNAMICS OF AUTOGENIC NEUTRALIZATION**

## PART IV.  BRAIN-DIRECTED MECHANISMS OF NEUTRALIZATION

## VOLUME I: AUTOGENIC METHODS

### PART I.  METHODS OF AUTOGENIC STANDARD THERAPY

# VOLUME IV:   RESEARCH AND THEORY

## PART I.   PSYCHOPHYSIOLOGIC CHANGES

# Foreword to Volume V

The content of this book and that of Volume VI is an attempt to present a psychophysiologically oriented synopsis of certain brain-directed processes which aim at functional readjustments when given an opportunity to do so.

The method which permitted the observations presented in this volume is called autogenic abreaction. This approach, which is a therapeutic extension of autogenic training, may be regarded as a brain-directed form of psychotherapy.

The text of this volume is divided into five parts. Part I comprises three sections which emphasize various aspects of autogenic discharge activity as occurring during the practice of autogenic standard exercises and their functional relation with processes of brain-directed neutralization during autogenic abreaction. Part II with six sections consists of a detailed discussion of the method of autogenic abreaction. Complementary to Part I and Part II, there follows a presentation of the different psychophysiologic modalities of autogenic neutralization in Part III. In Part IV the reader finds some information about the nature of the most frequently encountered mechanisms of brain-directed neutralization. A careful study of the different sections of Part IV appears to be of basic importance for appreciating the different neutralization-antagonizing and neutralization-facilitating forms of resistance discussed in Part I of Volume VI. Part V consists of the index of authors and the subject index.

The observations and hypotheses submitted in this book may be of particular interest to all those of my colleagues who are engaged in psychoanalytically oriented research and therapy. To others who are interested in psychosomatic medicine and in psychophysiologically oriented research, a general orientation in the vast area of brain-directed dynamics may be of stimulating value.

The purpose of this book is amply fullfilled in case it elicits productive criticism, stimulates further studies of the nature and therapeutic potentialities of brain-directed self-curative processes, and thus contributes to advance our understanding of certain normal and abnormal mental functions.

W. *Luthe*
*Montreal*
*July 1970*

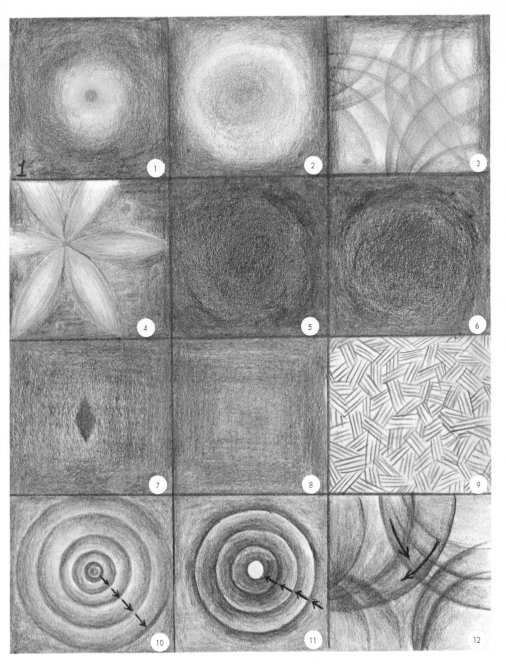

COLOR PLATE 1. Visual phenomena of elementary nature (AA 1, Case 84, p. 198f.).

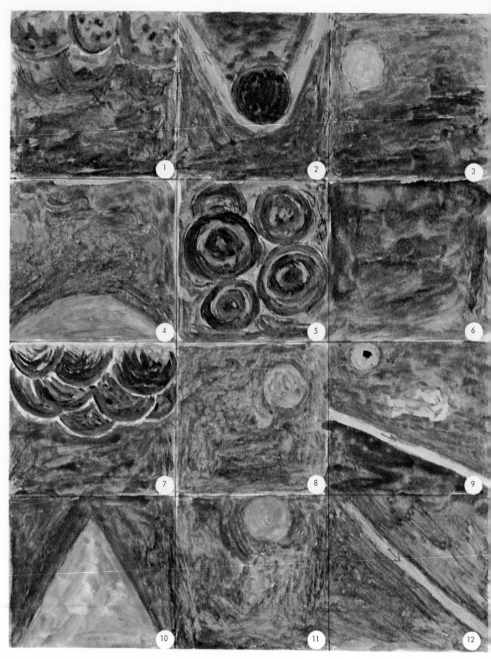

COLOR PLATE 2. Differences in brightness between initial (A) and terminal (B) sequences of visual elaborations restricted to elementary stages II and III (AA 8, Case 85, p. 198f.; see also Fig. 9C, p. 202; Fig. 10, p. 204; Color Plate 4).

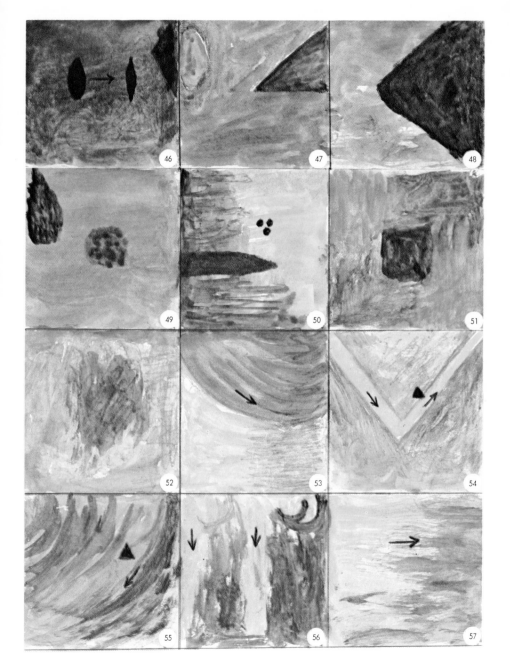

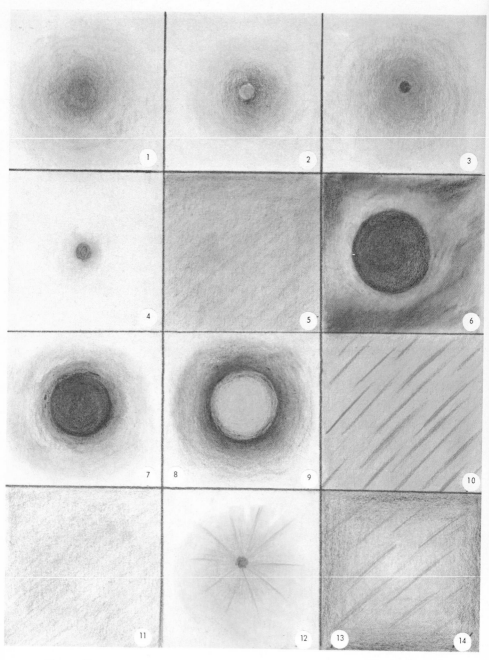

COLOR PLATE 3. Sequences of images (AA 3, Case 87, p. 207f.) with initial emphasis on elementary elaborations. Later appears a series of more differentiated reality-related images of symbolic nature which are characteristic for stage IV. Monothematic repetitions and antithematic sequences are evident.

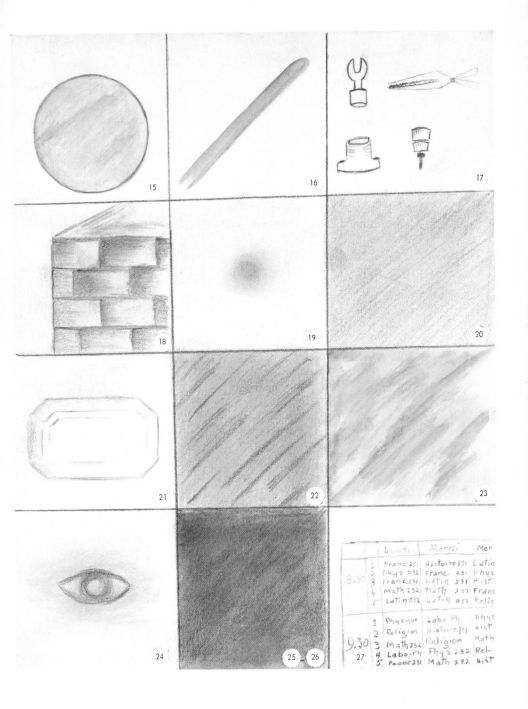

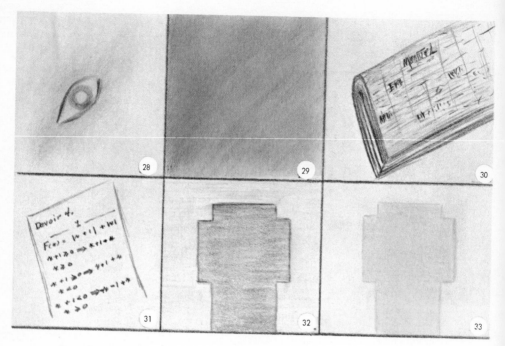

COLOR PLATE 3, continued

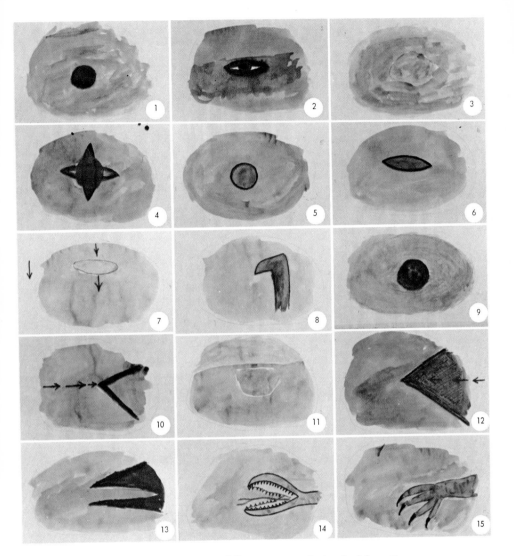

COLOR PLATE 4. Progressive differentiation of visual elaborations.

A. Initial abreactive phase (No. 1-12): structural, chromatic and dynamic components remain restricted to elementary stages of differentiation. A progressive development towards higher degrees of differentiation begins with No. 13 (see Case 88, p. 208-211f.).

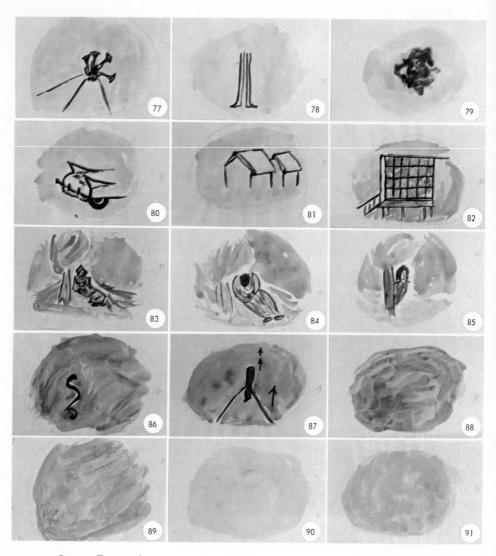

COLOR PLATE 4.

    B. End of central abreactive phase (No. 77-85), and terminal phase (No. 86-91): the images reach advanced stages of structural, chromatic and dynamic differentiation (e.g., No. 82-85) before a shift to elementary elaborations of the terminal phase occurs (see Case 88, p. 218-220; see also Fig. 8, p. 190; Fig. 19, p. 319).

# PART I.  BRAIN-DIRECTED ELABORATIONS DURING AUTOGENIC TRAINING

## 1. Introduction

The hypothesis that there exist biologically given self-regulatory brain activities which aim at a self-curative adjustment of functional disturbances resulting from neuronal material recorded or generated by parts of its own system is not new. Depending on the prevailing contemporary views and knowledge, a variety of neurophysiologically, psychologically, psychopathologically or strictly physiologically oriented efforts have been made to advance our understanding in this area.

The material, tentative conclusions and hypotheses presented in the following sections of this book and in Volume VI are another attempt to advance our understanding of mental functions and to enlarge our psychotherapeutic possibilities.

One of the elements which distinguishes this attempt from others is the assumption that the brain's own computer-like system knows best how certain functional disturbances have come about, where to find the disturbing material or systems,[2326] and what to do to reduce their patho-functional potency.

This assumption evolved partly from the well-known although clinically puzzling observation that the regular practice of passive concentration on autogenic standard formulas has helped to improve an unusually large variety of medical and psychologic disorders. Since it was difficult to believe that the verbal content and structure of the autogenic formulas in combination with passive concentration were alone responsible for bringing about a variety of significant functional adjustments, it seemed logical to conclude that self-regulatory activities of a variety of unknown brain functions participated in such improvements. In this connection it was furthermore assumed that passive concentration on autogenic formulas produced a mental state, the autogenic state, which permitted otherwise inhibited self-regulatory brain functions to engage in activities which aim at normalization of bodily and mentally oriented functional deviations. It was tentatively supposed that a change of cortico-diencephalic interrelations was involved.[1537]

Another category of observations which contributed to the formulation of the assumption that the brain knows best where the trouble is and what to do about it is related to systematic observations and studies of training symptoms (autogenic discharges) which had no apparent rela-

1

tionship to the thematic content and structure of the autogenic formulas used for passive concentration. It was the variety of sensory, motor, olfactory, psychic, visual and other spontaneously occurring training phenomena which clearly indicated that brain-directed self-regulatory mechanisms were actively engaging in the release of impulses from different parts of the brain.[7,20,32,33,35,38,42,72,73,74,75,81,141,149,160,208,212,286,307,363,409,]

[413,414,415,418,419,420,421,423,428,455,557,558,559,560,591,617,639,646,648,662,771,804,811,837,838,875,]
[876,881,882,886,887,888,891,893,894,895,897,899,903,904,931,932,933,977,994,1011,1012,1016,1032,1047,]
[1051,1067,1072,1080,1086,1169,1170,1175,1249,1258,1259,1273,1404,1416,1422,1524,1528,1531,1537,1541,]
[1566,1613,1653,1655,1796,1900,1906,1907,1921,1953,2014,2066,2068,2069,2070,2073,2076,2107,2117,2147,]
[2148,2200a,2221,2248,2284,2289,2994a,2326,2381,2390,2392,2393,2402,2423]

More detailed studies of these training symptoms indicated in many instances a close relationship to the patient's complaints, his actual clinical condition and certain events of his past.[875,876,881,882,886] Furthermore, there were indications that there were differences of autogenic discharge activity in different categories of patients.[887,888,891,899,977,2066,2068,2073,2076,] [2200a] These observations and the close resemblance of autogenic discharges with, for example, spontaneously released sensory and motor discharges during initial phases of O. Vogt's *"fractionirte Methode,"** phenomena described during "sensory isolation," occurring during certain stages of sleep (e.g., motor discharges, dreams, REM, D-state functions) or in connection with different forms of epilepsy,[72,73,74,75,888,891] and response obtained by direct stimulation of cortical and subcortical structures contributed to subsequent development.

It was assumed that there exists a central safety-discharge system (Centrencephalic Safety-discharge System), the self-normalizing activities of which are facilitated during the autogenic state.[875,876,881,882,886,887,] [888,891,894,895] In pursuit of the question of whether it would be possible to enhance the therapeutic effects of autogenic training by giving the brain better opportunity to elaborate or release according to its own self-cura-

---

* E.g., itchiness, feeling of coldness, "congestive" feeling of warmth, visual phenomena, laughing spells, crying, muscular twitches, trembling, swallowing, tearing and tension in certain bodily areas, feelings of weightlessness, sensations of floating or flying, palpitations, intruding thoughts. See:

Brodmann, K.: Zur Methodik der hypnotischen Behandlung. Z. Hypnotismus, 1897, VI, 1–10; VI, 193–214; 1898, VII, 1–35; 228–246; 266–284; 1902, X, 314–375.

Marcinowski, Dr.: Selbstbeobachtungen in der Hypnose. Z. Hypnotismus, 1899/1900, IX, 5–46.

Straaten, Th. van: Zur Kritik der hypnotischen Technik. Z. Hypnotismus, 1899/1900, IX, 129–176; 193–201.

Vogt, C. und Vogt, O.: Wie weit lassen sich schon heute bei Funktionsanomalien des Gehirns anatomische Besonderheiten nachweisen? Nervenarzt, 1950, 21, 337–339 (338).

tive principles, whatever modality is concerned, two technically related though different therapeutic approaches evolved: Autogenic Abreaction and Autogenic Verbalization (see Vol. VI).[32,33,35,38,415,418,893,894,895,897,898,901, 1528,1900,1906,1907,2200a,2284,2536]

Initially attempts at giving the brain a better opportunity to discharge consisted merely of prolongation of the standard exercises and of a subsequent study of the pattern of autogenic discharges from training protocols which the patient wrote after termination of such prolonged exercises. From pattern analyses of autogenic discharges recorded in this manner it became evident that the activity of those brain mechanisms which participated in autogenic discharge functions followed certain self-regulatory principles. For example, it became clear that unknown brain mechanisms permitted a *selective release* of neuronal impulses from various cortical areas of both hemispheres and that such selective processes of discharge also involved relevant subcortical and brain stem systems.

It was also noted that the brain-directed elaborations of autogenic discharges were well adapted to the trainee's level of physiologic and psychologic tolerance. Undue spreading of excitation as it may occur, for example during epileptic seizures, had not been observed.

Furthermore, autogenic discharges were usually of rather brief duration and always *self-terminating*. Such *self-starting* and *self-terminating* discharges also showed a strong tendency for periodic or serial *repetition*. The number of repetitions varied with each patient and the nature of the modality of the physiologic or psychologic discharge. In other words, there was an indication that the number of repetitions was determined by the participating (although unknown) brain mechanisms.

Also, different modalities of autogenic discharge (e.g., motor, sensory, visual, psychical) may occur simultaneously. This was considered as evidence that relevant *brain mechanisms can select and control the release* of neuronal material from different parts of the brain very efficiently.

It was also of clinical interest to note that the occurrence of certain types of discharges tended to decrease progressively and finally disappear. Various *patterns of alternating or rotating processes of discharges* were also observed. The dynamic and qualitative nature of these patterns led to the assumption that the brain-directed discharge activity follows a *brain-designed sequence of programming*.

---

* Vogt, O.: Die möglichen Formen seelischer Einwirkungen in ihrer ärztlichen Bedeutung. *J. Psychol. Neurol.* (*Lpzg.*), 1902–1903, I, 4, 146–160 (159).

Vogt, O.: Vorbemerkungen zu einer ätiologischen Klassifikation der Schizophrenie und anderer funktioneller Psychosen. *Psychiat. Neurol. med. Psychol.* (*Lpzg.*), 1953, 5, 112, 4–8.

More detailed studies of the specific qualities of various types of auto-genic discharge indicated that the brain tends to release sequences of small components of more complex material. This type of "splitting-up for release" was considered as *functional disintegration*. Furthermore, it was observed that such phenomena of functional disintegration may or may not be associated with variable degrees of *functional dissociation* and other manifestations of *functional modifications*.

Against the background of these observations, subsequent studies aimed at a systematic facilitation of brain-controlled release of neuronal impulses related to accumulated disturbing material.[2326] From the pur-suit of relevant hypotheses, a number of psychophysiologically and ther-apeutically oriented technical approaches evolved which proved to be effective in facilitating and promoting brain-directed self-normalizing discharge activities. The following technical elements are considered to be of therapeutic importance:

(a)  A mental shift from initial use of passive concentration on autogenic formulas to a spectator-like attitude, called "passive acceptance" (*carte blanche*).

(b)  Unrestricted verbal description of any kind of brain-directed elab-oration (e.g., sensory, motor, visual, intellectual, olfactory, psychic, gustatory, vestibular).

(c)  The psychophysiologically and therapeutically essential *principle of non-interference*, which is applicable to all patterns of *brain-directed neutralization*, and respects the implications of naturally given mechanisms of neutralization.*

(d)  Correct management of various occurrences of brain-antagonizing forms of resistance (requiring adequate knowledge and experience with normal patterns and with brain-antagonizing dynamics).

(e)  Adequate prolongation of the period of unloading in correspondence with dynamics indicated by the brain (e.g., self-termination).

When these technical approaches are correctly applied to trainees who have mastered the autogenic standard exercises, brain-directed processes of unloading of disturbing material (autogenic abreaction) unfold with an unmatched precision of biologic wisdom.

Progressive psychodynamic and psychophysiologic readjustments re-sult as the self-normalizing brain mechanisms are given adequate oppor-tunity to pursue their own program of multidimensional therapeutic activities.

---

* Not directed by the therapist, as is the practice, for example, with others using non-autogenic approaches[29,32,33,60,69,106,119,347,348,377,625,658,667,686,716,719,725,726,727,730,832,833,834,835,836,837,838,839,1108,1110,1629,1653,1655,1723,1725,1726,1728,1733,1755,1756,1829,2059,2170,2209,2302,2318,2341,2342,2422,2432] (see also Glossary, Vol. VI).

The nature of the prolonged, brain-directed process of neutralization during autogenic abreaction is essentially the same as discussed in connection with autogenic discharges (see above). However, as the patient remains passive and maintains the unrestricted implications of *carte blanche*, the sophisticated, computer-like dynamics of brain-directed processes of self-normalization become more evident.

Because of the close relationship between autogenic discharges occurring during autogenic training and the thematically more complex processes of brain-directed neutralization, a few selected data reflecting variations in autogenic discharge activity during the practice of standard exercises are briefly discussed in the following section.

# 2. Modalities and Patterns of Autogenic Discharge Activity

Since the beginning of autogenic training it has been observed by J. H. Schultz[1249,1258,1259,1273] and many others that passive concentration on autogenic standard formulas may result in bringing about two coexisting categories of responses: formula-related responses and formula-unrelated reactions. Formula-related responses are defined as psychophysiologic phenomena which are in direct agreement with the thematic content and topographic orientation of a given formula (e.g., "My right arm is heavy," "Heartbeat calm and regular"). Other physiologic phenomena which may also occur during the practice of autogenic exercises (e.g., tingling in the left foot, sensations of floating, borborygmus) are considered as formula-unrelated reactions. Formula-related responses may be considered as being largely the result of the *trainee-directed* functions of passive concentration on autogenic formulas, while formula-unrelated reactions may be considered as psychophysiologically associated changes which involve a variety of *brain-directed* self-regulatory activities which appear to be facilitated by the particular functional nature of different psychophysiologic stages of the autogenic state (see p. 3 ff./IV). Both categories of training phenomena are of therapeutic interest during treatment with various combinations of autogenic methods (see Vols. I, II, III and IV).

Formula-related sensations, such as heaviness and warmth, are phenomena which may vary from one autogenic exercise to the next. A number of patients may not experience any sensations of heaviness (see Table 1). During autogenic abreaction the feeling of heaviness is also variable. Certain phases of brain-directed neutralization may be associated with very intense feelings of heaviness (see Case 15, p. 64; Case 82, p. 184), while others are dominated by other modalities of brain-directed elaborations (e.g., turning, floating).[423] Such observationos indicate that the formula-related experience of heaviness sensations frequently associated with autogenic training appears to play a particular psychophysiologic role during the *induction phase* (see p. 38 ff.). However, during the abreactive period, the psychophysiologic significance of the sensation of heaviness seems to shift under the influence of brain-directed thematically related dynamics of neutralization (see Case 15, p. 64; Case 82, p. 184).

The formula-related experience of sensations of warmth also varies considerably during autogenic training (see Table 1). During autogenic

Table 1.  *Formula-related Sensations of Heaviness and Warmth during
Autogenic Standard Exercises*
(Psychosomatic and Neurotic Patients)

| Sensations of Heaviness, Warmth and Paradoxic Reactions | Autogenic Standard Exercises | | | | | |
|---|---|---|---|---|---|---|
| | I (N = 100) (%) | II (N = 96) (%) | III (N = 49) (%) | IV (N = 66) (%) | V (N = 46) (%) | VI (N = 48) (%) |
| 1. *Heaviness* (total) | 89.0 | 88.5 | 87.7 | 87.9 | 87.0 | 90.5 |
| (a) Cranial region | 27.0 | 17.7 | 16.3 | 13.6 | 13.0 | 14.3 |
| (b) Trunk | 36.0 | 63.5 | 63.3 | 60.6 | 60.8 | 64.3 |
| (c) Legs | 78.0 | 86.4 | 87.7 | 87.9 | 84.8 | 85.7 |
| (d) Arms | 86.0 | 86.4 | 83.7 | 87.9 | 89.8 | 85.7 |
| (e) Paradoxic reactions | 14.0 | 2.1 | 4.1 | 4.5 | 4.3 | 4.8 |
| 2. *Warmth* (total) | 77.0 | 92.7 | 95.9 | 89.4 | 91.3 | 90.5 |
| (a) Cranial region | 29.0 | 37.5 | 26.5 | 22.7 | 43.5 | 28.6 |
| (b) Trunk | 29.0 | 44.8 | 61.2 | 57.6 | 60.8 | 59.5 |
| (c) Legs | 46.0 | 70.8 | 87.7 | 86.4 | 87.0 | 83.3 |
| (d) Arms | 59.0 | 86.4 | 92.8 | 84.8 | 82.6 | 88.1 |
| (e) Paradoxic reactions | — | 29.2 | 26.5 | 16.7 | 21.7 | 26.2 |

abreaction the feeling of warmth seems to assume a particular psycho-physiologic significance therapeutically. Intensive feelings of warmth are usually reported after particularly disturbing subjective material has been released and significant progress in brain-desired directions has been made (Case 16, p. 71). A feeling of warmth is also frequently associated with elaborations characteristic for terminal phases (see Case 14, p. 63) and occasionally encountered during or after a "Bright Light Phase" (see Vol. VI). Since such developments tend to occur during later phases of the abreactive period, these reactions appear to be similar to those reported by J. H. Schultz in *Über Schichtenbildung im hypnotischen Selbstbeobachten* (1920),[1245,2379] and earlier observations by A. Döllken (1896).[2326,G/VI*] It is also apparent that the psychophysiologic mechanisms which lead to a formula-related experience of feelings of warmth are not exactly the same as those which promote a feeling of warmth during thematic neutralization.

Formula-related reactions to other standard formulas (see Fig. 1a,b,c) are also subject to considerable variations. Their occurrence during autogenic abreaction tends to vary with the particular nature of the topic under neutralization. The formula-related experience of coolness in the forehead area during autogenic abreaction is rare.

* See Glossary, Vol. VI

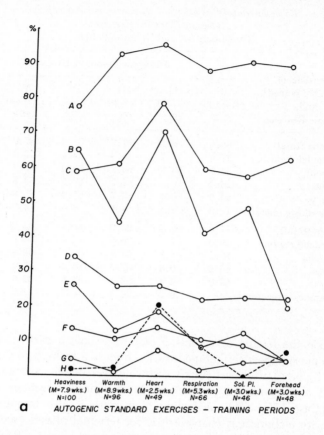

Fig. 1. Variations of discharge activity during autogenic standard exercises. Changes associated with the third standard formula (a), the fourth standard formula (b), and the fifth standard formula (c).

(a) Increase of autogenic discharge activity during the third standard exercise: feeling of warmth (A); circulatory sensations (B); visual phenomena (C); feeling of swelling (D); electrical sensations (E); perspiration (F); decrease of salivation (G); pain in left chest (H).

(b) Increase of autogenic discharge activity during the fourth standard exercise: feeling of tingling (A); feelings of anxiety (B); involuntary movements (C); feeling of detachment (D); changes of body image (E).

(c) Increase of autogenic discharge activity during the fifth standard exercise: twitching of muscles (A); pain-like sensations (B); intruding thoughts (C); feeling of pressure (D); feeling of tension (E); dizziness (F); borborygmus (G); feeling of warmth, cranial region (H); trembling (I); salivation increased (J); feeling of warmth, chest (K).

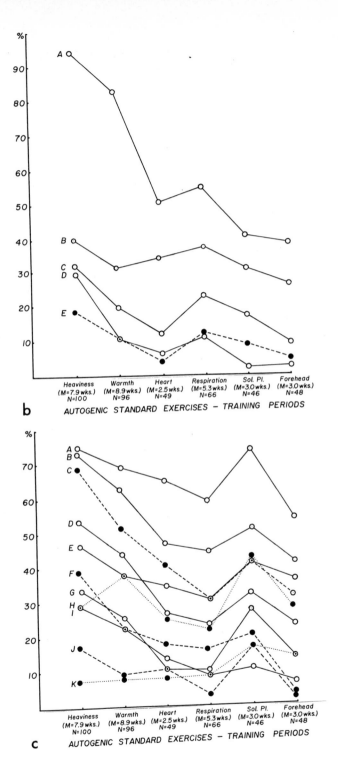

**b**  AUTOGENIC STANDARD EXERCISES - TRAINING PERIODS

**c**  AUTOGENIC STANDARD EXERCISES - TRAINING PERIODS

Of further interest in connection with the use of passive concentration on autogenic standard formulas as a preparatory phase (see *Induction Phase*, p. 38 ff.) for subsequent engagement in brain-directed dynamics of autogenic neutralization are certain sensory and motor reactions which were found to be associated with the third, fourth, fifth and sixth standard formulas (see Fig. 1). For example, in certain trainees, the third standard exercise (heart) was found to be associated with a significant increase of (a) decreased salivation, (b) difficulty in respiration, (c) onset of tachycardia,[455] (d) palpitations, (e) pain and disagreeable sensations in the left chest, (f) sensations of warmth in the trunk, (g) increase of circulatory sensations, (h) increase of disagreeable feelings in general and (i) increase of differentiated elaborations of visual phenomena (see Fig. 1a). During the fourth standard exercise (respiration), a significant increase of discharge activity was noted in the following modalities: (a) twitching in the cranial area and (b) involuntary movement (see Fig. 1b). In a number of trainees the solar plexus formula was associated with significant increase of (a) twitching, (b) salivation, (c) borborygmus, (d) sensations of warmth in the cranial area, (e) sensations of warmth in the abdomen and chest and (f) drowsiness (see Fig. 1c). The activation of these specific reactions in a certain number of patients indicates that the thematic content and topographic orientation of the standard formulas (e.g., SE III, SE IV, SE V) may participate in triggering the unloading of neuronal impulses from thematically related disturbing material.

To avoid such technically undesirable reactions in the beginning of autogenic abreactions, passive concentration during the induction phase (see p. 38 ff.) has been limited to the heaviness formulas of the first standard exercise.

The variety of autogenic discharges (formula-unrelated reactions) occuring during the practice of autogenic standard exercises (see Vols. I, II, III and IV) can be classified in groups according to their physiologic or psychic nature (see Table 2).

A high incidence and great diversity of autogenic discharges were found in psychosomatic and neurotic patients who had a history of severe accidents with injury to the cranial region (see Fig. 2)[875,881,882,886,887,888] and in an ecclesiastic group of patients who suffered from a variety of psychodynamic disorders, multiple psychophysiologic reactions and brain-disturbing consequences related to negatively oriented variables of religious education[428] in combination with chronic affective and heterosexual deprivation (see Fig. 2).[887,888,899,977,2066,2068]

A particularly great diversity and high frequencies of autogenic discharges were noted in patients who had suffered severe accidents and

TABLE 2. *Training Phenomena during Autogenic Standard Exercises*

| Categories | Modalities of Training Phenomena |
|---|---|
| **1. *Motor*** | |
| (a) Somatomotor | Twitching, jerking, trembling, involuntary movements, muscular tension |
| (b) Reflexmotor | Coughing, laughing, twitching of eyelids, sneezing, crying, swallowing, yawning, sucking, vomiting |
| (c) Visceromotor | Changes of respiration, heart action (e.g., palpitations, tachycardia, cramp-like sensations), gastrointestinal motor activity (e.g., cramp-like sensations, borborygmus), salivation, perspiration, urogenital functions (e.g., erection, ejaculation, orgasm, vaginal contractions, micturition) |
| **2. *Sensory*** | |
| (a) Somatosensory | Heaviness, warmth, coolness, burning, tingling, numbness, pain, pressure, circulatory sensations (e.g., pulsations, blood-flow), tension, electrical sensations, feeling of stiffness, lameness as if paralyzed, swelling, itching, restlessness, disagreeable feelings (nonspecific) *Changes of body image:* detachment of parts of body, disappearance of specific deformation of parts of body |
| (b) Viscerosensory | Pain and disagreeable sensations in throat, feeling of suffocation or strangulation, oppressed respiration, pain or other disagreeable feelings in the abdominal area, feeling of pressure or cramp-like sensations in the stomach, circulatory sensations in abdomen, nausea, feeling of hunger, urge to urinate, sensations in chest and cardiac area (e.g., pressure, tension, circulatory disturbance, pain, warmth) |
| (c) Other | Sleep, drowsiness |
| **3. *Vestibular*** | Dizziness, vertiginous sensations, turning, spinning, floating, sinking, flying, lopsidedness, displacement, falling, rocking, swinging |
| **4. *Auditory*** | Simple tones, noise, buzzing, music, voices |
| **5. *Olfactory*** | Agreeable, disagreeable sensations |
| **6. *Gustatory*** | Related to food, others (e.g., varnish, wood, sperm) |
| **7. *Visual*** | Uniform colors, cloud-like formations, shadows, simple forms, objects (static, dynamic), faces, differentiated images, film-strips, cinerama-strips |
| **8. *Affective*** | Anxiety, fear, depression, euphoria, longing for love and affection, feeling of loneliness, insecurity |
| **9. *Ideational*** | Intruding thoughts (difficulty of concentration), memories, planning |

12

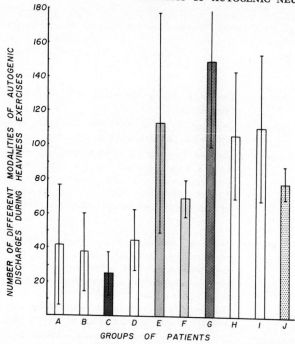

FIG. 2. Number of different modalities (diversity) of autogenic discharges noted during corresponding periods of heaviness training in different groups of patients.

Group A: 40 female patients (psychodynamic disorders, psychophysiologic reactions): M=41.20; S.D.=35.28.

Group B: 20 male patients (psychodynamic disorders, psychophysiologic reactions): M=37.40; S.D.=22.29.

Group C: 17 female and 3 male patients (moderate depressive reaction): M=25.45; S.D.=13.13.

Group D: 15 patients without severe accidents (control group for E): M=44.20; S.D.=18.40.

Group E: 15 patients who had suffered one or several accidents (anxiety reaction, multiple psychophysiologic reactions): M=113.93; S.D.=55.80.

Group F: 7 patients of Group E (non-ecclesiastic): M=71.30; S.D.=19.05.

Group G: 8 patients of group E (ecclesiastic): M=151.30; S.D.=53.85.

Group H: 25 male patients without severe accidents members of one specific order (psychodynamic disorders, multiple psychophysiologic reactions): M=105.68; S.D.=36.71.

Group I: 3 female and 25 male patients without severe accidents (members of various religious communities: psychodynamic disorders, multiple psychophysiologic reactions): M=110.83; S.D.=43.40.

Group J: 10 male patients without severe accidents (personality disorder, homosexuality): M=77.60; S.D.=10.20.

who also belonged to the ecclesiastic group (see Fig. 2). Low levels of autogenic discharge activity and diversity are usually observed in moderate to severe depressive reactions, with particularly low discharge activity in states of psychotic depression. Autogenic discharges are also less frequent in persons who enjoy a normal state of health and in others who have practiced autogenic standard exercises regularly over prolonged periods.

In schizophrenic patients the same modalities of autogenic discharges observable in psychosomatic and neurotic patients tend to occur.[2147,2148] Certain differences in the discharge profile between schizophrenic patients and others with psychosomatic and neurotic disorders appear to be influenced by ECT.[2073] The group of schizophrenics who had received ECT had a significantly ($P < .01$) higher rate of sensations of lameness, weakness and feelings of paralysis than other schizophrenics (without ECT) and psychoneurotic patients. The ECT group also reported a higher incidence of feelings of floating and sinking and significantly higher levels of feelings associated with distortions of the body image (see Fig. 8E, p. 49/III). It is of further interest that schizophrenic patients with ECT had an unusually low ($P < .01$; $P < .02$) rate of circulatory sensations (e.g., pulsation) than other groups of patients (see Fig. 8B, p. 49/III). Significant differences in circulatory discharge modalities were also noted between groups of patients with and without "ecclesiogenic syndrome" (see Fig. 6, p. 39/II). Other significant differences in sensory and motor discharge activity existed between groups with different degrees of sexual deprivation (see Table 8, p. 120/IV; Fig. 44, p. 122/IV).

Other studies have shown that the release of different modalities of autogenic discharges (e.g., motor, sensory) follows a phasic pattern (see Fig. 3, p. 20/III) in which certain modalities appear to assume thematic priority over others (see Fig. 3).

Although bilateral and generalized motor and sensory discharges do occur, the brain-directed discharge activities emphasize the release of sensory and motor modalities which are limited to topographically circumscribed areas. There are no apparent indications that the release of one specific modality (e.g., motor, sensory) always assumes general priority over others. In certain patients the general profile of autogenic discharge activity may show a clear emphasis on sensory discharges; in others there is a dominance of motor discharges; and in many cases no particular emphasis is evident (see Fig. 4A and B). More detailed pattern analyses do reveal that the discharge of certain sensory or motor modalities occurs in phases (see Fig. 3A and B; Fig. 7, p. 180; Fig. 3, p. 20/III). Thus, the sequence of release of specific discharge modalities fol-

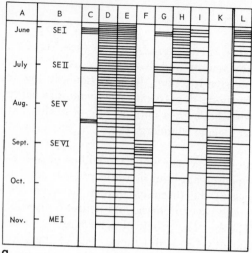

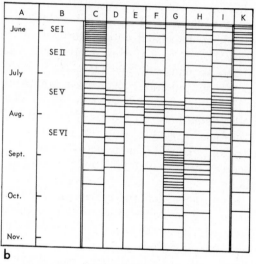

FIG. 3. Phasic patterns of progressively decreasing autogenic discharge activity during treatment with autogenic training in two psychomatic patients. *Code for Fig. 3a:* A. = Months of autogenic training. B. = Standard exercises practiced. C. = Motor discharges. D. = Circulatory phenomena. E. = Feelings of weakness and asthenia. F. = Borborygmus. G. = Other modalities. H. = Memories. I. = Visual landscapes. K. = Visual other reality images, faces. L. = Clinical symptoms.

*Code for Fig. 3b:* A and B as above. C. = Palpitations. D. = Feeling of numbness in cranial region. E. = Abdominal spasms. F. = Visual rural scenes. G. = Visual, monsters. H. = Feelings of anxiety. I. = Drowsiness. K. = Clinical symptoms. (Courtesy of S. Maeda, K. Aramaki, and S. Sato, Oskar Vogt Institute, Kyushu University, Fukuoka, Japan)[2076]

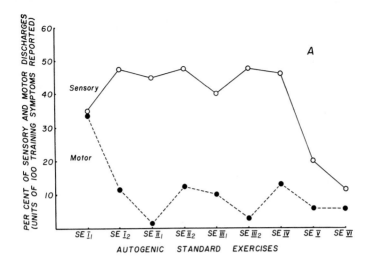

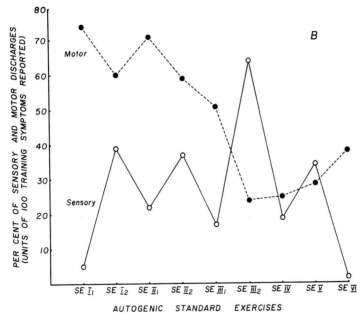

Fig. 4. Individual differences in motor and sensory discharge activity during autogenic training.

A. A 23-year-old female student (anxiety reaction, multiple psychophysiologic and phobic reactions) with dominance of sensory discharges (e.g., numbness, burning, itching, pressure pain, tingling).

B. A 49-year-old theologian (anxiety reaction, multiple psychophysiologic and phobic reactions) with a dominance of motor discharges during SE I-III, IV and VI.

lows a brain-designed pattern of thematic priority which varies from case to case. This agrees with observations of brain-directed dynamics which determine the release of more complex neuronal material during autogenic abreaction.

During the practice of autogenic training over prolonged periods, a general trend of gradually decreasing discharge activity can be noted (see Fig. 1, p. 8-9). A similar trend can be observed during autogenic abreaction. However, from a comparison of brain-directed discharge activity occurring during autogenic training with brain-directed processes of thematic neutralization during autogenic abreaction, it is evident that, in spite of many similarities, there are a number of therapeutically important psychophysiologic differences. Although the same sensory, motor, psychic and other modalities of brain-directed elaborations are released during autogenic training and during autogenic abreaction, the participating brain functions do not seem to operate on the same level of psychophysiologic integration and self-curative efficiency. It appears that the trainee-directed mental activity of passive concentration on autogenic formulas exerts a functionally restricting effect on brain-directed activities of self-regulatory normalization, and that under these circumstances (i.e., during AT) only a relatively limited amount of brain-disturbing neuronal impulses is accessible to the self-regulatory brain activities which aim at functional readjustment. In other words, during autogenic training, brain-disturbing material of a specific nature cannot be dealt with, and the brain-directed self-normalizing activities are obliged to emphasize disturbing material of a less specific nature which is more at the functional periphery of complicated and close-knit complexes of thematic material with particular disturbing potency. This assumption may in part explain why the therapeutic effects of autogenic training are variable in certain categories of functional disorders and relatively limited or unsatisfactory in others (e.g., those with history of severe accidents,[360,612,1758] sexual deviations). Other brain-restricting effects associated with autogenic training appear to be related to the fact that non-verbalized observations and engagement in brain-directed ideational processes which are not vocally expressed result in inhibitory effects which are not helpful to the psychophysiologic needs of those brain mechanisms which wish to engage in more complex and therapeutically more efficient processes of self-regulatory readjustment.

# 3. Autogenic Reactivity and the Beginning of Autogenic Abreaction

It has been emphasized often that the application of autogenic training is not only of value as a therapeutic approach in itself, but also that the method may play the clinically helpful role of a therapeutic filter (*therapeutische Siebfunktion*).[141,1796] In other words, the patient's reactivity during treatment with autogenic training and his therapeutic response may provide valuable information in determining the nature of a patient-adapted treatment program. It was, incidentally, in connection with the use of autogenic training as a transitional therapeutic support in certain cases which were thought to need psychoanalysis but where the final decision to employ it was postponed, that unexpectedly favorable improvements were noted and the original intention of applying psychoanalytic treatment was abandoned. In other instances the patient's collaboration during attempted treatment with autogenic training was so poor that only certain forms of clinical treatment (e.g., medication, hypnosis, subcoma insulin treatment, frontal lobe surgery) appeared to be the therapeutic answer. Other patients who collaborated well over longer periods but who did not show a desirable therapeutic response in certain areas of disturbances agreed more readily to engage in more specific and intensive forms of therapy.

In the field of autogenic therapy the patient's collaboration during treatment with autogenic training, his reactivity and his treatment response are particularly helpful in adapting, selecting, modifying and timing the application of special formulas or methods of autogenic neutralization.

When autogenic abreaction is applied, it is desirable that the patient practices autogenic standard exercises regularly and demonstrates that his therapeutic collaboration is reliable. His protocols, which are a preparatory task for more intensive therapeutic homework during later periods when autogenic abreaction is applied, are usually a valuable source of information in various respects. Those patients who do not find time to keep useful training protocols may find it even more difficult to engage in more time-consuming homework during treatment with autogenic abreaction. Unless it is practically possible to carry out a large portion of the therapeutic work under clinical conditions, it is suggested that autogenic abreaction should not be started with patients who are not able or not sufficiently motivated to contribute to their own therapeutic progress in a serious and reliable manner. The group of patients with

hysterical reactivity requires particular attention. Only after these patients have clearly shown that they are sufficiently motivated to help
themselves and that they have gained enough insight into their negatively
oriented dynamics to not use the treatment effort as another playground
for self-satisfying therapeutically destructive purposes can the application of autogenic abreaction be considered. In cases where autogenic
abreaction is applied to patients with hysterical personality who are not
motivated to contribute positively and who are allowed to extend their
negatively oriented maneuvers into the technical area of autogenic abreaction, formidable difficulties due to an unending series of patient-pro-
voked technical errors may be expected. However, once patients in this
category have decided for themselves that it is in their own interest to
collaborate in a positively oriented manner, very satisfactory progress is
possible.

The patient's training protocols are also a valuable source of information where changes in autogenic discharge activity are concerned. It is
in this respect that the general recommendation to postpone the introduction of autogenic abreaction (as long as therapeutic ground can be
gained through the beneficial effects of autogenic training) must be
adapted to the patient's reactivity during autogenic training. As long as
no particularly disturbing modalities of brain-directed elaborations are
noted, there is no particular technical reason to begin with autogenic
abreaction before the patient has learned all the standard exercises. However, depending on the patient's clinical condition and the brain-disturbing potency of the accumulated underlying material, the pattern of autogenic reactivity may include a progressively increasing number of disturbing phenomena before the trainee has learned all standard exercises.
Restlessness, vestibular modalities, pain, headaches, bursts of anxiety,
repeated episodes of disagreeable somesthetic sensations, inability to continue exercises as technically required, massive interference from intruding thoughts and progressively more frequent appearance of differentiated visual phenomena are some of the training phenomena which
indicate that the patient's brain presses for a more adequate opportunity
to engage in self-curative activity. When these brain-directed indications
of autogenic reactivity are not respected, the trainee may develop increasing resistance to autogenic training and abandon therapy. In about
10 to 15 per cent of psychosomatic and neurotic patients such brain-
directed developments become prominent within two weeks after the
beginning of autogenic training (see Table 3, p. 19), and the therapist
is confronted with the question as to whether autogenic abreaction can
be started or not. Under generally favorable circumstances such early

TABLE 3.   *Weeks of Autogenic Standard Training Preceding the Beginning*
*of Autogenic Abreaction*
(100 Psychosomatic and Neurotic Patients)

| Weeks of AT | 1–2 | 3–4 | 5–6 | 7–8 | 9–12 | 13–16 | 17–20 | 21–28 | 29–36 | 37–52 | 53–200 |
|---|---|---|---|---|---|---|---|---|---|---|---|
| Number of patients | 13 | 23 | 13 | 8 | 15 | 7 | 4 | 7 | 4 | 1 | 5 |

application of autogenic abreaction may be justified. In other instances it may be indicated that further advanced phases of autogenic standard training be reached before autogenic abreaction is applied. The temporary application of neuroleptic medication may help to achieve this goal. When autogenic abreaction cannot be applied for practical, technical or medical reasons, it is advisable to instruct the patient to practice longer series of very brief exercises (e.g., 10–20 sec./exercise) which makes it easier to maintain more adequate levels of formula-related passive concentration and thus give less opportunity to the brain to engage in disturbing discharges of formula-unrelated elaborations. In most of those cases supportive medication (e.g., meprobamate, chlordiazepoxide) is a valuable adjunct.

# PART II. METHODS OF AUTOGENIC ABREACTION

## 4. Preparatory Information

The actual technical introduction of autogenic abreaction as a complementary approach to autogenic standard therapy is usually preceded by a number of patient-adapted preparatory discussions. It is generally advisable to engage in such preparatory discussions at the earliest point which is clinically possible, when there is sufficient evidence (e.g., case history, diagnosis, reactivity to AT) indicating that it may be necessary or advantageous to apply autogenic abreaction at a later point.

In certain instances, for example, when the initial psychosomatic evaluation indicates involvement of complex psychodynamic disorders (e.g., homosexuality, severe accidents, anxiety reactions of long duration) and a patient expresses the hope that the practice of autogenic exercises may cure his difficulties, it is clinically important to dispel such over-optimistic and potentially frustrating attitudes. In these cases the helpfulness and basic importance of the regular practice of autogenic exercises should be emphasized, but it must be pointed out that the effectiveness of autogenic training has certain limits and that autogenic training is by no means a magic panacea. During such a clarification it is, however, equally important to encourage the patient by simply stating that complementary approaches specifically adapted to his particular therapeutic needs are available and may be used at a later point if necessary. At this point in the discussion many patients express their interest in the technical details of the contemplated approaches. While such interest may be welcome, it would be confusing and to the disadvantage of the patient to explain, for example, the technique of autogenic abreaction. As the patient is made to understand that technical details of the method are only explained at the time of its actual application, it may be useful to mention that the technique(s) contemplated is in certain respects similar to autogenic training, and that the regular practice of autogenic standard exercises is of basic importance and will be continued in any case. Depending on the patient's clinical situation, his practical possibilities and his intelligence, one may go on to explain that after an initial learning period, and as the patient shows reliable collaboration, he may be allowed to carry out the major portion of that treatment phase at home; and in that case a tape recorder[294] might be a valuable instrument which greatly facilitates therapeutic work at home.

In some instances it also may be helpful to mention that many patients are sufficiently motivated in advancing their own treatment and in economizing on medical expenses to work 10, 15 or more hours a week at home with the help of a tape recorder. The patient's further questions about the exact purpose of the tape recorder, the type of tape recorder needed and other technical details should be referred to a specific discussion at a later date.

Although the use of a tape recorder is very helpful for the therapist and many patients, treatment through autogenic abreaction may be conducted without recordings, by simply taking notes or writing summaries after termination of an autogenic abreaction. A patient should not be left with the impression that successful treatment is impossible without the help of a tape recorder.

Where such technically non-specific preparatory discussions are conducted in the course or toward the end of the patient's initial psychosomatic evaluation, it is therapeutically important to maintain all possible flexibility and to point out clearly that at this time it is very difficult to predict the patient's therapeutic progress, and that the discussion only deals with a possibility which may or may not be considered as the treatment progresses.

In many cases it cannot be foreseen whether or not autogenic abreaction may be needed at a later point, and relevant preparatory discussions may only be considered after several weeks or months of autogenic standard training.

## General Orientation

When autogenic abreaction is therapeutically indicated but cannot be applied for various reasons (e.g., unreliable collaboration, unfavorable circumstances interfering with regular medical control and therapeutic homework), the method should not be mentioned.

Under clinically and otherwise favorable circumstances, when the actual introduction of autogenic abreaction is planned for the near future, a well-timed preparatory discussion of a more specific nature is indicated. In the course of such a discussion and after it has become clear that the patient is sufficiently motivated to engage more actively in his treatment, the following changes in the therapeutic pattern may be included in preparatory discussion:

1. *Changes related to frequency and duration of appointments.*

Since a patient who is proceeding through the six standard exercises of autogenic training is usually seen once a week or once every two weeks for about 30 to 60 minutes, it is important to explain to him that the "new approach" (AA) requires more time. In the beginning, as the trainee proceeds through a learning phase, the appointments last about 60 to 90 minutes (sometimes longer) and are spaced at intervals of about 7 to 14 days. Only in relatively few instances unexpected developments may temporarily require two appointments per week. During later phases, when the patient has repeatedly demonstrated that he can engage in autogenic abreactions in a technically satisfactory manner, he may be asked to carry out unsupervised autogenic abreactions at home (see below, see p. 23 f.). About 45 per cent of a group of 200 patients suffering from various psychodynamic disorders were able to perform autogenic abreactions at home after less than 10 supervised sessions, another 20 per cent after 15 AAs, 15 per cent needed between 16 and 30 AAs to arrive at a satisfactory level of technical management, and about 20 per cent required longer series of supervised autogenic abreactions. Depending largely on the nature of the clinical condition and the patient's intelligence, a variable 10 to 15 per cent cannot be give permission to engage in autogenic abreactions without medical supervision.

The duration and frequency of office appointments for patients who are permitted to engage in unsupervised autogenic abreactions at home varies largely with the intensity and quality of each patient's therapeutic homework. A patient who manages to carry out three or four autogenic abreactions at home within a week obviously requires more time to discuss his work during the next control appointment than another patient who has only managed one autogenic abreaction within ten days.

During further advanced phases of treatment with autogenic abreaction, experienced and reliably working patients may require control sessions at intervals from two to four weeks.

As a number of patients prefer to continue the practice of autogenic abreactions after their treatment is considered as being terminated, and as there are experienced cases who require long-term maintenance programs, the frequency and duration of control appointments may eventually be adapted to the patient's wishes and suggestions.

2. *Changes related to the pattern of therapeutic homework.*

This phase of the preparatory discussion is limited to a general discussion of time and the circumstances required to carry out the therapeutic homework in connection with autogenic abreactions. Specific technical details of the nature of the patient's therapeutic homework are only given *after* the first AA has been performed in the therapist's office (see p. 27 ff., p. 96 ff.).

During the learning phase, when autogenic abreactions are only carried out in the therapist's office, most patients (with tape recorder) may need about four to six hours of therapeutic homework per week (e.g., transcript of AA, commentary; see p. 103 ff.) in addition to their habitual pattern of practicing autogenic training regularly. However, as the nature of therapeutic homework varies with the nature of the pattern of different types of autogenic abreactions and the working capacity of each patient, there are many variations. In certain cases it may be of therapeutic advantage to eliminate therapeutic homework altogether, or to limit the patient's contribution to relatively simple and easily performed tasks (e.g., "Perhaps you can make some notes about what you think of this autogenic abreaction").

When patients are technically far enough advanced to do autogenic abreactions at home, it is largely up to the patient to decide how much time he would like to spend in advancing the progress of his treatment. Since advanced patients can see what their brain produces and how processes of autogenic neutralization work to their own advantage, many patients become sufficiently motivated to work 10 to 15 or more hours per week to make further progress.

3. *Environmental requirements.*

Therapeutic homework in connection with autogenic abreaction is difficult or impossible to carry out unless the patient can retire into a room where he can work undisturbed and talk aloud without having to worry that someone may overhear him. This requirement demands the understanding collaboration of other persons living in the same household. Where this requirement cannot be met, autogenic abreactions cannot be carried out at home, the frequency and duration of office visits must be increased, and various other therapeutically unfavorable consequences tend to arise. For these reasons it might be better in many instances not to start treatment with autogenic abreactions unless sufficiently favorable environmental circumstances have been arranged (e.g., change of apartment).

It is also important to explain to the patient that during the learning period, or until the patient has demonstrated repeatedly that he has obtained sufficient technical knowledge to be able to manage satisfactorily during brain-directed neutralization without the therapist's assistance, it would be medically inadvisable to plan journeys or vacations which might last longer than five or eight days. This recommendation was adopted after unfortunate experiences were reported by patients who were unexpectedly confronted with certain brain-directed developments while being far removed from the therapist and having no opportunity to ask his advice or to follow an adequate pattern of control sessions. Generally it is recommended to plan a three to four month period during which an uninterrupted and well-controlled learning program can be carried out.

Since it is therapeutically desirable that a patient acquires satisfactory working knowledge with autogenic abreaction as early as possible, it is also to his advantage to arrange his occupational activities in such a manner that he has sufficient time and energy to work productively on his autogenic abreactions. Autogenic abreactions should not be started with patients who are confronted with a period of work overload or demanding and time-consuming activities.

Another factor which requires some preparation is related to the technical necessity that all material related to treatment with autogenic abreaction must be securely locked and protected at all times. The file or box containing the AA reports should be labeled with instructions that the content is of strictly personal nature and is to be turned over unopened to the therapist in case of an accident or on the patient's request. In cases where this security measure is not observed, therapeutically unfavorable complications may easily result from brain-antagonizing forms of resistance during autogenic abreaction.

4. *Other facilitating items.*

Whenever possible and indicated it is of great therapeutic and economic advantage to use a tape-recorder[294] during treatment with autogenic abreaction. While a technical discussion of the exact therapeutic nature of the role of the tape recorder is postponed until the actual introduction of autogenic abreaction, it is necessary to specify certain technical requirements and perhaps make some specific recommendations as to the usefulness of certain types and brands of tape recorders. In particular the following specifications need to be considered:

(a) *uninterrupted* recording time of at least 90 minutes,
(b) portability,
(c) operation on both batteries and power outlets,
(d) earphones and foot control,
(e) reliable repair service, which will not leave the patient without his machine for longer than about one week.

Furthermore, it is recommended that the patient be encouraged to learn or to improve his typewriting abilities and to secure a typewriter. Without going into the details of the future homework program, it may be stated that valuable time can be saved at home and in the office where the patient can use a typewriter (see item 4d: foot control). Many patients who initially insist that they can write faster by hand then with a typewriter, later decide on their own that even a poorly typed transcript of an autogenic abreaction is better than a handwritten one.

5. *Premature and inadequate information.*

Patients who express a wish to read about autogenic methods, and particularly autogenic abreaction, should be advised not to do so at this point. Later, however, when the patient's brain has unfolded its pattern of neutralizing dynamics, intelligent patients may be encouraged to read up on the method and engage in discussions which will help them to gain a clearer understanding of their therapeutic work.

Occasionally patients try to obtain more information about autogenic abreaction by discussing it with other patients who already have some experience with the method. Information obtained this way tends to be confusing for the inexperienced patient. Not knowing that each brain follows its own peculiar program and pattern of neutralization the inexperienced trainee then incorrectly expects his brain to engage in elaborations which are similar to those described by another patient. Such preconceived orientations easily result in nonautogenic patient-directed maneuvers which interfere unfavorably with or even block the normal development of autogenic dynamics and brain-directed programming of thematic neutralization. It is for this reason that it is in the patient's interest to begin autogenic abreaction in an unbiased open-minded manner and for the therapist to advise him to avoid sources of information which are not helpful.

Only in relatively rare instances does treatment with autogenic standard training develop in such a manner that spontaneous brain-directed dynamics cause episodes of acute anxiety or very disagreeable periods of bodily symptoms (e.g., severe headaches, vivid visual elaborations of a disagreeable nature, multiple accident-related disagreeable discharges, chains of disturbing dreams), and the therapist is confronted with the decision whether to use sedative drugs and/or autogenic abreaction to obtain quick relief. In such situations, when the application of autogenic abreaction appears feasible, there is usually no time for lengthy preparatory discussions and simple technical explanations (see below) are indicated.

The possibility exists that a therapist may use the habitual practice period of autogenic standard exercises as an opportunity to direct an unprepared and unsuspecting trainee into the complex dynamics of autogenic abreaction. Under such undesirable circumstances there is a high probability that unfavorable complications of therapeutic management may follow. Therefore an unprepared therapist-directed conversion of autogenic training into autogenic abreaction should be avoided.

Particular problems of therapeutic management may be encountered when the method of autogenic verbalization is introduced to trainees who have no experience with dynamics of autogenic abreaction, and a spontaneous conversion into autogenic abreaction occurs (see Vol. VI).

# 5. The Beginning of Autogenic Abreaction

When the patient and the therapist have agreed that the "new method" will be initiated at the next appointment, a number of technical aspects require consideration. Although the first autogenic abreaction takes about 15 to 30 minutes in most cases, it is not possible to foresee how much time will be required. In about 20 per cent ($N = 200$) more time was needed to avoid premature termination (see p. 87 ff.) and undesirable after-effects (see p. 93 ff.). On relatively rare occasions unexpected developments may force the therapist to continue for two hours or longer until the brain-directed dynamics indicate that a satisfactory level of neutralization has been reached (see p. 78 ff.) and the autogenic abreaction can be terminated without leaving the patient in a precarious condition. Partly for these reasons, about 90 minutes should be reserved for the introductory session, which is preferably scheduled in such a manner that the therapist has enough flexibility in his program to add more time in case unusual developments require his presence for a longer period. Particularly during a patient's first autogenic abreaction it is considered a technical error to interrupt pressing brain-directed dynamics prematurely because of lack of time, thus leaving a technically helpless patient in an unstable state of mobilized semi-neutralization.

Since states of fatigue are known to interfere unfavorably with dynamics of autogenic neutralization (Vol. VI), it is helpful to suggest to the patient to be well rested for the next appointment. Furthermore, it is therapeutically favorable that certain tasks of therapeutic homework are carried out directly after the autogenic abreaction. For this reason it is advisable that the patient has a few hours at his disposal after the next appointment. When a tape recorder is available to the patient, he should be encouraged to use the interval to become familiar with its technical features.

The structure of the therapeutic session during which the first autogenic abreaction is carried out is in many respects similar to the sequence of procedure which has been adopted as a standard pattern of office work during subsequent phases of treatment with autogenic abreaction (see p. 147 ff; p. 200/I).

After the patient has been invited to report certain happenings which occurred during the interim, to describe his complaints, his observations and to discuss actual problems (see p. 147), technically more specific aspects related to the practice of autogenic training are focussed upon (see p. 155 ff.). After the discussion of these matters have ended certain technical aspects of the method of autogenic abreaction are explained.

To avoid occasional frustrating and time-consuming interruptions at a later point, patients who have brought their tape recorder are asked to set up their machine and ensure adequate recording by direct testing. In about 30 per cent (N = 200) various difficulties of manipulating the tape recorder are encountered in spite of the patient's affirmation that everything is well prepared and they are familiar with their machine.

Technical explanations are then given. As such presentations must be carefully adapted to each patient's situation and his capacity and need for adequate understanding, a flexible, simple and clear approach is indicated. The information given usually centers around the following points:

(a) Practice of passive concentration on the heaviness formulas (e.g., RAH, LAH, BAH, RLH, LLH, BLH, ALH) of the first standard exercise for an initial *induction period,* with possible use of a supportive formula (see p. 29 f.) added when the trainee has not started his verbal description of training phenomena and other brain-directed elaborations (see b and c).

(b) A mental shift from initial use of passive concentration on the various heaviness formulas composing the first standard exercise of autogenic training to a spectator-like attitude, called "passive acceptance" (*carte blanche*).

(c) Continuous verbal description of any kind of brain-directed elaborations (e.g., sensory, motor, visual, intellectual, olfactory, psychic, vestibular).

(d) The psychophysiologically and therapeutically essential *principle of non-interference,* which is applicable to all patterns of *brain-directed* neutralization occurring during autogenic abreaction.

(e) Correct management of various forms of brain-antagonizing resistance.

(f) Adequate prolongation of the period of brain-directed unloading until an adequate level of autogenic neutralization (as indicated by relevant brain dynamics) has been reached.

(g) Avoidance of therapeutically unfavorable premature termination through sudden interference or other inadequate maneuvers directed by an inexperienced patient.

(h) Correct termination of autogenic abreaction in the usual three-step manner (i.e., flexing both arms vigorously, taking a deep breath, opening the eyes).

Simple instruction may be limited to emphasizing that the new approach is designed to give the brain more freedom to engage in more efficient neutralization of disturbing material. For this purpose the new exercise (AA) will be prolonged for 15 minutes or longer, and instead of writing a training protocol after the exercise it would be therapeutically more efficient to describe whatever the brain chooses to elaborate directly during the exercise. For technical reasons, the period of passive concentration would be limited to the series of heaviness formulas which the patient used during the initial learning phase of autogenic training (i.e., RAH, LAH, BAH, RLH, LLH, BLH, ALH) and that the verbal description should begin as soon as the trainee notices that training symptoms or other brain-directed elaborations have started. The verbal description should consist of continuous reporting, similar to a reporter who is describing a football game. Even in case nothing particular seems to occur, it is technically necessary to continue the description (e.g., "Absolutely nothing is going on . . . I don't know what to describe . . . I think this is stupid . . . it is all dark . . . nothing in particular . . . this is really a waste of time . . . I don't know what to say anymore . . . my head seems to be empty . . . I find this boring . . . ."). To facilitate the beginning of this technique, the therapist will recite the heaviness formulas for the trainee and stop his recitation as soon as the trainee begins to describe. In case the patient does not start to describe while the therapist recites the heaviness formulas, a supportive formula may be added at the end of the series of heaviness formulas. The supportive formula may take the form of "And now you imagine that you are in a meadow and you describe how the meadow looks today or whatever else you see or feel or think." In this connection, however, it is technically important to emphasize that the word "meadow" was chosen, since description should start at this point, because a meadow is a relatively neutral thing which may serve as an object of description. The patient should not make an effort to force himself to imagine a meadow, and whether or not there is a meadow is not important. Furthermore, the word "meadow" has a technical significance which in certain respects is similar to the word "heavy" used in the heaviness formulas. In many instances there is no feeling of heaviness: about 12 per cent of larger groups of trainees never experience any sensation of heaviness, and in others this training phenomenon is quite variable. In the same sense, it is actually not important whether or not a meadow is imagined. The most important thing is to remain completely passive, to adopt an attitude roughly like that of someone who watches a television program: not to interfere with the brain's own programming system, but simply to describe what is going on. Whether the brain's elaborations make sense or are pure fantasy, whether they are logical or absurd should not be a matter of concern. What really counts is that a stream of verbal description continues while maintaining the passive attitude of a spectator.

It is also important to ask the patient to indicate when he wishes to terminate this new exercise, and where the wish for termination occurs at a technically favorable point, the habitual three-step termination procedure should be used (i.e., flexing both arms vigorously, taking a deep breath, opening the eyes).

At this point of the technical introduction it is frequently necessary to explain to the patient that for certain technical reasons which he will come to understand a little later, it is not an advantage for him to terminate whenever he wishes, but that the termination procedure must be adapted to the brain's own performance (see p. 76 ff.). For this reason it may be advantageous not to terminate at the moment the patient indicates his desire to do so, but to continue perhaps for a few minutes until a technically more favorable phase has been reached; then the therapist may indicate that this is a good opportunity for termination.

While these instructions are sufficient for many patients who have already had advanced experience with various brain-directed phenomena which tend to occur during autogenic standard exercises, more elaborate explanations may be required in other cases. A number of patients wish to have more information about the phenomena they are expected to describe. During such discussions it is often helpful to explain that every brain is different and that one cannot foresee what the brain is going to do. The best approach for the trainee is to be completely open-minded and simply describe whatever is going on. Sometimes there are so many things going on that complete description is impossible, and one just does his best. In other instances one may have the impression that one's mind is blank, nothing is going on. During such periods it is generally helpful for the patient to consider the inner visual field as a convenient area of description because "there is always something to describe." Even when the inner visual field seems to be "empty," "just dark" or "blank," it is easy enough to describe just that. Sooner or later progressively more differentiated elaborations in the inner visual field tend to develop (see p. 187 ff; Color Plate 3 and 4; see also Table 33, p. 188). To facilitate productive description it is frequently helpful to mention that three major aspects of visual elaborations may be described: (a) chromatic, i.e., dark, light colors, (b) structural, i.e., shadows, forms, outlines, and (c) dynamic features, i.e., direction and nature of movements.

However, when brain-directed elaborations of visual nature are discussed, the patient should not be left with the impression that he is expected to limit his description to visual phenomena (*iatrogenic* resistance.). Such a one-area orientation may easily inhibit the brain in the elaboration of other areas which may be of therapeutically greater importance. Again it is important to repeat that a completely passive, open-minded, *carte blanche* attitude with continuous description of whatever comes up is the most desirable manner to proceed.

Other patients wish to have more information about the correct application of the termination procedure (see p. 77 ff.). In this connection it is also important to state that one cannot foresee how the patient's brain will respond. But to be helpful, a random example may be used to assist the patient's understanding: "Let us assume your brain starts elaborating a dream-like story. You are walking on a beach. A giant comes and puts you into a cannon. You feel uncomfortable and wish to terminate at this point. But as you see, the story is just beginning, and it would be unfavorable to interrupt your brain here. Therefore it is better to go on. Then, you are shot toward the moon, you drop on the moon, fall through the moon, and as you come out on the other side you feel really uncomfortable and would like to stop. But again it is technically too early. It is better to remain completely passive and let the brain do its job. You fall toward the earth, you see the water, you are afraid that you will die on impact and you wish to terminate. But nothing bad is going to happen to you, simply let yourself die, since this is a technical brain-directed maneuver to neutralize anxiety related to the topic of death. You remain passive, describe how you disintegrate and perhaps how your corpse is swallowed by a big fish. You continue describing the story until you perhaps find yourself again on a peaceful sunny beach, where you feel comfortable and you can relax. Then, as you realize, it is a good point to terminate. But this was only an example, which actually has nothing to do with the work your brain is going to perform. Anyway there is really nothing to worry about, I am here to help you and to show you when and how to terminate."

When all relevant questions have been answered, the patient is invited to lie down comfortably in horizontal training posture, to clip the microphone to his shirt and to start the tape recorder for uninterrupted recording.

This *preparatory* phase is followed by the *inducton phase* during which the therapist recites the sequence of the heaviness formulas for the patient (i.e., "My right arm is heavy . . . My right arm is heavy . . .

My right arm is heavy . . . My left arm is heavy . . .".). The therapist stops reciting the heaviness formulas as soon as the patient starts describing. Otherwise the therapist continues until the last heaviness formula "My arms and legs are heavy," or the additional supportive formula (i.e., "And now you imagine you are in a meadow and you describe how the meadow looks today or whatever else you see or feel or think") has been reached.

Most patients start describing toward the end of the induction phase before the supportive formula is reached, or within a few seconds after the therapist stops talking (see Table 9, p. 42). Only a relatively small percentage of patients remain silent for more than one minute (see Table 10, p. 46). In these cases, it is the therapist's task to be patient and to wait until the patient does begin to describe. During this *latent phase of non-verbal reactivity,* after several minutes of waiting, it may be indicated in certain cases to encourage the patient by asking in a low voice "Can you try to describe what is going on." Generally, however, it is therapeutically favorable to avoid such interferences during the latent phase and to remember that very productive autogenic abreactions have been observed in patients who gradually overcame their initial resistance (Vol. VI) and who began describing after unusually long latent phases, lasting up to eight minutes (see Table 10, p. 46).

As the patient maintains a spectator-like attitude of passive acceptance and as he keeps describing a variety of brain-directed elaborations, progressively more differentiated and therapeutically, positively oriented dynamics of neutralization develop (see Case 14, p. 60; Case 15, p. 63; Case 17, p. 72; Color Plate 2; Color Plate 3; Color Plate 4). Since the participating brain mechanisms concentrate on neutralization of accumulated psychophysiologically disturbing material, and since the use of non-disturbing agreeable material appears to be limited to interjections of neutralization-supporting antithematic dynamics (see p. 308 ff.), a large proportion of each autogenic abreaction is frequently experienced as relatively difficult and periodically as outrightly disagreeable (see Table 4, p. 33). Relatively neutral, more agreeable or very positively oriented antithematic elaborations may be viewed as brain-desired self-facilitating stimuli which tend to encourage the patient to continue through the next difficult or disagreeable phase of neutralization (see Case 17, p. 72; Case 118, p. 274). As the principle of non-interference (see p. 28) is respected by the therapist and the patient, and the brain is allowed to continue undisturbed with its work according to its own program of thematic priorities (see p. 251), a *terminal phase,* with brain-

TABLE 4. *Impressions of Psychosomatic and Neurotic Patients after their First and Second Autogenic Abreactions*

| General Impression of Nature of AA | After AA 1 (%; N = 100) | After AA 2 (%; N = 96) |
|---|---|---|
| (a) Agreeable | 38.0 | 36.4 |
| (b) Somewhat disagreeable | 16.0 ⎫ | 22.9 ⎫ |
| (c) Disagreeable | 20.0 ⎬ 50% | 20.8 ⎬ 55% |
| (d) Very disagreeable | 14.0 ⎭ | 11.4 ⎭ |
| (e) No particular comment | 12.0 | 8.3 |

directed indications (see p. 76 ff.) that the autogenic abreaction can be terminated will be reached. At this point, the patient usually feels calm, relaxed and comfortable. To avoid the technical error of premature termination (see p. 87), and when the patient has not expressed his feelings, the therapist should inquire "How do you feel?" or "Do you feel comfortable?" An affirmative response is then followed by the *standard termination procedure*:

*Dr.*: Do you feel comfortable?

*Pt.*: Yes, quite comfortable and calm.

*Dr.*: All right, everything is comfortable, and now you can terminate in three steps.

[*Pt.* Flexes his arms, takes a deep breath, opens eyes.]

*Dr.*: Fine, so, just stretch a bit, move a little bit and get up slowly.

[*Pt.* Stretching, moving arms and legs, sits up slowly, remains sitting on the couch for a little while, gets up and ready for the postabreactive discussion.]

Following the technical termination of the autogenic abreaction the *postabreactive period* begins with the *immediate postabreactive phase* (see p. 93 ff.) during which psychophysiologic after-effects are observed and the case-adapted nature of the patient's therapeutic homework (see p. 96 ff.) is discussed. As the patient leaves the therapist's office, the initial phase (about 6–8 hr.) of the *interim period* begins (see p. 120 ff.).

Each of the phases of the three major periods (i.e., preparatory, abreactive, postabreactive) is characterized by certain therapeutically significant dynamics which, depending on the nature of the patient's autogenic abreaction, require case-adapted consideration and technically adequate management (see also Vol. VI).

TABLE 5. *Periods and Phases during Treatment with Autogenic Abreaction*

| Periods of the Therapeutic Program | Sequence of Therapeutic Phases | General Explanatory Comments |
|---|---|---|
| *Preparatory period* (in office) | General discussion phase | Interim: events, observations, problems |
| | Autogenic training phase | Training protocols, observations, difficulties, discussion of intentional or organ-specific formulas; introduction of new standard formulas; dreams; (control and discussion of autogenic verablization, see Vol. VI) |
| | Thematic mobilization phase | Reading of transcript and commentary of last AA(s), explanatory and preparatory discussion |
| | Immediate preabreactive phase | Getting ready for AA (tape recorder, bathroom, lying down) |
| *Abreactive period* (in office) | Induction phase | Passive concentration on heaviness formulas (supportive formula), shift to passive acceptance (*carte blanche* attitude) |
| | Latent phase | Non-verbalized reactivity, "silent" phase |
| | Initial abreactive phase | Beginning of description of brain-directed elaborations, thematic adjustment |
| | Central abreactive phase | Description of brain-directed elaborations, various patterns of thematic neutralization |
| | Terminal abreactive phase | Description of brain-directed elaborations characteristic for self-regulatory brain-desired termination (forms of premature or delayed termination); application of standard termination procedure |
| *Postabreactive period* (in office) | Immediate postabreactive phase | After-effects, psychodynamic and psychophysiologic reactivity |
| | Postabreactive discussion | Technical errors, resistance, homework, supportive medication, etc. |
| *Interim period* (at home) | Initial interim phase | Delayed after-effects, listening to and transcription of AA, autogenic training |
| | Central interim phase | Rereading of transcript, commentary on AA, drawings, AT, AT protocol, note on dreams, (AV) |
| | Preappointment phase | Rereading of transcript, commentary on AA, AT, AT protocol, notes on dreams, preparation of material for appointment, (AV), sufficient sleep |

# 6. The Abreactive Period

To facilitate the progressive understanding of the complexity and variability of brain-directed processes of autogenic neutralization, the following discussion of the abreactive period with its different phases is intentionally limited to information intended for general orientation. More specific information about the variety of psychophysiologic modalities which participate in processes of autogenic neutralization is found in Part III. Furthermore, to avoid repetitions, the specific dynamics of brain-directed mechanisms of neutralization are referred to, but are not discussed in detail. For this reason it may be helpful to consult those chapters dealing specifically with relevant mechanisms of autogenic neutralization (Part IV; Vol. VI). Also specific discussion of brain-antagonizing and brain-facilitating forms of resistance have been omitted since they are presented in Part I, Vol. VI.

For research purposes, technically oriented discussions and practical reasons it has been found useful to consider the time between *the beginning of the induction phase* (see p. 38) and *the end of the standard termination procedure* (see p. 33) as the abreactive period.

Within the abreactive period it appeared practical to distinguish five major phases: (a) the *induction phase,* with passive concentration on heaviness formulas and mental shift to passive acceptance, (b) the *latent phase* or silent phase during which autogenic reactivity exists but is not described by the patient (see p. 46), (c) a relatively short *initial abreactive phase,* during which dynamics of brain-directed neutralization start unfolding (see p. 48), (d) the *central abreactive phase* with therapeutically progressive dynamics of neutralization taking up the major portion of the abreactive period (see p. 56 ff.), and (e) a usually very short *terminal phase* which includes the standard termination procedure (see p. 76 ff.). Each of these phases of the abreactive period has its own peculiar features of psychophysiologic dynamics and may confront the therapist with particular problems of management. In this connection it must be emphasized again that the following chapters are designed for purposes of orientation and that a more adequate understanding of a variety of technically and therapeutically oriented implications can only be expected at a later point, when a more comprehensive view of the dynamics of autogenic neutralization has been obtained.

The duration of the abreactive period varies greatly. In some cases it may be advisable to terminate the autogenic abreaction after about ten minutes, and in other instances the nature of the brain-directed dynamics may oblige the patient and the therapist to continue for longer than two hours. During the initial learning period, about 15 to 45 minutes are required by 70 per cent of psychosomatic and neurotic patients (see Table 6).

As the method of autogenic abreaction is based on the hypothesis that the patient's brain mechanism knows much better than the therapist how certain functional disorders came about, where to find the disturbing material, how to assign thematic priorities and how to co-ordinate, alternate, camouflage, adapt and terminate self-curative processes of neutralization, it is considered a basic technical requirement for the patient and the therapist to adopt the passive spectator-like attitude throughout the abreactive period (excluding application of the termination procedure). This requirement, which respects any kind of brain-directed elaboration in its broadest psychophysiologic sense, is called the *principle of non-interference.* The principle of non-interference is particularly important to allow the patient's brain mechanisms to follow the most efficient path of neutralization, as this is elaborated by the brain's own programming system. It is in this connection that the principle of non-interference might be misunderstood and lose its psychophysiologically oriented brain-supportive significance when various forms of brain-antagonizing resistance (see Vol. VI) repeatedly interfere with the process of neutralization and no technical support is given. Particularly in the beginning of treatment with autogenic abreaction, when patients still have certain difficulties in maintaining an attitude of passive acceptance and do not understand the "language of their brain-computer system," specifically adapted and well-timed supportive interventions by the therapist may be essential to help the patient's brain mechanisms continue their work along a thematic dimension, the nature and direction of which had been clearly indicated by preceding brain elaborations. However,

TABLE 6.   *Duration of the First and the Second Autogenic Abreaction*
*(Psychosomatic and Neurotic Patients)*

| Autogenic Abreaction | Duration in Minutes | | | | | | | | |
|---|---|---|---|---|---|---|---|---|---|
| | 1–10 | 11–20 | 21–30 | 31–40 | 41–60 | 61–80 | Over | M | S.D. |
| AA 1 (N = 100) | 8 | 20 | 28 | 15 | 21 | 5 | 3 | 32.7 | 20.717 |
| AA 2 (N = 96) | 4 | 15 | 18 | 26 | 22 | 7 | 4 | 37.3 | 18.409 |

even in instances where phenomena of brain-antagonizing resistance are evident, a minimum of support should be given, and only after the patient's brain has repeatedly tried in its own way to overcome or circumvent the inhibitory resistance in question (see Vol. VI). Apart from rarely used very specific supportive interventions, it may be necessary, particularly with beginners (see Table 7), to provide occasionally well-timed non-specific support. Such non-specific supportive interventions are occasionally required when patients stop describing for longer periods (e.g., "Can you continue to describe?"; "Can you try to describe what is going on?") or, depending on the type of resistance, one may supportively interject: "Can you describe that in detail?", or "Can you repeat that again?" As the patients advance in treatment with autogenic abreaction and as they become more familiar with the dynamics of their brain, there is a progressively decreasing need for supportive interventions.

Generally two major categories of autogenic abreaction can be distinguished: (a) monothematic and (b) multithematic. Where the patient's brain adopts a *monothematic pattern* of neutralization, variations of the same theme dominate the initial, the central and a large portion of the terminal phase. Such patterns are frequently encountered in patients who have suffered severe accidents (e.g., hit by a car with loss of consciousness, drowning with subsequent resuscitation), in obsessive-compulsive conditions, in cases suffering from ecclesiogenic syndrome when the brain engages in neutralization of anxiety dynamics related to damnation and hell, and in certain types of depressive reactions when very positively oriented antithematic dynamics dominate from the beginning to the end.

TABLE 7. *Number of Supportive Interventions during the First and the Second Autogenic Abreaction*
*(Psychosomatic and Neurotic Patients)*

| Autogenic Abreaction | Number of Supportive Interventions | | | | | | | | | M |
|---|---|---|---|---|---|---|---|---|---|---|
| | 0 | 1 | 2–5 | 6–10 | 11–15 | 16–20 | 21–30 | 31–40 | Over | |
| AA 1 (N = 100) | 23 | 10 | 25 | 11 | 8 | 7 | 9 | 5 | 2 | 9.1 |
| AA 2 (N = 96) | 21 | 9 | 15 | 18 | 13 | 7 | 7 | 1 | 5 | 10.9 |

When *multithematic patterns* of neutralization are adopted, a large variety of thematic combinations can be observed. Such multithematic processes frequently follow a pattern of thematic rotation with repetitions of versions involving the same topics. Less frequently are multithematic patterns which evolve in clearly distinguishable phases. In these cases the brain mechanisms tend to repeat versions of the same theme a certain number of times before a thematic shift to the next (related or unrelated) topic occurs.

In many instances, particularly during advanced treatment with autogenic abreaction, a stratifunctional organization of thematic neutralization characterizes the pattern of brain-directed dynamics. For example, for an initial period (e.g., 40 min.) the brain concentrates on neutralization of well-known "old" material subsequently more emphasis is given to repetition of "more recent" material (e.g., 25 min.); and as this phase advances, new elements tend to appear sporadically, gradually leading up to an emphasis on the neutralization of "new" material (see Table 42, p. 256; Table 43, p. 257).

Whatever the pattern of neutralization may be, one invariably notices brain-directed dynamics aiming at thematic repetition. It is for this reason that brain-directed dynamics of thematic repetition may be considered as the vehicle of neutralization (see Part IV).

THE INDUCTION PHASE

After the patient has assumed the horizontal training posture and says that he is ready for autogenic abreaction, the induction phase is initiated as the patient closes his eyes and begins passive concentration on the standard series of heaviness formulas. In agreement with technical principles applied during autogenic standard training (see Vol. I, p. 13 ff.), the sequence of heaviness formulas varies with the handedness of the patient. With right-handed trainees the following sequence is applied: "RAH, LAH, BAH, RLH, LLH, BLH."

In cases of left-handedness it is appropriate to use: "LAH, RAH, BAH, LLH, RLH, BLH."

During the learning period of supervised autogenic abreactions, the patient's mental shift from passive concentration on heaviness formulas to a mental attitude of passive acceptance is initially facilitated by repetition of the formulas by the therapist. Later, after the patient has gained experience with autogenic abreaction, it is therapeutically desirable that the induction phase of (silent) passive concentration on heaviness formulas is performed by the trainee himself.

In the course of the average induction phase, each heaviness formula is repeated three to five times. In restless and evidently nervous and tense patients it may be advisable to prolong the induction phase by increasing the number of repetitions for each formula. In the beginning the duration of the induction phase varies largely between two to three minutes. Later, as the treatment with autogenic abreaction advances, an increasing number of patients tend to start describing within about 60 to 90 seconds after the beginning of formula-related passive concentration (see Table 8).

In the beginning, during the first and the second autogenic abreaction, about 6 to 12 per cent of trainees tend to interrupt the therapist's recitation of heaviness formulas (see Table 10, p. 46) by starting to describe various modalities of brain-directed elaborations, most of which have already occurred repeatedly during the patient's preparatory practice period of autogenic standard training (see Case 1).

*Case 1:* A 24-year-old male student (anxiety reaction, moderate depressive reaction). During recitation of the heaviness formulas (i.e., RAH, LAH, BAH, RLH, LLH, BLH) the patient interrupted the therapist at the beginning of "Both legs are heavy." The patient's following descriptions indicate that dynamics of brain-directed elaborations had already started shortly after the beginning of the induction phase.

"For about a minute its turning, turning as if I am on a turntable. Somewhat later I saw the sun going down . . . it seems to be near St. Joseph Oratory . . . and there was a car which crashed into a tree and there was a big fire . . . and the tree is on fire and the car too . . . it seems that I am the tree, and the branches turn . . . and it is as if my arms are turning . . . it's still turning like on a turntable . . . and as if a voice of somebody is crying . . . somebody who is falling into a well. . . ."

Occasionally the induction phase is interrupted by, for example, onset of massive motor discharges, laughing or crying spells (see Case 2, p. 40; Case 3, p. 40). In such instances inexperienced and surprised patients may open their eyes and sit up or engage in other maneuvers which automatically terminate the induction phase. In such instances,

TABLE 8. *Duration of the Induction Phase for the First and the Second Autogenic Abreaction (Psychosomatic and Neurotic Patients)*

| Induction phase | AA 1 (N = 100) | | AA 2 (N = 96) | |
|---|---|---|---|---|
| Minutes | $M = 2.65$ | $S.D. = 1.028$ | $M = 2.67$ | $S.D. = 1.167$ |

after the patient has become calm again, it ought to be explained that the sudden onset of such brain-directed processes of unloading are medically very helpful, and that any brain-antagonizing interference (e.g., opening eyes and sitting up) or efforts at suppression will only lead to an increase of inner tension and other undesirable functional reactions (e.g., headache). The best way is to remain completely passive, to maintain a *carte blanche* attitude and to permit the brain to discharge whatever it wishes to unload. When these instructions are followed, such episodes of massive discharges invariably subside after a while (see Case 2). As this is observed, a direct approach (e.g., "Can you try to describe what is going on?" aiming at the continuation of unfolding of brain-directed dynamics may be applied. However, in many cases it is technically preferable either simply to continue with the recitation of heaviness formulas or to start over again with the induction procedure.

*Case 2:* A 39-year-old businessman (anxiety reaction). Shortly after lying down and the beginning of passive concentration on "My right arm is very heavy," the patient started having massive motor discharges mainly involving the trunk, the shoulders and neck, with the face assuming a contracted mask-like appearance. While these motor discharges continued (36 major contractions), the patient started describing the visual field.

"I'm getting this impression again with these rotating wheels like on the tape-recorder and the tubular nose in between [end of motor discharges] . . . my field of vision is sort of a mushroom gray with so . . . eh . . . sweeps. . . ."

The association between these massive motor discharges and the symbolic elaborations of penis and testicles in the visual field reflect recently prominent dynamics of thematic neutralization related to (a) castration anxiety (feelings of guilt, fear of punishment, wish of having no penis) related to masturbatory activities during puberty and (b) latent homosexuality and relevant dynamics involving the patient's relationship with his mother and father.

During the first few autogenic abreactions the majority of patients prefer to wait for the beginning of their description until after the end of the therapist's pronounciation of the induction formulas (see Table 10, p. 46; see Case 3).

*Case 3:* A 41-year-old engineer (anxiety reaction). A series of motor discharges started about 30 seconds after the beginning of the induction procedure (see passages below). However, the patient did not start to describe during this period but waited until the end of the induction phase.

"I seem to see a couple of slitted eyes . . . very heavy eyelids . . . the eyes are barely slit . . . it's sort of a mask, and in a way it's like three spokes of a wheel . . . my field of vision is sort of a grayish color . . . *I have had several twitches when I first lay down and started listening to you,* but I feel quite twitchy as a matter of fact today . . . my ear is quite uncomfortable, it keeps blocking and unblocking, from time to time my hearing keeps changing . . . it's getting to be a metallic gray, a dark metallic gray . . . I have a bit of a pain in my forehead, aside of the discomfort of my jaw below my ear. . . ."

The supportive formula "And now you imagine being in a meadow, and you describe how the meadow looks today, or whatever else you see or feel or think" may be added in instances when the patient does not start to describe during or at the end of the therapist's recitation of the heaviness formulas. The thematic structure of this supportive formula is intentionally designed to provide (a) a facilitating specific, however relatively neutral, element of departure (i.e., meadow) and (b) to provide all necessary elements of functional flexibility (i.e., ". . . or whatever else you see or feel or think") to avoid psychophysiologically unfavorable unilateral fixation on the meadow theme with undesirable brain-restricting emphasis on visual elaborations. Considering the wide range of modalities of autogenic discharges occurring during autogenic standard exercises and the even larger range of brain-directed elaborations during autogenic abreactions, the second part of the supportive formula "or whatever else you see or feel or think" is well adapted to the brain's need for engaging in unrestricted multidimensional processes of neutralization according to the thematic priorities of its own programming system. The thematic content and verbal structure of this thematically and functionally unrestricted supportive formula was adopted after observations showed that a simpler thematically and functionally restricted meadow formula (i.e., "And now you imagine being in a meadow and you describe how the meadow looks today") as for example, used by C. Happich,[G/VI] H. Leuner[832–839,2059,2318] and others[69,377,686,730,1108,1110,2209,2341,2342] during the application of therapist-designed non-autogenic approaches[60,106,119,278,347,348,625,667,716,719,725,1629,1653,1655,1726,1728,1733,1755,1829,2422] appeared to exert inhibitory effects on autogenic dynamics of psychophysiologically multidimensional processes of brain-directed neutralization.

To ensure that brain-restricting effects related to the meadow theme of the supportive formula are avoided as much as technically possible, the supportive formula should not be applied without a patient-adapted discussion of its purpose. During such a discussion it is useful to emphasize repeatedly that the word "meadow" was chosen because something relatively neutral had to be said at that point; and actually it is of no importance whether or not the brain elaborates images related to a meadow. The patient must clearly understand that, as during the standard exercises, all kinds of brain-directed elaborations are of equal importance, and that he should never force himself to imagine a meadow or to restrict his description to elaborations in the inner visual field.

In the beginning a relatively high percentage of patients prefer not to interrupt the therapist's recitation and rather wait with the beginning of their description until the induction phase (including the supportive formula) has ended (see Table 10). Initially a relatively large number of patients find the meadow theme a convenient point of departure for their description (see Table 9). However, it usually takes less than three minutes until progressively unfolding brain-directed dynamics follow their own program of elaborations (see Case 9, p. 51; Case 14, p. 60). As the treatment with autogenic abreaction advances, a progressively decreasing number of patients react to the meadow theme.

As during autogenic standard exercises, a variety of autogenic discharges tend to occur while the therapist is reciting the heaviness formulas. Motor discharges, as for example, muscular twitches in the extremities, of the face, generalized jerks and contractions, fluttering of eyelids, tears and certain changes of the respiratory rhythm are readily noticed (see Case 2, p. 40; Case 3, p. 40). However, the therapist cannot notice the release of other forms of brain-directed modalities, such as feeling of nausea, headaches, abdominal cramps, pain in the left chest, palpitations, vestibular phenomena (see Case 1, p. 39) or visual elaborations. Since the occurrence of such discharges

TABLE 9.   *Initial Response during or after the Induction Phase for the First and the Second Autogenic Abreaction*
*(100 Psychosomatic and Neurotic Patients)*

| Autogenic Abreaction Initial Response | AA 1 (No. of Patients) | AA 2 (No. of Patients) |
|---|---|---|
| (a) Supportive formula not used | 6 | 12 |
| (b) Description involving a meadow or other elaborations which were in some way related to a meadow | 57 | 45 |
| (c) Description of differentiated visual elaborations not related to a meadow | 8 | 26 |
| (d) Description of other modalities of brain-directed elaborations usually associated with elementary form of visual elaborations | 35 | 25 |
| (e) AA discontinued | — | 4 |

is closely related to accumulated brain-disturbing material of a more complex nature (see Case 4), it is of therapeutic importance that the patient feel free enough to start describing as soon as such symptoms of autogenic reactivity occur (see Case 5). To facilitate the patient's task in starting to describe during the recitation of heaviness formulas, it is essential that the therapist observe the patient's face throughout the induction period and that he stops talking as soon as he thinks that the patient is about to start reporting. However, about 20 per cent of patients with more advanced experience in autogenic neutralization tend to maintain their preference of waiting to begin their description when the standard induction procedure is terminated (see Case 9, p. 51; Case 5, p. 44; Case 4).

*Case 4:* A 36-year-old housewife (anxiety reaction, multiple psychophysiologic reactions). After terminating recitation of the heaviness formulas, the patient started describing and elaborating on images which flashed by earlier during the induction phase. The subsequent pattern of neutralization confirmed that these brief visual elaborations which occurred during the induction phase were essential elements in the brain's program of thematic neutralization during the central phase of the abreactive period.

"While you were talking, about four or five scenes flashed by, one after the other, very fast. One was driving back to Dr. X with my daughter, when I was telling her in the car, I forget what led to it exactly, it was: 'Don't compare with what others do; thing to do is the best you can do with the capacity you have. If you have to do ten percent of the work, if you are equipped to do it, do it. And the more you are equipped with, the more responsibility you have and the harder it is to accept it sometimes. . . .'" The second one was the living-room when my husband said: 'You won't have that problem or trouble much longer. . . .' He said later: Yes, I want separation, the children' . . . I forgot what the third one was. Was it at the hairdresser's? Tuesday? Aggy? She has twins. I know we talked about the children at one point . . . and all these scenes were in color . . . and it is the three of them . . . Lise on the left, I was going to say in her maroon coat . . . now it is coming back, Saturday. . . ."

While various forms of brain-antagonizing resistance (see Vol. VI) which may interfere with the normal development of autogenic reactivity during and after the induction phase require a detailed discussion at a later point, certain manifestations of *intentional resistance* should be mentioned. Of particular interest at this point are those maneuvers which a patient carries out intentionally to avoid engagement in certain topics and which are designed to side-track the therapist. They may involve unilateral continuous description of all kinds of bodily phenomena, be unusually slow descriptions with many silent intervals, or be simple repetitions that nothing is happening. More experienced and intelligent patients try to get away from the feared topic (already announced by the brain) by not beginning to describe immediately as requested, but by waiting until the end of the supportive formula. Then they attempt to use the meadow theme as an evasive point of departure (see Case 5). However, even in most of these instances the sophisticated mechanisms of the patient's brain will gradually introduce elements and dynamics which are designed to approach the unpleasant topic in a progressive and well-camouflaged manner as the patient keeps describing. When such patterns are observed, it is necessary to explain the unfavorable implications of the patient's resistance during the postabreactive discussion period and to ask the patient to engage in specifically designed tasks of therapeutic homework (see Case 5).

*Case 5:* A 35-year-old salesman (reactive depression). This case illustrates the importance of instructing a patient (a) to start describing the elaborations of his brain as soon as they start during the induction period, (b) to mention in his commentary if any particular elaborations or reactions had occurred during the induction period. Furthermore, the passages below and the patient's comments also illustrate various implications of avoiding the brain-selected theme for neutralization by intentionally interfering with brain-directed programming (see *Direct Intentional Resistance,* Vol. VI). In spite of the early onset of brain-directed elaborations during the induction period, the patient permitted the therapist to continue with the recitation of the heaviness formulas and even the supportive meadow formula (which in this instance was intentionally misused by the patient as a welcome support for thematic evasion). Then, after a 10-second interval, the patient started to describe elaborations which are initially clearly related to the meadow theme.

"I guess I should start off with, that when you were going through the formulas I had a bit of trouble . . . just concentrating on it . . . the tree [an item which came up during previous AAs] looks like . . . something which is in the distance, and right now I'm standing quite away from it, there are green bushes on the left of me, and just a few moments ago it seemed that there was someone in, what seemed to be a painting or a picture that somebody had photographed or painted . . . this is what I appear to see at first. . . ."

*The patient's comments (homework):*
"I would say there was a significant reason for the initial lack of concentration at the start. It is a series of small incidents which start with the age of about eight or nine. I was with another boy at the time, and we were quite far away from home. I think it was on Ninth Avenue. We walked toward Royal Street about 12 blocks away. A fellow on a bicycle asked us if we wanted a lift, we agreed. The other fellow went on the carrier at the back of the bike. I went on the front, and the fellow who gave us a lift started feeling about my genitals. I permitted him to do this, and I don't know what my

reactions were at the time. I don't think there was an erection or anything like that. I remember telling the other fellow what had happened. When I was in Quebec at the age of 20, I had my bicycle with me. One day I took a ride along the road. I stopped near a group of very young people, I think it was three boys and a girl. I offered the little girl a ride and she refused. I think it was in my mind to explore the little girl physically, although I am quite sure, say 95 percent to 99 percent, that it was nothing more than that. The utter stupidity of what I tried to do and my reasons for doing this are recalled from time to time. *I think all this came to my mind when the formula was being said, and it bothered me.* Also, later the idea of incest came to my mind. Certainly there was no intention of having intercourse with the five- or six-year-old girl. Yet the whole idea of just asking the little girl with the intention of touching her, physically, so near to molestation, had been recalled many times. At the time, I had no physical knowledge of a woman."

*Remarks:* While reading and discussing the patient's commentary, he stated that he felt embarrassed about the topic and other actual activities of similar nature. *He did not wish to talk about this, and therefore had not interrupted the therapist and had tried to use the meadow formula as an artificial point of departure.* His attempt in this direction (see initial passages of the patient's AA) convey an unusual pattern (in his case) of brief duration. Subsequently, the brain shifted toward topics involving tension and anxiety producing material of heterosexual nature.

Frequently the question has been asked whether the induction period must be limited to passive concentration on heaviness formulas and if it is permissible to include other standard formulas before engaging in autogenic abreaction. An answer to such a question requires consideration of certain psychophysiologic aspects and relevant technical implications. Psychophysiologically, a mental shift from passive concentration on autogenic standard formulas (SE I-VI) to a spectator-like attitude of passive acceptance and verbal description of brain-directed elaborations is always possible. However, it is of practical advantage to establish a pattern of procedure which clearly distinguishes between the habitually practiced pattern of standard formulas used for autogenic standard exercises (i.e., SE I-VI) and the pattern of formulas applied for an initial period of passive concentration (i.e., all formulas of SE I), with subsequent shift to passive acceptance and promotion of dynamics of autogenic neutralization. As a consequent distinction between RAH, LAH, BAH, RLH, LLH, BLH, ALH as used for the AA induction phase, and the series of standard formulas applied for autogenic training (i.e., ALH + W, HCR, IBM, SPW, FC) is observed and the trainee maintains an adequate level of passive concentration in each instance, he tends to be less prone to be bothered (during AT) by technically undesired interference from brain-directed dynamics pressing for engagement in autogenic abreaction. In case such a technical distinction of procedure is not observed during the application of autogenic abreaction and during the daily practice of autogenic training, patients undergoing treatment with autogenic abreaction tend to report increasing difficulties with brain-directed interferences during the practice of autogenic training. Furthermore, there is some evidence that the thematically and topographically more specific nature of the formulas of SE III-VI may influence the orientation of specific brain dynamics in thematically predetermined undesirable psychophysiologic directions (e.g., heart formula; see Fig. 1, p. 8 f.). Such possibilities are excluded as the formulas used during the induction phase remain categorically limited to the thematic, relatively non-specific series of heaviness formulas.

THE LATENT PHASE

The period between the end of the induction phase (i.e., ALH or supportive formula) and the beginning of verbal description by the patient is called the *latent phase*. When the verbal description has already begun during or directly after termination of the induction phase, the latent phase of non-verbal reactivity is practically non-existent. In the beginning of treatment with autogenic abreaction, about 85 per cent of psychoneurotic and psychosomatic patients react in this therapeutically favorable manner (see Table 10). During more advanced treatment periods, when the patient has gained a better

TABLE 10.   *Duration of the Latent Phase of Non-Verbal Reactivity*
*for the First and the Second Autogenic Abreaction*
*(100 Psychosomatic and Neurotic Patients)*

| Latent Phase | AA 1 (No. of Patients) | AA 2 (No. of Patients) |
|---|---|---|
| Beginning of description: | | |
| (a) During or right after termination of the *Induction Phase* | 84 | 85 |
| (b) Within less than 20 sec. after termination of the *Induction Phase* | 7 | 1 |
| (c) Within 21–40 sec. | 1 | 2 |
| (d) Within 41–60 sec. | 6 | 5 |
| (e) Within 61–120 sec. | 1 | 2 |
| (f) Within 121–540 sec. | 1 | 1 |
| (g) Did not wish to continue AA | — | 4 |

understanding of the brain-directed dynamics of autogenic neutralization, the latent phase is absent in about 93 per cent of psychoneurotic and psychosomatic patients.

Provided that the patient has understood the preparatory technical instructions correctly, a delayed onset of verbal description, particularly when the latent phase exceeds about 20 seconds, is in many instances related to interferences resulting from various forms of brain-antagonizing resistance (see Vol. VI). It is in this connection that the duration of the latent phase is of particular clinical significance concerning the therapeutic management of a relatively small percentage of patients.

Undue prolongation of the latent phase (i.e., over 20 sec.) may involve a variety of factors. In some cases such a delay may be related to an unsatisfactory discussion period at the beginning of the therapeutic session when the patient has forgotten or had no opportunity to mention some problem which is of particular importance to him. While experienced patients might start out correctly by expressing their concern or question at the beginning of the *initial abreactive phase,* less experienced patients may find themselves in doubt, because they think that the matter in question has actually nothing to do with their habitual pattern of autogenic neutralization. To avoid such inhibitory brain-disturbing forms of resistance, it is technically important that (a) a patient is given adequate opportunity to discuss his actual problems and questions during the initial part of the therapeutic session (see p. 147 ff.), and (b) that even the most trivial concern which may appear during or after the induction period is promptly expressed.

In other instances prolonged latent phases may be related to a brain-directed shift of thematic neutralization to a dimension which is new to the patient. This, for example, is the case when the habitual pattern of cinerama-like visual elaborations, which the patient expects on the basis of his previous experiences, does not occur; because the brain-designed program of thematic priorities has shifted to a need, for example, for the expression of verbal aggression. Similarly, the onset of description may be delayed because the patient's brain started thematic elaborations concerning the therapist (e.g., aggression, sexual desire), and he does not feel free to express and neutralize such transferential dynamics.[208,415,418,601]

Prolonged periods of silence may also occur as a result of a lack of passivity and the patient's technically erroneous attempt to direct his brain instead of leaving the programming of thematic priorities to relevant brain mechanisms. However, as the patient learns that his own autogenically working brain mechanisms are more sophisticated and efficient than he initially thought, such technical errors become less frequent.

Sometimes a delay of the verbal response is related to what may be called a "storm of rapid and confusing thematic elaborations," and the patient simply does not know where to begin with his description, and is waiting until this overproductivity subsides.

The attempt to suppress a need for crying, already felt during the induction phase, is sometimes another reason for prolongation of the induction period. Closely related are other maneuvers of *thematic avoidance* (see Vol. VI) which are designed to change the orientation away from one or several brain-directed thematic elaborations which appear undesirable to the patient.

Only occasionally it may occur that forms of *indirect psychophysiologic resistance* (see Vol. VI) such as a sudden need to urinate or a particularly marked deficiency of sleep, may participate in undue prolongation of the latent phase.

As a general rule it is advisable for the therapist to remain passive and patient and not to interfere with questions or therapist-directed maneuvers when the silent period of the latent phase is extended beyond the habitual period of time. It is therapeutically favorable to leave the initiative to begin description to the patient. Only in particular instances, after waiting at least two minutes, one may perhaps ask in a low voice: "Can you try to describe what is going on?"

To elucidate the underlying forms of resistance and to facilitate a more adequate response during the subsequent autogenic abreaction, the patient's reluctance to start describing during or directly after the induction period should be discussed (see Case 5, p. 44).

## THE INITIAL PHASE

The initial phase of the abreactive period commences as soon as the patient starts describing either during the induction period or after a latent period of variable duration. Since the variability of brain-directed elaborations is great, and since it is in most instances impossible to predict a brain's programming of thematic priorities and the closely related pattern of neutralization, it is difficult to limit the duration of the initial phase to a specific period of time. However, on the average about 5 to 12 minutes may be required until brain-directed dynamics attain a functional pattern which is largely characteristic for the *central phase* of the abreactive period.

Generally it may be said that the initial phase may begin with descriptions of any of those phenomena which compose the spectrum

of autogenic discharges habitually encountered during autogenic standard training (e.g., heaviness, numbness, tension, abdominal discomfort, vestibular sensations, visual or psychic elaborations). The particularly high frequency of intellectual elaborations which tend to interfere as "distractions" with passive concentration on standard formulas during autogenic training, the high incidence (59.0-70.0%) of spontaneous elaborations of visual nature during standard exercises (see p. 143/I), and the large variety of bodily oriented motor and sensory modalities of autogenic discharges are also the elements which, according to their functional dominance, determine the nature of initial phases of autogenic abreaction. Therefore it may be appropriate to make a tentative distinction between four large groups of initial patterns of dynamics of autogenic neutralization:

A. Patterns of predominantly intellectual elaborations which may or may not be associated with sporadically occurring visual phenomena or other bodily oriented modalities of discharges.
B. Patterns dominated by a variety of sensory (viscerosensory) an motor (visceromotor) phenomena with or without sporadically i terjected intellectual or visual elaborations.
C. Patterns in which visual elaborations assume central importa and bodily oriented phenomena or intellectual elaborations are secondary nature which may or may not participate occasiona
D. Mixed patterns in which all known modalities of brain-dir elaborations may participate with variable intensities.

Patterns characterized by predominantly intellectual elaboratic quently emphasize dynamics of neutralization which focus on ing material related to the patient's daily or professional activit Case 6, Case 7).

Case 6: A 42-year-old business executive (anxiety reaction, hy teremia, subclinical hypothyroidism) started his autogenic abreact scribing frustrating situations in his company, money problems, inc of employees, and unsolved financial problems endangering the his family. The first crying spell occurred after about 3 minut other crying episodes followed later as this pattern of intellectua continued for about 25 minutes, and a brain-directed thematic s'

Case 7: A 38-year-old male teacher (anxiety reaction, mild d tion) virtually burst into violent attacks against the educational tions of unprintable and aggressive tirades against almost ever intendent, the School Board, the students, certain colleagues, ' a thematically related depreciation of himself. After about nine

directed thematic shift toward topics of a sexual nature with interjected visual elaborations took place.

Initial phases with dynamics emphasizing vestibular modalities, feelings of motion, falling, spinning, dizziness, motor discharges, pain and other modalities of sensory nature are frequently encountered in patients who suffered severe life-threatening accidents (see Case 8).

*Case 8:* A 33-year-old housewife (anxiety reaction). The following passages covering the first six minutes of the AA, are characteristic for a non-visual pattern, dominated by diffuse feelings and specific sensations. A slight occipital headache and the feeling that an old boy friend was close to her started soon after the beginning of the induction phase.

"There is a bit of a headache at the back of the head. Just before the end of the exercise, I thought of or I felt Dick quite close. Visually there is nothing . . . it is black or emptiness, no limits, no shape to it . . . I have the feeling I am outside . . . I had a few waves of dizziness . . . they are increasing . . . it is not quite the oscillating movement that I have felt before, but it is the sensation of being on something that is propelling me . . . I don't know which way I am going . . . I feel the worst of it in the head . . . I am trying to identify movement. I think whatever I am on is moving counterclockwise and I think I am stationary on it . . . yet I have the sensation of movement . . . I am definitely moving . . . speed is fairly fast . . . I have the feeling that my shoulders want to go to the right and what I am on is going clockwise . . . I think that is it but not positive . . . it is still going on, it seems to go in a crescendo and then . . . either I am not aware of it as much as I thought . . . it is not as fast as the previous times I felt or had that sensation . . . and seems to . . . I think I said it, the head is where I feel it the most, almost like a vertigo . . . it is a picking up speed, I don't know if it is in rotation or carrying me away. There are very mild oscillations with it . . . it is slightly nauseating . . . just outside of the eyes, there is that mixture of blue and mauve. . . ."

*Remarks:* While trying to work out a commentary at home, the patient felt unable to associate the different thematic elements of this initial phase with any specific event. She felt that the following possibilities exist: water skiing, water skiing accident 11 years ago, drunkenness, or perhaps an incident at age 18, when she was carried away by a fast current and almost drowned when she got caught in the weeds while trying to reach the river bank. The details concerning the latter incident developed later during the central part of the abreactive period.

Initial phases with emphasis on differentiated visual elaborations are encountered in 65 to 70 per cent (see Table 37, p. 194) of psychosomatic and neurotic patients during their first and second autogenic abreaction (see Table 38, p. 195). Most of these patients have already experienced such spontaneously occurring visual phenomena during the practice of autogenic standard exercises (Table 6, p. 143/I). For

these patients the suggestive elements of the first part of the supportive formula (i.e., "And now you imagine being in a meadow," etc.) appears to be of facilitating value for beginning their description. However, even during the first autogenic abreaction the meadow theme remains only a transitory one of departure which soon is transformed or simply overruled by the brain's own programming system (see Case 9).

*Case 9:* A 37-year-old male technical assistant (anxiety reaction, sexual deviation, ecclesiogenic syndrome) who for quite a while felt dissatisfied and unhappy with his work. He complained about a number of grievances and other difficulties at work.

"I see a meadow . . . the meadow looks like a projected square . . . now it disappeared . . . I see my boss . . . he stands there in a posture ready for putting . . . and he does not move . . . his head turned upward toward the sky . . . he looks at me . . . I am somewhere up in space . . . he is holding his golf club in his hands . . . ready to hit . . . but there is no ball on the grass . . . he is still looking at me . . . and one has the impression that he is waiting for a signal to hit . . . he occupies only a small part of the landscape, his face is too small to describe in detail . . . nothing is moving . . . the situation changes and I find myself at level with his belt . . . and now I see him in his actual size . . . I have the impression that I should like to jump on him and beat him to pulp. . . ."

*Case 10:* A 42-year-old housewife (hysterical personality, anxiety reaction, moderate depressive reaction). During her first ten autogenic abreactions this patient started the initial period on six occasions with visual elaborations related to the meadow theme (see examples below). In each instance the meadow theme is associated with particular features and symbolic elements which (a) reflect the patient's actual condition and (b) forecast thematically significant dynamics of thematic neutralization which tend to develop in greater and progressively more realistic detail during the central phase of the abreactive period.

*AA 1:* "I keep seeing the traffic on the street; buses, trucks, a yellow schoolbus and a big moving truck; little volkswagens, people trying to cross the street—but there is no traffic light . . . then I was thinking of the circular traffic that you have in Turkey—you have to keep circling—in Dorval also . . . I never know which exit to take. They are gone because I don't want to slow down and then I usually take the wrong exit and get on the circle again; I usually hate traffic circles. . . .

*AA 2:* "The meadow is dark . . . there is going to be a storm . . . there is one tree, very crooked, it has no leaves, just very crooked branches . . . and . . . there are a few bushes . . . it is getting very windy . . . getting darker and darker . . . you look up . . . it is gray . . . the clouds are coming . . . and you look around, you don't see a person . . . there is just one person standing there, watching the clouds . . . and . . . the grass is all dry . . . all you can do is to sit in a raincoat if you have one . . . it is going to rain. . . . Off the meadow,

there is a small forest . . . some pine trees . . . a little path and dry bushes . . .
there are no animals . . . no horses . . . no cows, just a very crooked tree . . .
that's all. . . . There is a railway line behind the meadow that you can see
from where you stand. You can see the railway tracks with a train coming . . .
once in a while . . . once a day it stops. A little bit further there is a tourist
house . . . I stayed in the tourist house once. . . .

AA 3: "The meadow looks sunny today. Trees with yellow leaves and the
wind blowing . . . the grass is still green . . . and the meadow is pleasant
today. . . . But in the meadow . . . there is a fish . . . on the meadow . . . all
the day today I was thinking of that fish . . . it's a red fish . . . I had a nightmare and all night I was trying to . . . I can see the red fish and I can see that
it is in two pieces . . . I am standing there holding it in my hands . . . but it
did not start with the fish . . . I was driving a car . . . I had this ghastly fat
red fish . . . it is a red fish . . . it is very fat and sort of short . . . and . . .
except that I know it is not a fish . . . the spoon and the inside of the fish is
black full of . . . caviar . . . and with . . . dirty little bits and pieces . . . and
there is just this scraping and scraping . . . the scraping of the fish reminds
me of . . . when you are just scraped out from inside. . . .

AA 4: "The meadow is rainy today . . . just as it is outside . . . but I am
still thinking . . . I can still see this old picture of my father . . . it never before
occurred to me that he looks like Hitler . . . and I often think that I remember
him . . . I was three I think when he died . . . I definitely remember the house
where we lived then . . . it was a tiny tiny village . . . just one short street . . .
at this end of this street was our house . . . and my father was the notary . . .
and I remember the time when he was very sick . . . he was in bed all the time
. . . the doctor used to come and it was always a big commotion . . . somehow
they had to take water out of him . . . I don't know how, but it was with a hose
and everybody was running around with buckets . . . my mother thinks I probably don't remember it because I was too young . . . but I can see it very
vividly . . . and then I remember best of all the cemetery where he was buried
. . . and I did not even know whose funeral it was . . . they told me it was my
father's but it did not mean anything . . . and I can see the ribbons and the
wreaths and flowers but I didn't know it was my father . . . or that I had anything to do with him. . . .

AA 5: "The meadow is sunny, somehow there are a lot of people . . . I can
see the orthodox Jew with a long beard, black hat and long coat . . . and . . .
there are all sorts of animals running around . . . there is something happening
. . . only I don't know what. It could be a parade . . . or it could be a some
sort of . . . a sort of demonstration . . . still in the meadow . . . they are march-
ing to some building now. . . .

AA 6: "I don't see anything. It is completely dark . . . I see somebody in a
white hospital gown . . . it is a little girl watching on the top of a bed . . . in a
hospital. It is a big room . . . there are lots of beds in the room. Lots of people
in the room . . . there must be 14 or 16 of them . . . and . . . and . . . there is
a woman in one of the beds . . . she starts screaming . . . and she jumps out
of the bed and through the window . . . and. . . .

*AA 7:* "Well the meadow is very empty . . . dark . . . it is a little bit misty and rainy . . . you can't see to your right or to your left because it is very dark. . . . No . . . there is a half of a skeleton and there is a man with a knife . . . a short pointed one . . . the kind you use for peeling potatoes . . . he is peeling the arm of the skeleton . . . pulling down to the elbow . . . and then he goes back to the shoulders with the knife . . . and there is another layer . . . he pulls it down and lets it hang on the hand. . . .

*AA 8:* "I don't see the meadow at all today. . . . I see a small warm lake. There are wooden buildings around it. In the water there are benches . . . you can sit on them . . . they are just deep enough so that your arms . . . rather your head sticks out. I am sitting there often . . . my brother used to come with me . . . he used to push me under the water . . . he used to push me to the bottom and . . . I had the feeling that I will never get to the sur- face . . . I'd be out of breath. . . .

*AA 9:* "It feels very heavy, the meadow is foggy . . . and then there is the river . . . with a number of bridges. There is the river bank . . . and there are stairs going up and then there is a streetcar line. A streetcar is going on it. Then there is a wall . . . and . . . the sidewalk is over the wall . . . there is a coffee-house close by, and I have a fight with my husband . . . I ran toward the sidewalk . . . and I want to kill myself in the river. I jump off the wall . . . and . . . it's a high wall . . . but now there is no streetcar coming. . . ."

*AA 10:* See p. 66; see also the patient's commentary to AA 10, p. 104.

In the group of patients who initially respond with a description of visual phenomena, various degrees of structural, chromatic and dynamic differentiation as occurs during the practice of autogenic standard exer- cises (see Table 7, p. 145/I) may be encountered. During the first autogenic abreaction 62 per cent ( N = 108 ) of psychosomatic and neurotic patients begin the initial phase with a dominance of *filmstrips* (stage IV; see Table 7, p. 145/I) or *multichromatic cineramas* (stage VII; see Table 33, p. 188). Such differentiated brain-directed processes of neutralization may be composed of sympolic elements, or they may emphasize reality features which are more directly related to accumu- lated brain-disturbing material (see Case 11, Case 12).

*Case 11:* A 32-year-old priest (anxiety reaction, multiple psychophysiologic reactions, ecclesiogenic syndrome, vocational conflicts). In this case the begin- ning of the initial phase started with a complex pattern involving cinerama- type elaborations with *direct active self-participation* (see Table 44, p. 296), auditory associations and emotional reactions.

"I see the image of my father and I am very small . . . and I look at him, at his big eyes . . . and I am afraid of him . . . his eyes look angry and hard . . . I am afraid of him . . . I am afraid of him . . . I am afraid that he is going to be angry with me . . . his eyes are threatening . . . they are not friendly . . . I am afraid of him . . . I am afraid he is going to beat me . . . and he is talking in a loud voice and harsh voice . . . and his eyes are frightening . . . and I see the cardinal . . . and I see my father . . . and his eyes are terrifying . . . I am afraid of him . . . I am afraid of being punished . . . the cardinal is looking at me . . . and I am in the big church . . . and I am reciting the Credo . . . it is my ordination . . . and everybody is there . . . and I am advancing toward the cardinal . . . and everybody is happy and applauding . . . and I feel embarrassed, I have the impression I don't belong here . . . I do not want to become a priest . . . I want my liberty . . . the cardinal with his big eyes . . . I am afraid of him. . . ."

*Case 12:* A 29-year-old housewife (posttraumatic reaction). Rather unexpectedly, during AA 5, brain-directed dynamics confront the patient with elements of a car accident which occured five months earlier.

"I see nothing . . . a car . . . I am tense all over . . . I think this will not work . . . the whole accident was there . . . [starts crying] . . . [sobbing] . . . the street corner . . . not dark . . . and so many cars . . . [continues sobbing] . . . so many people . . . [continues crying] . . . lately I did not think at all of the accident . . . now its all there . . . the street corner . . . many cars . . . many people . . there are so many cars and the ambulance . . . and the police . . . and I see this man in front of me . . . medium size . . . unpleasant, imposing . . . [crying very loudly] . . . and the telephone . . . now its all farther away . . . I am in the hospital . . . [continues crying]. . . ."

When the initial phase is dominated by less differentiated visual elaborations, as for example *objects* (stage IV, see Table 33, p. 188), various developments can be expected (see p. 206). When the patient's brain prefers to remain at the level of stage IV (objects), an initial emphasis on relatively slow elaborations of symbolic objects tends to become progressively less symbolic. As the frequency (per min.) of object elaborations increases toward the end of the initial phase and during the central phase, an increase of reality-related elements and interjected dynamic features preparing for a shift toward stages V and VI (see Table 33, p. 188) is usually noted (see Fig. 5).

In 19 per cent of a group of 108 psychomatic and neurotic patients who emphasized visual phenomena in their description during the initial phase of their first autogenic abreaction, the visual elaborations remained at a low level of differentiation (stages I-III; see Table 33, p. 188). Such elementary elaborations tend to gain in chromatic and structural differentiation as the patient's brain mechanisms are permitted to pursue their own program of therapeutic action (see Case 87, p. 207). Eight patients who started out with descriptions of *static uniform colors* (stage I) or *dynamic polymorph colors* (stage II) progressed during the central phase of the abreactive period toward significantly more differentiated and visually less symbolic elaborations characteristic for stages III to V (see Case 87, Case 88) and occasionally very quickly to stages VI and VII (see Case 13).

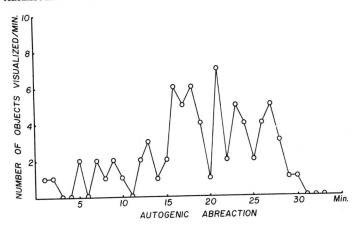

FIG. 5. Frequency of objects visualized during an autogenic abreaction by an 11-year-old schoolboy (posttraumatic reaction). After an initial period of relatively slow elaborations, the brain-directed dynamics appear to be significantly facilitated after about 15 min. After 28 min. frequent yawning and a slowdown of visual elaborations indicated that the termnial phase had been reached. During the last 3 min. no structured visual elaborations were reported, and the standard termination procedure was applied.

*Case 13:* A 43-year-old housewife (anxiety reaction). In this case the pattern of the initial phase is characterized by a rapid transition from elementary forms of visual elaborations to multichromatic cinerama (stage VII) with *passive observation* (see Table 44, p. 296). These initial passages contain essential elements related to brain-disturbing material accumulated while piloting her own aircraft (e.g., problems of coming in, possibility of crash and death). Later, after the patient realized how much disturbing material her brain had accumulated in connection with flying, she decided to discontinue this sport.

"Visually, there is absolutely nothing, not even atmospheric. . . . My varicose veins are pulling, burning. . . . I said there was nothing visually, there is not but there are limits as if it were I don't know if it is a square or rectangular starting from . . . of the back of the temple, projecting toward, I don't know how far . . . in that, it is black . . . it is not blocked off nor a screen . . . it is emptiness or it has perspectives. Now I feel . . . at the bottom it is opened, there is light . . . I feel apprehensive, I don't want to block it . . . I think it's lake X . . . I don't see enough to identify it . . . it must be feeling . . . atmosphere . . . I see . . . see or think the blue of the lake . . . the island . . . the white of the sand . . . I think . . . either we were coming in or there was an aircraft just turning . . . it was downwind, in the turn for base . . . I think it was white with red trim . . . it was definitely a high wing . . . now it seems to be more . . . it came in, on final, I just saw it over the trees . . . there was the tower, the hangar. . . ."

## The Central Phase

Although it is relatively rare that one finds a distinctive limit between the initial phase of the abreactive period and the beginning of the central phase, it is generally easy to see certain case-specific differences of brain-directed dynamics which distinguish the central phase from the initial phase. In the same way as the dynamics of the central phase progress, there is usually a gradual development toward what has been called the *terminal phase* (e.g., Case 16, p. 72). In other instances the dynamics of the central phase lead to developments which relevant brain mechanisms tend to terminate in a rather unexpected, abrupt manner (see Case 14, p. 63). The variability of the thematically and functionally determined nature of the initial and the terminal phases precludes exact measurements of duration of the central period. Generally, however, the central phase occupies about 70 to 90 per cent of the duration of a given autogenic abreaction.

During this period the brain follows its own program of thematic neutralization of brain-disturbing material. Unknown systems in our brain make use of highly sophisticated and efficient functions (see Table 12, p. 58, Table 14B, p. 65) which invariably aim at decreasing the unfavorable potency of functional interferences resulting from accumulated brain-disturbing material. As the functional capacity of relevant self-regulatory mechanisms of neutralization is limited, such brain-directed processes of self-curative action progress in sequences of phases of thematic neutralization which require a series of autogenic abreactions. Depending on the functional situation of a given brain and depending on the nature (e.g., quantity, disturbing potency) of the accumulated disturbing material, adequate neutralization may require a variable number of thematic repetitions within the same autogenic abreaction and over longer series of autogenic abreactions. As the patient's self-curative brain mechanisms are given technically adequate opportunity to pursue their work according to their own program, a number of positively oriented, therapeutically desirable changes can be observed (see Table 11).

The positively oriented changes of psychophysiologic brain dynamics are not based on insight. They result from brain-designed combinations of self-regulatory functions which are adapted to the self-curative requirements of thematically specific combinations of brain-selected and brain-programmed neuronal records. In cases where a brain is not permitted to follow its own program of thematic priorities (see Table 12), a variety of functional difficulties and therapeutically undesirable psychophysiologic reactions tend to result (see Vol. VI). It is in this

TABLE 11.  *General Trends of Psychophysiologic Changes Resulting from Dynamics of Autogenic Neutralization During the Central Abreactive Phase*

| | |
|---|---|
| Dominance of symbolically disguised elaborations | Dominance of less disguised elaborations |
| Remoteness from reality | Increase of reality features |
| High incidence of antithematic elaborations | Lower frequency of antithematic elaborations |
| High rate of brain-antagonizing forms of resistance | Low rate or no brain-antagonizing forms of resistance |
| Frequent lack of passive acceptance with, inadequate trainee-directed maneuvers | Decrease of trainee-directed interferences and technically favorably *"carte blanche"* attitude |
| Frequent periods of anxiety, apprehension and tension | Decrease or disappearance of anxiety, apprehension, and tension with dominant feeling of calmness and relaxation |
| High incidence of morbid and negatively loaded elaborations | Low incidence or disappearance of negatively oriented elaborations with increase of healthy and positively oriented elements |
| Dominance of disagreeable feelings | Dominance of agreeable or relatively neutral feelings |
| Great need for affective discharges | Decreased or no need for affective discharges |
| Relatively low levels of structural dynamic or chromatic elaborations of visual phenomena | Increasingly more differentiated structural dynamic or chromatic features of visual elaborations |
| High frequency of dark, "dangerous" or morbid colors | Increasing rate of more agreeable, lighter shades of chromatic elaborations |
| Relatively low levels of self-involvement (high degrees of dissociation) | Progressive development toward direct participation (low degree of dissociation) |
| High incidence of interferences with normal verbal expression | Progressively more normal verbal expression |
| Frequent occurrence of thematic shifts or "distractions" related to disagreeable bodily symptoms | Progressive disappearance of disagreeable bodily symptoms with increase of feeling of bodily well-being |
| High incidence of thematic dynamics aiming at neutralization of brain-disturbing material related to inadequate identification with others | Progressive decrease of themes related to inadequate identifications with progressive emphasis on dynamics related to the authentic self |
| Frequent and intensive dynamics aiming at neutralization of the destructive effects related to inadequate negatively colored religious education | Progressive evidence of more naturally and positively oriented needs and attitudes related to spiritual dimensions |
| High incidence of aggressive, destructive dynamics | Increase of elements and dynamics of productive, constructive nature |

connection that a thorough understanding of brain-directed mechanisms of autogenic neutralization is of basic importance. To facilitate the understanding of these basic dynamics it seemed appropriate to make extensive use of case material in connection with a discussion of each of the self-regulatory mechanisms listed in Table 12 (see below) and in Part IV of this book (p. 249 ff.).

In many instances, particularly during more advanced phases of treatment with autogenic abreaction, the case-specific combination and sequence of brain-directed functions of thematic neutralization tend to pass quite rapidly through a brief initial phase and unfold in a progressively more flexible and dynamic manner (see Case 14). Depending on the brain-determined thematic priority, monothematic or multithematic patterns composed of progressively changing versions of thematic repetitions may be observed. The functional dominance of brain-directed elaborations, i.e., (A) *intellectual,* (B) *sensory, motor,* (C) *visual,* (D) *mixed* (see p. 49) may vary considerably and undergo periodic changes as the central phase proceeds or may be quite restricted to a limited number of psychophysiologic dimensions (see Case 8, p. 50). Visual elaborations may occur as secondary associated features and assume variable degrees of differentiation (e.g., elementary, uniform colors, filmstrips) and clarity ((e.g., vague impressions, microscopic clarity) or may not participate at all because the brain-determined thematic priority emphasizes other dimensions (e.g., intellectual, motor, crying, sensory). However, in the majority of cases visual elaborations eventually tend to assume a guiding role

---

TABLE 12.  *Autogenic Abreaction: Mechanisms of Neutralization*

---

*Classification of Self-regulatory Brain Mechanisms*
*Responsible for the Elaboration of the following:*

1. Thematic programming and general adaptation
2. Thematic determination, selective release, and inhibition
3. Thematic repetition and confrontation
4. Thematic modification
   (a) Thematic disintegration
   (b) Thematic dissociation
   (c) Thematic distortion
5. Thematic analogies
6. Thematic antitheses
7. Thematic anticipation
8. Thematic regression and progression
9. Thematic resynchronization and integration
10. Thematic verification
11. Thematic termination

during the central phase. In a high percentage differentiated visual elaborations tend to occur during the initial phase (see Table 13) of the first two autogenic abreactions. During later treatment a variable five to ten per cent of autogenic abreactions remain without significant participation of visual elaborations. The high incidence of associated or of functionally dominant visual elaborations during autogenic abreaction has occasionally led to various misunderstandings. For example, certain patients conclude that the dynamics of autogenic neutralization are necessarily associated with images and that autogenic abreaction is not effective without visual elaborations. Such erroneous ideas may easily lead to thematic exclusion of other material which the brain cannot release because of the patient's overly directive emphasis on the "production" of visual elaborations. To forestall the development of such inhibitory, brain-restricting attitudes, the therapist should occasionally repeat his initial explanation, namely, that *carte blanche* means passive acceptance and open-mindedness of any kind[1829] of brain-directed elaboration.

The recurring dominance of visual elaborations during the central phase is of particular interest for advancing our understanding of brain-directed dynamics and the functional nature of psychodynamic and psychophysiologic disorders. The variety of processes of autogenic neutralization appears to support a number of hitherto accepted psychoanalytically oriented views and hypotheses. However, in many other instances the brain's autogenic dynamics appear to suggest the necessity of reevaluating certain perspectives of therapeutic management and theoretical thinking. It is in this connection that the variety of dynamics encountered during the central abreactive phase are of particular interest (see Case 14; Case 16, p. 66 ff.; Case 41, p. 109 ff.; Cases 34–38, p. 201 ff./I; Case 36, p. 79 ff./III).

TABLE 13. *First Appearance of Differentiated Complex Images during the First and the Second Autogenic Abreaction* (*Psychosomatic and Neurotic Patients*)

| Appearance of Differentiated Visual Elaborations | Minutes after Termination of the Induction Phase | | | | | |
|---|---|---|---|---|---|---|
| Autogenic abreaction | Less than 1 min. | 1–5 | 6–10 | 11–15 | 16–20 | 21–30 | None |
| AA 1 (N = 100) | 63 | 13 | 3 | 4 | — | 4 | 13 |
| AA 2 (N = 96) | 70 | 8 | 4 | 4 | 3 | — | 7 |

*Case 14:* A 37-year-old theologian (anxiety reaction, personality disorder, asthenic personality, sexual deviation, multiple psychophysiologic and phobic reactions, ecclesiogenic syndrome). During the central abreactive phase the dynamics of the patient's first autogenic abreaction focus largely on neutralization of transsexual material with subsequent emphasis on heterosexual and autosexual activities. Homosexual elements remain relatively camouflaged and do not lead to engagement in relevant activities (see Fig. 6).

Of further interest are brain-directed (a) transformation, (b) preparatory symbolically disguised elaborations, (c) antithematic dynamics (e.g., masculinity–femininity), (d) associated olfactory and auditory elaborations, (e) positively oriented terminal adjustment (i.e., "I have become a perfect man—quite suddenly I become myself again"), (f) self-termination (i.e., "Nothing . . . some drawing-like pattern on a dark background . . . that is all") and (g) the immediate postabreactive remark: "I feel very warm all over."

"I see white bordered by black . . . I see myself sitting in a meadow . . . and there is a big castle in the back . . . I have my arms crossed, I feel exhausted, it is cold and late at night. . . . [*Is there anything you would like to do?*] . . . No . . . I feel a sort of movement in my head. . . . I see an airplane very high up in the sky, it is night . . . and I see the white stripes running parallel on the dark background . . . [*Can you investigate the castle?*] . . . It is a huge castle of the Middle Ages . . . a big empty corridor . . . very dark . . . it is autumn

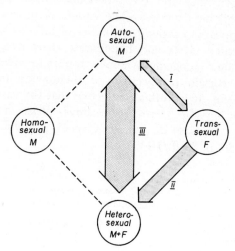

Fig. 6. Schematic presentation of the quantitative and directional aspects of the intricate thematic alternations and interactions between the four major sexual components as elaborated by Case 14. Active engagement in heterosexual activity is achived via the transsexual component (I, II). Autosexual elaborations alternate with heterosexual activity (III). Active engagement in homosexual activity is avoided (IV).

and there is quite a bit of fog . . . I am alone in the castle and it sounds empty
. . . I penetrate further and walk along the corridors and start running and cry
. . . I feel sad . . . and there are the big huge windows with the small bars . . .
outside it is foggy. . . . [*Can you look around a bit?*] . . . There are statues with
halberds . . . about sixteenth century . . . they are motionless . . . they do nothing . . . I am still in one of these big corridors with the big barred windows . . .
it is sad and dark. . . . [*Are there any doors?*] . . . No . . . well there is a big
room . . . a library . . . and a fireplace . . . the fire is burning . . . bright and
yellow . . . I am there alone . . . now I feel quite at ease and look over the
books . . . and I am walking a bit around . . . I am very happy . . . there are no
problems . . . and near the fire it is very comfortable . . . the room is dark
except for the fire. . . . [*How about visiting other parts of the castle?*] . . . I go
to one of the towers and go up . . . I am up . . . it is a beautiful afternoon . . .
the scenery is boundless and beautiful . . . there is a nice breeze and it is a bit
cool . . . the scenery is very beautiful, the fields, the lakes, a farmer . . . extremely peaceful. . . . He is plowing the field . . . and the earth breaks up like
a wave and falls to both sides leaving the open furrow. . . . I am walking on
the roof of the castle and look around . . . it is late in the afternoon . . . extremely charming . . . I am alone and very calm . . . beautiful clouds are
drifting along . . . it is getting darker . . . I am walking on the roof and it is
almost night. . . . I hear a train . . . and I see the train . . . and lights are
lighting up . . . I am very happy and feel very well . . . I see the train entering
a tunnel . . . the train enters the tunnel and there is some smoke . . . I am still
on the roof and I stay there . . . it is now night . . . the image of the train going
into the tunnel and the smoke is always coming back . . . again . . . again . . .
again . . . and again. . . . And I am walking on a wooden sort of gangway
(*passerelle*), it is night and there is an agreeable breeze. . . . Now I see something like drawings, white crosses on a dark background . . . now white stripes
on dark background . . . and now there is nothing at all . . . it is very calm . . .
and again there are the same drawing-like things, white on black . . . I am still
on the roof and I am walking around . . . now I see the number '4' . . . and now
nothing at all. . . . I go back down a long spiral staircase . . . it is quite narrow
and goes in circles as I go down . . . it is like a huge dungeon and sometimes
I look out of the small windows . . . very interesting . . . a black tieplate on
white . . . I am still going down very slowly and calm . . . and I arrive in the
kitchen and the servants bow and greet me very politely and I inhale . . . it
seems they prepare a very good supper, it smells good . . . and I talk to the
people and it is quite pleasant. . . . I feel like being the master of the house,
and I feel like a woman, like the lady of manor, and I inspect the kitchen . . .
I have a wig on my head and long hair . . . suddenly I have quite a bad pain
in my abdomen . . . I talk to the servants . . . and I feel excited in view of the
big banquet to come . . . and I walk around and make some jokes and everybody is in good spirits. . . . I am half a woman and the metamorphosis continues
. . . I am laughing like a woman, my fingernails are painted and I have large
red lips and silken lady's stockings and feet like a woman, a small white blouse,
a simple skirt, a big necklace made of precious stones, rich jewelry, a big

ring . . . and I play with it, take it off my finger and put it back, sometimes I put my hands up to my face and I laugh and talk to the cook . . . I really feel like the chatelaine. . . . Suddenly I am again outside on the meadow, on my knees and I weep . . . like a forgotten woman, like a prostitute . . . and I am very sad . . . I feel like a woman who has been thrown out of the castle and I feel quite depressed . . . on my knees . . . in a very sad mood . . . I feel extremely depressed . . . and I do not know what to do, I feel abandoned . . . and I stay there . . . with my skirt, the long hair, the silk stocking and lady's shoes . . . and I feel rather peculiar . . . and my transformation into a woman seems to go on, and I feel like a young girl, very pretty and I raise my face against the wind and my long blond hair flutters in the wind . . . and now I am again a man and I get up . . . and I am now again a beautiful girl . . . I am standing and feel more confident than a little while ago . . . I make my toilet, fix my hair, rearrange my skirt and feel extremely refined (delicate, dainty) and my shoulders and my body and everything is quite feminine . . . like Greta Garbo and I am extremely beautiful . . . I am outside alone, abandoned but self-confident and I see the lights of the castle . . . the banquet has started . . . rich people arrive . . . and I hear the music, they are playing a waltz . . . it is very nice inside . . . and I am outside . . . the lights are creating a warm atmosphere . . . and I am dressed like a lady with a skirt and a blouse, lady's stockings and pretty shoes . . . I listen to the music and I feel in harmony with everything . . . I am very beautiful and I let my delicate fingers run through my beautiful blond hair . . . I have delicate fingers, long and round fingernails and feel completely myself . . . my hair is long and curled, I have nice and pretty shoes and I feel very well . . . the party is going on in the castle . . . and there is the moon, a summer night, peaceful and calm. . . . And now I am walking in a forest, the scenery is a bit foggy and the moon is shining on my face and hands . . . I sit down . . . the trees of the forest look dark . . . there is the moon, it is night . . . there is the forest and the castle is further away . . . the feeling of loneliness is more intense . . . I am still a beautiful woman with a skirt, a blouse, silk stockings, pretty shoes, long beautiful blond hair and jewelry . . . I am sitting and look around at the moon and the forest and I am very gay and happy and I feel protected by the moon. . . . Now there seems to be something threatening or dangerous in the wood . . . and I see cannibals with spears and shields, they are coming closer, their faces are painted with big white patterns, it looks terrible . . . I am very much afraid and I cry and I run and they follow throwing spears and shooting arrows at me, I am surrounded by them and they are pointing their lances at my throat and they are tatooed all over . . . they grab me and I am very much afraid and I cry . . . I look and see their spears directed toward me . . . they have red eyes . . . I see their eyes . . . but there are too many . . . about 1,000 cannibals and they have their hands on me . . . I am a naked woman and they want to slaughter me . . . I am a woman completely naked . . . and I start dancing and the cannibals start laughing they drop their spears and begin to dance . . . they seem to disappear and only one stays there . . . he is still holding his spear but turned downward . . . and we dance . . . this is very funny . . . and I am all white and he is black and we dance and he is pressing me against him and dances with me and I feel warm . . . hot all over . . . and we have intercourse in upright position and he is holding his spear in his hand but pointing it downward . . . that is all . . . I feel very satisfied . . . the pleasure of love-making is very agreeable . . . we muse and play and he plays with his sex organ which is erect . . . and he is a cannibal and sometimes he enters his organ into me . . . and I am a white woman . . . and sometimes I become a cannibal and I play with my male sex organ . . . and the cannibals have fun in front of me . . . he is still playing with his sex organ . . . this is extremely sensual and I feel very excited . . . and there is the clearing and the forest . . . and the moon is shining and it is very attractive . . . and they jump on me as if to kill me . . . and he plays with his sex organ and the scene continues . . . it still continues . . . and he plays with his sex organ and this goes on and on . . . and I feel the movements in me and this is very agreeable and pleasant . . . sometimes I feel like the cannibal and at the same time a woman . . . the cannibal and the woman . . . I am both, I am the cannibal in all his masculinity and I am the woman with all its pleasure (*je suis la femme dans la jouissance*) . . . this seems to be over . . . the cannibal is suddenly afraid, he wants to run away, looks all around, he wants to kill me before . . . I am now cannibal myself, tattooed, in the wood and I have become a perfect man . . . quite suddenly I become myself again . . . nothing . . . some drawing-like pattern on a dark background . . . that is all . . . I feel comfortable . . . ." [42 min.; standard termination]. Immediately after termination the patient remarked: "I feel very warm all over."

When the initial phase is characterized by an emphasis on description of elementary visual elaborations, and this pattern continues, it is important to remember that the patient's brain has reasons for proceeding in such a manner. Any supportive interference, except for repeated evidence of brain-antagonizing forms of resistance (e.g., suppressed need for crying, swearing; see Table 14, p. 65; see Vol. VI), is contraindicated (see Case 15). In such cases, the brain appears to engage in functionally important preparatory work which, in spite of its restricted range of elaboration is therapeutically effective. As the brain is permitted to continue this type of pattern through a number of autogenic abreactions (participation of brain-antagonizing resistance excluded), one can observe a slowly progressing increase of dynamic flexibility, a trend toward higher degrees of differentiation in visual elaborations and widening of the range of elements preparing for more complete processes of multithematic neutralization (see Case 15; Case 88, p. 208).

*Case 15:* A 26-year-old social worker (anxiety reaction, moderate depression, multiple psychophysiologic reactions). During her first autogenic abreaction (see below) this patient described visual phenomena limited to elementary stages of differentiation (see Table 33, p. 188). However, as her slow description continued, a progressive development from stage I to higher degrees of differentiation (i.e., stage IV) occurred. After 24 minutes her description slowed down. During the twenty-seventh, twenty-eighth and twenty-ninth minute the patient remained silent. The standard termination procedure was applied after 30 minutes. In this case 11 autogenic abreactions were needed before the patient's brain became able to engage in sufficiently differentiated (e.g., stages VI and VII), functionally multidimensional and thematically flexible processes of autogenic neutralization.

"I feel my heart beating more strongly than usual and my face is quite warm. . . . The visual field is quite dark . . . there is something like a half of a circle . . . now I see a white dot . . . there is a sort of illumination . . . and now I see a big white circle . . . the circle is still there . . . and now another small circle passed and disappeared . . . the background is dark and in the distance there is a small circle which appears and disappears several times. . . . I see something like four fingers . . . lower part is dark and the upper part is less dark . . . now it is less dark and the white is still there. . . . My fingers are numb. . . . The black and the white are separated by a diagonal line, the white is on the right side . . . now I see something like a small curved line, the line has the shape of an S . . . there is a sort of illumination effect like northern lights in white . . . now there is a white circle, the circle is not static, it is oscillating . . . now I see a white circle with rays . . . the rays are only on the right side . . . now I see the rays without circle . . . now the rays are only at the left side . . . several small white dots pass rather fast from right to left . . . now I see a white pine tree . . . now this is a triangle pointing down . . . and now there is a sort of mountain with a sharp top, the mountain is white . . . there is a nose, now the nose is black and the rest is white . . . now I see only half a pine tree on the left side of the visual field . . . this has disappeared and now I see a curved line . . . and there again I see the side of a pine tree . . . there is a white point toward the left . . . my arms feel stiff . . . it feels as if I have the arms full of lead . . . I thought I saw toes but this was not very clear . . ." (30 min.; standard termination).

The management of patients during the central phase may require the therapist's undivided attention when various forms of brain-antagonizing resistance (see Table 14; Vol. VI, Part I) interfere with the brain's program of thematic neutralization. Particularly in the beginning (see Table 7, p. 37) when the patient is learning to understand the language of his brain and when he has difficulty in maintaining an attitude of passive acceptance, well-timed and thematically correctly adapted technical support is required (see initial phase of Case 14, p. 60; see Case 16; Case 50, p. 127 ff.). Such technical support is designed to help the brain in continuing its dynamics of neutralization along dimensions or in a direction which the brain has already indicated repeatedly. As such carefully adapted technical support respects and facilitates its own program of action, and as such interventions are kept to a minimum, the basic principle of non-interference is maintained. Even when technical support is indicated, each intervention should be as neutral as possible, given the circumstances. Only rarely is thematically very specific support (see Case 16) necessary, and in such instances the specific nature of the support should be based on thorough knowledge of the patient's pattern of neutralization and his pattern of resistance-reactivity as it has become evident during preceding autogenic abreactions. The careful use of such supportive interventions should not be misunderstood as a technical encouragement for therapist-designed maneuvers which are actually aiming at producing, revealing and clinically interesting experiences, which are more satisfying to the therapist than to the patient's brain mechanisms which are being managed in a technically camouflaged but rather careless manner.

Correct timing of well-adapted support requires adequate experience with brain-facilitating and brain-antagonizing forms of resistance (see Table 14; Part I/VI). Since certain features of normally progressing dynamics of neutralization may be easily misinterpreted as brain-antagonizing resistance it is considered important that the beginner in the field of autogenic neutralization acquires a good understanding of

TABLE 14. *Autogenic Abreaction: Brain-antagonizing and Brain-facilitating Forms of Resistance*

| A | B |
|---|---|
| *Antagonizing Forms of Resistance* | *Facilitating Forms of Resistance* |
| 1. Intentional resistance | 1. Counter-resistance |
|   (a) Direct intentional resistance |   (a) Promoting counter-resistance |
|   (b) Indirect intentional resistance |   (b) Arresting counter-resistance |
| 2. Thematic exclusion |   (c) Terminating counter-resistance |
| 3. Thematic evasion | 2. Preparatory antithematic resistance |
| 4. Premature disengagement | 3. Program-related resistance |
| 5. Repetition resistance | 4. Integration-promoting resistance |
| 6. Associative resistance | 5. Compensatory resistance |
|   (a) Missed association | 6. Recuperative resistance |
|   (b) Inadequate response | 7. Protective resistance |

| C | D |
|---|---|
| | *Indirect Psychophysiologic Resistance* |
| | 1. Side-effect resistance |
| | 2. Circumstantial resistance |
| *Essential Forms of Resistance* |   (a) Intrinsic concomitant factors |
| 1. Anticipatory resistance |   (b) Extrinsic concomitant factors |
| 2. Presentation resistance | 3. Pharmacodynamic resistance |

normal mechanisms of brain-directed neutralization (see Table 12, p. 58; Part IV). Furthermore, it may be remarked that a clear distinction between certain brain-facilitating forms of resistance and certain forms of brain-antagonizing resistance may be difficult or even impossible for an experienced therapist. To facilitate the understanding of these dynamics, it seemed useful to present detailed discussions and illustrative case material in a systematic manner in Part I, Volume VI.

*Case 16:* A 42-year-old housewife (anxiety reaction, moderate depressive reaction; see initial phase of this patient's first nine AAs on p. 51 ff.). The following autogenic abreaction (AA 10, 74 min.) shows almost all essential dynamics of mechanisms of autogenic neutralization (see Table 12, p. 000). The pattern of multithematic neutralization revolves largely around anxiety and aggression involving death, various operations (including a traumatic postoperative experience), negatively oriented elements of religious education, specific sexual problems, and a variety of other traumatic situations and brain-disturbing confrontations. The cinerama-type pattern is occasionally associated with auditory, gustatory, vestibular and other sensory (viscerosensory) elaborations.

During the nine preceding autogenic abreactions, the patient had great difficulty in maintaining an attitude of passive acceptance and frequently interfered (e.g., thematic evasion, abortive engagement, repetition resistance; see Table 14, p. 65) with the brain's program of thematic neutralization. For this reason, for instructive purposes and to avoid a reoccurrence of previously encountered post-abreactive difficulties, an unusual amount of technical support was given (see Table 7, p. 37). In each instance the support respects the thematic orientation already indicated by the brain, or known from dynamics which dominated preceding autogenic abreactions.

The particular pattern of thematic repetition with progressively advancing neutralization was also seen during previous autogenic abreactions.

The terminal phase contains several elements indicating advanced and successful neutralization: (a) increase of reality features, (b) brain-directed facilitating maneuvers, as for example: "My bed starts lifting up, . . . disintegration," (c) remaining calm during elaborations that had been previously disturbing, (d) feeling relaxed and peaceful, (e) feeling of intense warmth, (f) brain-directed indications in the visual field (e.g., "All I see is whiteness").

"I think of a big eye. It is a red eye and there is red paint around . . . and it is a huge eye with red veins running across it . . . [*Can you describe that?*] . . . It is oversize, it is on a filmscreen . . . it is red all around . . . and the eye is very bloodshot . . . it is very red . . . running all over . . . and . . . there is something, a splinter or something in the eye . . . and there is a hand with pincers trying to get the splinter out of the eye. . . . [*Please keep describing*] . . . I saw it . . . I went yesterday . . . I went to an industrial exibition . . . I don't know what it had to do with office equipment, but there it was on the screen. I watched it for a minute or so and then I walked away, but I kept thinking of it. Very bright red, and the eye is almost swollen up . . . sort of bulging eye . . . I didn' t see the eyelid and the eyelashes . . . they were pulled up . . . it looks dead . . . the eye looks dead but . . . not around it, because it is very bright red. . . . Now there is somebody peeling potatoes . . . sitting on a stool, there is a bucket underneath . . . and holding a sharp knife . . . and peeling it without breaking the peel to pieces, it just comes down in a long, long, long stream and drops into the bucket . . . potatoes . . . it is a very sharp knife [see initial phase AA 7, p. 53]. I don't know who it is, I don't know why I see it. I haven't been peeling potatoes for a long time. But it is such a contrast to the big red eye . . . they are small white potatoes. Brown peels running down. There is blood running down from the eye . . . but the eye is looking at me . . . [Please keep looking at the eye and describe what you see] . . . it is changing and I didn't see the whole eye because somebody was holding the pincers to take the splinter out . . . and half-covered the right corner of the eye . . . but now probably the splinter is out . . . there is just this big eye . . . looking at me. . . . It is like . . . we used to learn about God and the priest or nun told us to draw a triangle on the blackboard . . . a triangle and a big eye stretching from one end of the triangle to the other. Teaching us that God's eyes see everything. But that was not a red one. It was white chalk. And . . . this one is very bloody . . . and bigger . . . even the eyelashes are red . . . it doesn't blink . . . it is immobile on a screen . . . as if somebody was standing behind . . . there are blood drops . . . running from the corner . . . it's again like the big red heart we used to draw of Jesus. His heart is bleeding if you are bad. Once I went to an exhibition of Salvador Dahli's moving jewels and there was a mechanical heart, "the pulsating heart," that is all swollen and shiny . . . shiny red . . . and it moves: swells and shrinks and then again . . . the bloody eye and the red heart and the peeling of potatoes . . . opening up one's heart . . . it is your heart . . . somebody takes it out with a small sharp knife . . . opens up your chest . . . and takes out the heart . . . and puts it on a table . . . then goes on pulsating . . . pumping . . . you are lying on the table . . . your chest all cut up, your heart is on a paper towel . . . on a table beside you . . . and I am not dead because my heart is still there. Potentially . . . it works. Except that somebody ought to put it back . . . I try to . . . I imagine that I lie there and I know and see my heart pumping . . . I am still alive. . . . If they took your brain out, it would be different . . . they could cut your head, spoon the brain out and put it in a mug [see initial phase of AA 3, p. 52] . . . then you wouldn't even see it, because you can't see . . . then you can't see . . . when they put it back . . . they could put it back any odd way . . . then you would be mad . . . and all mixed up . . . like a puppet . . . which is crude and just hooked up dangling in front of a window, or the strawman. The strawman from the wizard of Oz, whose head was all full of straw. He had no brain . . . just dangling . . . not even a puppet, a rag-doll, that's more like it . . . it is soft it has no bones, no brain, can't walk. You would just get off the operating table and you would fall . . . and you wouldn't even know that you fell . . . they would be just staring at you and let you walk or crawl away . . . whichever. . . . Once I was wheeled out from the operating table . . . and I had difficulty waking up. And that was a time I was not sure if I was dead

or not. I kept hearing the nurse saying: you have to wake up . . . and . . . uncross your legs . . . your blood circulation will never work. And I couldn't . . .
uncross my legs. I felt so . . . deep on the bottom of a well that I wasn't sure
if it was I who was hearing or thinking . . . or just the spirit of mine . . . somewhere. . . . I feel dizzy . . . it is a strange feeling that you are on the bottom of
a deep hole and they are throwing earth on you . . . and I am lying in a hole
but I can't see earth, just hear this metallic voice: 'You have to wake up. . . .'
I couldn't think . . . I wasn't sure if I could or would wake up. . . . I am sinking now . . . the bed is going . . . down, down . . . if it goes down it has to
reach the bottom . . . I am on the bottom of the hole and I see the big red
eye . . . it is on the top looking down at me . . . it's almost as big as the opening of the hole . . . [Just look at the eye and describe what you see] . . . I
close my eyes . . . but I can see it even with my eyes closed . . . It's long,
almond-shape, but bulging . . . it is almost like a big round ball . . . I see the
eyelids that are red and underneath and in the corner it is all red . . . the
eyeball is white with red veins . . . there is just a black point at the middle . . .
it doesn't have any color . . . I see not only the surface of it. It seems that I
can see the back of the eye too. It is just very loosely set in the eye-opening
. . . when it turns around then it is completely white . . . like a potato . . .
no veins because they are on the other side . . . or a peeled apple . . . even
the red side was better than just seeing the white . . . I am lying on the bottom
of the pit on my back. I am a lot smaller than the eye . . . I would like to come
up but I can't. . . . [Please keep describing] . . . It is a long climb and I would
try if it weren't for the eye . . . if I had a knife, I could climb up and cut it
up . . . to cut the eye and then it couldn't see . . . there would be just liquid
coming out. . . . [OK—do all that] . . . I have to get up and climb on the wall
of the hole . . . it is crumbling . . . it is hard to get a hold . . . I use my
fingers and my feet . . . I have my shoes on. I climb closer and closer . . . and
. . . then I stop thinking that it would do something, if I get any closer. But
it doesn't. And I have a knife . . . a little  potato-paring knife. And I get up
and I hold on with my left arm, and I put the knife into the eye and then the
earth is crumbling and I fall down on the bottom . . . and . . . a white jellied
sort of liquid keeps coming down from the eye . . . it is spraying on me . . . I
can't see anything only the cut-up film of the eye. It's huge and the . . . this
liquid just covers me. It's slippery . . . and I am still where I was. . . . [Please
describe that] . . . I just wish I could stop this . . . this stuff. It is cold, it is
almost transparent white . . . and there is so much of it . . . and I keep wiping
it off. . . . [Don't fight it, describe it] . . . I can't . . . it is very unpleasant. . . .
[Alright—describe how it is unpleasant] . . . it is just cold and slippery as if
someone has emptied a big lot of . . . I don't know . . . Jello or sperm on you
. . . and it is on my head . . . on my face . . . then it keeps dripping onto the
ground [Can you taste it?] . . . No! . . . [For technical reasons—go ahead—taste
it] . . . it's bitter and bitter and slimy and it makes me nauseated . . . it is the
same as getting sperm into your mouth and . . . I spit it out . . . and I don't
like the smell of it . . . it still comes dripping on me . . . [Alright, then drink it
all up] . . . No! . . . [For technical reasons please go along with the brain—

*otherwise we'll have trouble*] . . . crying . . . [*Don't fight it, just go along with what the brain wants you to do*] . . . But there is such quantity of it . . . if I take it all in my mouth, I start throwing up. . . . [*Maybe the brain wants you to drown in that. So do it. Don't fight it—keep describing*] . . . All right, the smell itself is nauseating . . . I keep throwing up and it gets mixed up with this horrible white stuff . . . and I keep sweeping it off myself but then it comes higher up on the ground, it comes up to the top of the bed. . . .[*So let yourself drown in it*] . . . because I don't want to step into it, I don't move at all . . . I stay on the bed . . . it is coming up to my hands. And I don't try to grab it . . . I just let it flow over my hands . . . It is coming higher up . . . I am lifting my head up to keep out of it . . . [*Please don't fight it*] . . . I close my eyes, my mouth . . . I don't want to get it in my mouth . . . and then it comes into my nose also . . . I can't breathe any more . . . it's not heavy . . . it just fills up everything inside me . . . it covers my forehead and my hair and then it is quite . . . [*Please go on*] . . . I don't breathe any more. I lie there dead . . . [*Can you describe that?*] . . . I am all covered with the white stuff. I don't see anything any more . . . just whiteness . . . an opaque kind of whiteness. I don't feel anything any more . . . it is cool, it feels cool . . . [*Please describe the whole story again*] . . . So I fell down on the bottom of a pit . . . I lie there looking up. On top of the well I see nothing but a huge, huge eye, as big as the top of the hole itself, it's longish . . . it has wrinkled eyelids and red long eyelashes . . . the eye has no color . . . just a black dot at the middle . . . the eyeball is full of veins . . . tiny, tiny tree-shaped blood vessels . . . it is looking down at me and I keep looking up . . . and I don't dare to move . . . then the eyeball turns around in its socket and it becomes completely white . . . huge white ball . . . full of liquid . . . then I remember that I have my potato knife . . . I get off the bed. I start climbing on the wall of the pit . . . it is completely vertical, very loose earth . . . crumbling . . . and I climb . . . bit by bit . . . looking up at the eye to see if it does anything. I reach the wall close to it . . . I grab my knife and push it as far as I can . . . deep into the eyeball with it . . . then my left hand lets go and I fall . . . fall, fall down to the bottom of the pit. And the stuff from the eye starts coming down . . . in big splashes . . . it flows all over me . . . and I feel it on my lips and it tastes bitter-sour . . . it tastes exactly like sperm . . . then I throw up . . . I get very sick. The stuff keeps coming . . . it is building up on the floor . . . it comes up to the level of the bed . . . up to my hand, to my elbow and I don't want to get up . . . I don't want to do anything . . . I want to stay quiet so it would reach up quicker and would be finished . . . it reaches my lips . . . now it goes slowly, it takes a while before it covers my face, my nose and my hair . . . I hold my breath for a while. There is pressure in my head . . . then I give up . . . I don't breathe any more . . . [*Please describe how it is now*] . . . Very quiet . . . no noise at all . . . it is sort of like floating in a very cool, white substance. You can't swim in it because it is too thick . . . so you just float . . . [*All right, so then let's do this over again*] . . . I am lying on a bed. Start to sink and sink and it sinks way, way down . . . it stops on the bottom of a pit . . . I am falling with the bed . . . it stops . . . I stay on my back . . . my eyes are open

and I look up . . . there is a huge eye looking down at me . . . I see the red
. . . eyelids . . . wrinkled and very red . . . very bright red, long eyelashes . . .
underneath the eye it is also red . . . it is like solid red paint . . . and in this
eye-opening I see the eyeball . . . it looks loose in its socket, and . . . it is full
of red veins . . . it doesn't move at all . . . I look up and it looks down at me.
Then the eyeball turns in the socket . . . it becomes completely white . . . it is
the size of a big balloon, but it is white . . . it is the size of a potato or a peeled
apple . . . I start to feel very hot now . . . and after looking up for a while, I
remember that I have a knife and decide to climb up and kill the eye . . . I
climb up . . . looking up at the eye ever so often to see if it does anything . . .
my fingers are sore . . . as I grasp . . . the earth crumbles . . . and then I get
up to the top . . . I can't get hold of the edge of the hole, because the eye is
covering it completely . . . so I hold on to a hole in the earth . . . I stab the
eye very very hard . . . the knife goes in and my fist and my arm as far as my
elbow . . . and with this big push I fall right back down onto the bed . . .
and then the skin of the eye opens up . . . it rips completely . . . and this jelly
. . . white jelly-type of stuff comes down, flowing on me . . . if falls on my face
. . . I taste it . . . and I don't like the taste, it makes me sick in the stomach
. . . I throw up, it is cool and it is slimy . . . it tastes bitter and sour . . . it
tastes like sperm . . . and I have such a quantity in my mouth that I know I
can't swallow it and I get tears in my eyes . . . I can't swallow it and quick
enough because it comes down in such quantities . . . [Can you swallow it? That
is what the brain wants] . . . I keep swallowing it . . . after a while I don't
feel the taste at all . . . I am afraid that I would choke on it . . . I open my
mouth while swallowing it as wide as I can . . . I don't smell and I don't
taste it anymore . . . [Just keep swallowing it] . . . I feel that my stomach is
almost bursting . . . I know if I have to swallow much more, my stomach will
swell up completely and then it will burst . . . [Just continue to swallow, the
liquid goes down through your intestines and comes out the other end, that's
all right] . . . I do . . . but I have a stomach ache . . . finally it is as if I have
a hose running through me and the stuff comes in and runs out through the
hose . . . I will be drowning . . . it builds up on the floor . . . and after I
swallowed it, it starts to swallow me . . . [Go ahead] . . . and my stomach is
aching, it is like swallowing acid . . . it starts to burn, and as it comes out it
comes up higher and higher . . . it is almost up to my chin . . . then I don't
swallow any more . . . I just keep my mouth open . . . it keeps coming down.
I am full inside . . . outside it filled up over my head and I just disintegrate in
it . . . I become part of it. There is nothing left . . . if you looked down, all you
would see would be a sort of large jellied pool . . . [Let's repeat it] . . . My
throat is sore too . . . [That's all right, just go on] . . . I am on the bottom of a
pool . . . not pool, hole . . . together with the bed and I am lying on the bed . . .
completely quiet and immobile . . . I look up and way, way above me on the
top of the pit, there is a huge eye looking down . . . no, no . . . it turned into a
huge penis . . . I don't . . . [Please keep describing] . . . it's different . . . [Keep
describing] . . . still red . . . [Please remain passive and keep describing] . . . I
keep quiet and I look up at it . . . I don't like the sight of it . . . [Can you

*describe it in detail?*] . . . it almost fills the whole opening of the pit . . . it's completely full of blood, and from where I lie . . . I can just see the end of it . . . shiny red . . . again it looks like a bulging eye . . . it's rather purple than red . . . and I close my eyes several times because I don't want to see it . . . I can't resist though . . . I keep opening my eyes, I keep seeing it . . . [*How does it look?*] . . . it is fantastically huge because it covers the whole opening . . . I see it coming down . . . the foreskin is all wrinkled . . . the end . . . the way I see it from where I am . . . turns into violet red with veins running all across . . . I feel very dizzy . . . I feel as if my bed were lifting up . . . floating up . . . if I go up any higher . . . I am going to reach it . . . I reach it . . . I take it to my mouth and feel the same taste . . . I am floating in the air . . . and I turn my head away . . . [*No, don't do it, keep describing, otherwise we will have to come back*] . . . I keep my head straight . . . I take the penis into my mouth and I am choking . . . it is so big . . . it fills my mouth and throat and I want to go down but I can't or I don't want to . . . I stay there . . . first I don't taste anything . . . then it gets swollen in my mouth and I have to swallow the sperm . . . it keeps coming . . . and when I think that I am going to get sick . . . my bed falls back down . . . but the stuff keeps flowing at me . . . it still comes up and up from the bottom until I am covered completely . . . then I can't see anymore . . . but I smell it . . . [*Just keep describing*] . . . now I feel terribly hot . . . [*Please keep describing*] . . . I am still alive . . . I am holding my breath . . . I am completely full up to my mouth and up to my nose . . . and then the pressure builds up in my head, I get a headache . . . my head is bursting, my stomach is bursting . . . then I think I won't fight anymore . . . I lie very quietly and my eyes are closed . . . and I don't think of anything any more . . . as my eyes are closed, I am getting less and less hot . . . getting cool . . . and peaceful . . . through my eyelids *all I see is whiteness . . . whiteness everywhere around* . . . then I rest . . . [*Can you describe it again?*] . . . I am falling down again, the hole is round . . . I am lying on a bed . . . the bed is falling down . . . not too fast . . . it is rather sinking slowly and I am not scared . . . it floats . . . sinks down quietly . . . it stops on the ground . . . like a well . . . just a long round hole . . . I am going down . . . I look up, way way above . . . at the top of the pit where I came in and where there was air and blue skies before . . . I don't see anything, just a huge penis . . . it fills up the opening of the pit completely . . . I look up . . . up . . . I want to see it in detail . . . I see the hair, the wrinkled skin, very red . . . as I look up I see it almost as thick as the hole in which I am . . . I look at it . . . hands are now getting very hot . . . almost burning . . . I think my hands are burning because I want to go closer and see and touch it . . . [*Do that*] . . . and as if by magic, my bed starts lifting up . . . I go close to it . . . at first I touch it. . . it is very thick . . . I can't get my hands around it . . . it feels much cooler than my hands . . . then I try to get it to my mouth but I can't because it is huge . . . I still hold it . . . then all of a sudden the sperm starts flowing into my mouth . . . a thick, strong stream . . . I don't taste it . . . not any more . . . it pushes me and the bed down . . . it keeps pouring on me . . . I look up at it . . . it has not changed in any way and the white stuff keeps coming . . . I drink it . . . as much as I can . . . it is flowing on my face . . . it is coming out of me . . . until it builds up . . . goes up and up and very slowly covers me . . . I close my eyes . . . this stuff fills me up inside and covers me outside . . . *and I feel relaxed and peaceful* . . . just slowly start disintegrating . . . pieces of me just float in the jelly . . . I become nothing . . . I can't see anything anymore . . . *all I see is whiteness.* . . . [*Can you describe?*] . . . To describe what I did or what I see now? . . . [*Describe that*] . . . *all there is is whiteness* . . . *whiteness* and I can't see anything . . . my hands are still very hot . . ." [74 min.; standard termination]. The patient's commentary is presented on page 104 ff.

Of particular clinical interest are patients who are known to have accumulated considerable quantities of brain-disturbing material and who start out with an autogenic abreaction which is delightfully pleasant and agreeable (see Case 17; Case 118, p. 274). When such positively oriented antithematic dynamics (see p. 308 ff.) dominate the central phase of the first autogenic abreaction, it may be expected that a brain-directed shift toward thematic neutralization of very disturbing material with unpleasant confrontations may occur during the second autogenic abreaction. After a number of cases reported the onset of depressive manifestations with increase of anxiety and various psychophysiologic reactions within about two to five days after such "very pleasant" antithematic beginnings, it seemed appropriate to give more detailed consideration to the probability of the development of such unfavorable reactions. As a general rule, to forestall the development of therapeutically disturbing reactions during the interim period, it has been found helpful to shorten the interim period by scheduling the next appointment for the second autogenic abreaction within three to four days and to invite the patient to call at any time he did not feel well, and that an earlier appointment would be arranged to accommodate the needs of his brain (i.e., neutralization of mobilized material). When early appointments are practically impossible and the interim period is longer than five days, it is in many instances advisable to prescribe supportive medication (e.g., antidepressive, tranquilizing) to forestall and to reduce the variety of disturbing reactions which usually result when adequate neutralization of mobilized material cannot be carried out.

*Case 17:* A 36-year-old mother of 8- and 4-year-old boys, separated 18 months from her alcoholic husband because of frequent acts of violence. The overworked patient (foreman in a shoe factory) complained about nervousness, excessive sensitivity toward noise, inferiority feelings, her impatience with her children and the temptation to punish them too severely, tiredness, frequent crying spells, occasional suicidal ideas, constipation and frequent headaches. After 11 weeks of autogenic standard training (heaviness, warmth) the patient felt much better but still had some difficulty in controlling aggressive impulses toward her children. The first autogenic abreaction (see below) was started after a brief introductory discussion.

"I see a green meadow and trees and the sun is shining . . . it is agreeable . . . I am sitting in the grass and my children are playing around me and there is air and I imagine a fire . . . and it is smelling good and fresh . . . it is a wonderful day . . . not too warm, not too cold . . . with a blue sky . . . the children are playing in the fresh air and I let them do so. . . . Now I am on the beach but I do not go into the water . . . we are alone and there is no noise . . . I can hear the water . . . the birds . . . and there are insects . . . I observe them and I have a collection of caterpillars . . . the trees are beautiful with nice leaves and a rough bark . . . a little bit farther, there is a road and I can hear some little noises . . . now we are dining on the grass . . . the children are happy . . . laughing . . . shouting and talking . . . my children look younger than they are actually . . . and now it is time to go home and I would like to stay here . . . the children are not too tired yet . . . now I see my oldest son at the age of three, now eight . . . an airplane is passing by and distracts us . . . the children are happy to see an airplane . . . there still is nobody around . . . all is quiet except the noise of the airplane and of a car passing far away . . . now it is darker and less warm . . . we put some wood into the fire and we can hear the wood crackle . . . and it is smelling good . . . we are still looking at the fire . . . I observe the work of the ants and I explain it to the children . . . my son is playing in the water with small boats . . . some people are coming and it is not nice anymore . . . I do not feel like staying anymore . . ." [20 min.; standard termination].

*After-effects:* "I feel fine, sort of refreshed."

*Postabreactive discussion:* The patient felt that she needs something like that and that this was easy for her. "I easily go off dreaming things like that, I imagine nice trips to New York or Quebec or elsewhere. This was really pleasant and much cheaper too. I also used to do this particularly during the difficult periods I had with my husband." The patient felt that this was a sort of very helpful evasion from disagreeable circumstances of her everyday life.

Positively oriented very pleasant antithematic beginnings may be considered as a form of resistance related to thematic avoidance (see Vol. VI). However, the brain-designed nature of such positively oriented antithematic dynamics and the spontaneity of multidimensional (e.g., visual, olfactory, auditory; see Case 17) elaborations rather indicate that the brain for some reason wished to avoid a direct confrontation with very disturbing material, and for its own purposes found it facilitating to begin with preparatory encouraging, very nice, antithematic dynamics. It is in consideration of these aspects that brain-directed antithematic elaborations are not classified as brain-antagonizing forms of resistance (e.g., thematic avoidance; see Vol. VI, Part I).

Occasionally difficult problems of management are encountered in relatively inexperienced patients when the central phase is dominated by dynamics involving attempts at neutralization of severely disturbing material (e.g., car accident, plane crash, drowning). The generally disagreeable nature of brain-directed elaborations and the inexperienced patient's difficulty in remaining passive and giving *carte blanche* to his brain are frequently associated with multiple occurrence of various forms of brain-antagonizing resistance (see Vol. VI, Part I). Since the brain mechanisms wish to follow their own program of thematic priorities, and as these brain-programmed dynamics are blocked through patient-directed interferences, functionally more complicated and subjectively more disagreeable situations (e.g., headache, stomachache, heart pain) tend to result. While it is possible in many instances to readjust such functional complications through precise application of brain-supportive interventions, it is not usually possible to arrive at adequate levels of neutralization. The disagreeable dynamics of the central phase are strenous, patients tend to feel exhausted, and often a technical termination during a relatively neutral phase is indicated (see Case 29, p. 91; Case 125, p. 286). In such cases a carefully conducted postabreactive discussion (see p. 94 ff.) and specific suggestions concerning the patient's homework (see p. 96 ff.) are of particular therapeutic importance.

The central phase of the first and occasionally the second autogenic abreaction is frequently composed of varying kinds of elements which on first sight may appear as incoherent. However, in the course of thematic analysis of longer series of autogenic abreactions, it becomes evident that many, if not all, essential topics of neutralization which evolved in greater detail during later autogenic abreactions had already been present as "incoherent thematic elements" in the central phase of the first (and sometimes the second) autogenic abreaction. This suggests that the first (or first and second) autogenic abreaction forecasts, as in a table of contents, the major topics of future programs of neutralization. While it is technically not advisable to discuss these aspects with inexperienced patients, a careful study of the first autogenic abreaction might be very instructive for the therapist.

As brain-directed dynamics tend to become more active during the central phase and more acutely disturbing material is mobilized, a patient's motor behavior may be affected in significant ways. Crying spells, occasional wiping off of tears, minor motor discharges (e.g., twitching, trembling) and other thematically related motor activity (e.g., gesticulating while describing, banging the mattress while un-

loading violent aggression, lifting the pelvis during dynamics of intercourse, sucking motions associated with episodes of breast feeding) do
not interfere with the dynamics of neutralization (see Table 15). It is,
however, technically necessary to maintain the horizontal posture. Major
changes in posture, such as sitting up suddenly, turning around, opening the eyes and looking around tend to interrupt processes of neutralization and should be avoided. In case such motor behavior occurs, the
patient should be asked to resume the horizontal training posture. A
sudden onset of massive motor discharges involving the trunk and the
extremities is particularly disturbing to the inexperienced patient.
When the patient is asked to maintain the training posture and to let
the brain unload whatever it wishes to discharge, it has been occasionally helpful to recite the heaviness formulas again for a brief period
until the patient is again calm and can continue to describe.

When brain-directed dynamics are associated with feelings of nausea
indicating the probability that vomiting might be technically desirable,
the necessary equipment for dealing with such an event should be
ready by the couch. Experienced patients, who know that everything
is ready, manage to keep their eyes closed and continue describing

TABLE 15. *Motor Behavior during Autogenic Abreaction Characteristic
for Advanced Phases of Treatment\**
*(50 Psychosomatic and Neurotic Patients)*

| Motor Behavior | Male (N = 25) | Female (N = 25) | Total (N = 50) | (%) |
|---|---|---|---|---|
| 1. No movements in extremities, no change of posture | 18 | 22 | 40 | 80 |
| 2. Major changes in posture (e.g., sitting up, turning, lifting trunk) | 4 | 2 | 6 | 12 |
| 3. Thematically related gesticulation | 1 | 4 | 5 | 10 |
| 4. Occasional movements | | | | |
| (a) Lower extremities | 3 | 7 | 10 | 20 |
| (b) Upper extremities | 4 | 6 | 10 | 20 |
| (c) Head | 5 | 7 | 12 | 24 |
| (d) Trunk (e.g., pelvis) | 5 | 2 | 7 | 14 |
| (e) Oral (e.g., sucking, biting) | 3 | 2 | 5 | 10 |
| 5. Occasional motor discharges (e.g., jerks, twitches) | | | | |
| (a) Generalized | 3 | 1 | 4 | 8 |
| (b) Localized | 6 | 2 | 8 | 16 |
| 6. Crying spells | 8 | 13 | 21 | 42 |

\* Compare with motor behavior during the first and the second autogenic abreaction,
Table 39, p. 226.

after sufficient vomiting has occurred. Inexperienced patients tend to be disturbed, and a good deal of reassurance is necessary before continuing the autogenic abreaction. In these cases it is necessary to return to the standard induction procedure. The central phase is sometimes interrupted by an increasing need to urinate (see *Circumstantial Resistance*, Vol. VI). While experienced male trainees prefer a urinal in order not to interrupt the autogenic abreaction, premature termination may be indicated in other cases. In such situations it is strongly suggested that undesirable after-effects be avoided by continuing the interrupted autogenic abreaction (i.e., application of standard induction procedure) after the patient has returned from the bathroom.

## THE TERMINAL PHASE

The functional transition from a pattern of neutralization which is characteristic for the central phase of the abreactive period to a pattern of the terminal phase may be gradual or may come about in a rather abrupt manner. Depending on how the brain wishes to terminate, the terminal phase may last less than one minute or, and this is more frequently the case, extend over a period of several minutes. Although the nature of the brain-directed elaborations which occur when processes of autogenic neutralization approach their end are distinguishable from the dynamics which dominate the central phase, it is often not possible to determine the exact point of transition between the central and the terminal phase.

The terminal phases of different patterns of neutralization, i.e., (A) intellectual, (B) sensory and motor, (C) visual, (D) mixed (see p. 49) are generally characterized by (a) a decrease of negatively loaded elaborations, (b) an increase of neutral or positively oriented elements, (c) a slowdown of brain-directed elaborations which may come to a complete halt, (d) agreeable feelings of relaxation, comfort, warmth, frequent desire to rest or sleep and a number of specific changes in visual elaborations which may be considered as signals that the brain has terminated its program of neutralization for the time (see Table 17, p. 83). In case the standard termination procedure is not applied at such a time, there is little probability that therapeutically favorable phases will follow (see p. 84 ff.). In many instances progressive transition toward sleep appears to be a natural manner of termination.

In many ways there is a functional similarity between the self-regulatory dynamics of thematic termination as they tend to occur during the central phase (see Part IV, p. 329) and the dynamics of the terminal phase. However, the generally less drastic indications of thematic termination which intermittently occur during the central phase are followed by a thematic shift and continuation of undiminished processes of neutralization.

Occasionally even experienced therapists may have some difficulty in understanding whether the brain's indications mean "thematic termination" with intent to bring about a program-related thematic shift with continuation of neutralization or whether the brain's elaborations signify the end of the abreactive period. In such instances of doubt it is instructive to wait and see how the brain continues. In cases where the brain really wishes to terminate, it will repeat its signals and discontinue the previous pattern of neutralization (see p. 78 ff.). But where the brain's message has not been correctly understood and a silent interval, which actually is a preparatory phase for a thematic shift, is considered as an indication for application of the standard procedure, the situation is still in agreement with the principle which guides the application of *premature technical termination* (see p. 87 ff.).

The termination procedure is essentially the same as during autogenic standard training: (a) flexing both arms vigorously, (b) taking a deep breath, (c) opening the eyes. However, during supervised autogenic abreactions, particularly when the patient is still in the learning phase, the standard termination procedure should always begin with the preparatory question: "Do you feel comfortable?" Only after the patient has said that he does feel comfortable is the usual three-step termination procedure applied (e.g., "Yes, then we can terminate, and you can terminate as usual," the patient flexes his arms, takes a deep breath and opens his eyes). After this, it is helpful to encourage the patient to stretch, to keep his eyes open and to flex his limbs on the couch before sitting up. Patients who sit up or stand up too quickly after termination of autogenic abreactions tend to feel dizzy and occasionally experience several minutes of blurred vision.

Under certain circumstances, particularly when premature termination is necessary, a case-adapted modified termination procedure may be indicated (see p. 87 ff.).

As a general rule, it is therapeutically favorable to adapt the termination of autogenic abreactions to the self-regulatory, self-terminating dynamics of autogenic neutralization as carefully as possible. *Brain-directed terminations* (see p. 78 ff.) are significantly more favorable than well-adapted *premature technical terminations* (see p. 87 ff.). *Premature requested terminations* (see p. 89 ff.) or inadequate patient-directed terminations are usually followed by disturbing emotional and psychophysiologic reactions, resulting from mobilized dynamics which were not permitted to undergo adequate neutralization.

TABLE 16.   *Termination of the First and the Second Autogenic
Abreaction in Psychosomatic and Neurotic Patients*

|  | Autogenic Abreactions | |
|---|---|---|
| Termination of AA | AA 1 (N = 100) | AA 2 (N = 96) |
| (a) Premature termination requested by the patients | 17 | 17 |
| (b) Particular difficulties of termination | 1 | 4 |
| (c) Adequately timed termination without technical difficulty | 82 | 75 |

Difficulty in termination occurs rarely (see Table 16). In some instances where patients stop describing and appear to have fallen asleep, it is advisable to allow the patient to sleep. After five or ten minutes of rest, one may interject in a low voice: "Can you continue to describe what is going on?" Usually patients tend to react, and perhaps it then may be useful to add: "Please continue to describe." After the sleepy patient has attempted to do so, one may progress toward the application of the standard termination procedure. There are very few occasions in which patients did not respond to this approach and remained silent. However, the desired response occurred after another period of up to 20 minutes of sleep.

In several other instances when technical termination was found necessary, there simply was no favorable opportunity to terminate, and up to 50 minutes went by before the standard termination procedure could be applied.

Occasionally it happens that even experienced patients are convincing in their affirmation that they feel comfortable and then terminate before the therapist has a chance to intervene. Such unusually quick patient-directed terminations are frequently a manifestation of brain-antagonizing resistance. The patient usually hopes to avoid, for example, a thematic shift or a crying spell. However, these patients soon discover that such maneuvers are not to their advantage (e.g., the crying spell started at full force right after premature termination) because they continue to feel miserable during the postabreactive period (see p. 90 ff.).

## Brain-directed Termination

The arsenal of sophisticated maneuvers a brain may use to indicate that its work of self-curative neutralization has ended is perhaps one of the most impressive categories of phenomena which distinguish autogenic neutralization from other forms of treatment. Particularly instructive are studies of various types of visual elaborations with features which clearly convey the message of termination (see Table 17, p. 83). Arrest of dynamic cinerama features with transformations of a lively image into a postcard-like picture which moves farther and farther away and finally disappears in the distance is only one brain-directed way of termination. Cessation of differentiated visual elaborations with production of intensive "almost blinding" light (see Case 18, p. 79; Case 19, p. 79 f.) which appears to have some similarities with the Zen phenomenon of enlightenment[793,810,1036,1037,1038,1039,1903,2015,2070,2074,2098,2193] is usually an impressive experience for the patient. Progressive fading away of image, "folding up" or "rolling up" of complex scenes are unmistakable elaborations, particularly when these terminal phenomena are associated with a strong sensation of warmth, agreeable feelings, for example "being cleaned" (see Case 19, p. 79) and comfortable relaxation (see Table 17, p. 83). Visually elaborated processes of dissolution, disintegration, shrinking (see Case 16, p. 66 ff.) and other brain-designed maneuvers of making things disappear are common features of terminal phases (see Cases 20, 21, p. 80).

*Case 18:* A 29-year-old female social worker (anxiety reaction, depressive reaction, situational stress reaction, hyperthyroidism). After a relatively long (43 min.) central phase emphasizing neutralization of aggressive material accumulated during a non-consummated marriage with a sexually and affectively frustrated partner, the patient finds herself with a brain-produced, ideal partner. The subsequent dynamics are related to the patient's state of affective and sexual deprivation which culminates with the experience of orgasmic sensations. Immediately following this, a *Bright Light Phase*, usually indicating the end of a successfully accomplished phase of thematic neutralization occurs.

*Terminal passages:*
"The hay looks whitish-gold and the sky is blue, blue, blue . . . that is all what one can see . . . I would like to do nothing . . . just letting things go . . . as if I am just ready to receive something . . . well, I think I would be very happy . . . he would feel it . . . and he would be also quite happy . . . now it is as if there is, inside of my body . . . it is as if something is penetrating . . . I think I feel something like an orgasm . . . I see only something like a very strong light . . . a very intensive white light . . . it is almost blinding . . . now . . . I really feel good . . . I would like to sleep . . ." [standard termination].

*Case 19:* A 36-year-old housewife (anxiety reaction). Toward the end of a relatively long (60 min.) reality-related multithematic cinerama-type pattern of neutralization, the terminal phase begins with several elementary, symbolic elaborations, which are followed by a characteristic *Bright Light Phase*.

"The rods are still coming slightly but they don't close, they don't squish or squash and they don't recede to the background, they stay there . . . I think the screen is a sky . . . I don't want to block, I don't want to stop it . . . that had an awful lot of perspective . . . I felt . . . I think there is a sun somewhere

. . . light . . . the sun was at the horizon . . . I don't know if it was sunset or a sunrise . . . it gave an awful lot of light . . . then there was a bit of a hint of the turquoise blue . . . [*Do you feel comfortable?*] . . . Yes, I feel as if something has just been completely cleaned . . . light gray, as if just wiped . . ." [standard termination].

*Case 20:* A 26-year-old nun (anxiety reaction, obsessive-compulsive disorders with sado-masochistic manifestations, multiple phobic and psychophysiologic reactions, ecclesiogenic syndrome). After about 50 minutes of uncensored brain-directed cinerama-type neutralization of heterosexual dynamics (sexual deprivation), autogenic termination occurs in the following manner.

"And then he starts sucking my breasts . . . and I let him do that . . . I deeply enjoy that contact again . . . and he takes me into his arms and he embraces me as strong as he can . . . my whole body is pressed against his . . . we cannot embrace each other more strongly than that . . . and one may say, I am still interested in his penis, it is as if I still have the desire to caress it, to touch it . . . and he lets me go ahead . . . and I take it again into my hands and I touch it in all directions and I have again this need to pass it over my face, to rub my face against it . . . and I keep doing it. . . . And I have the impression that this desire evaporates, I feel less attracted . . . even the image is getting vague, becomes blurred . . . now it is completely gone . . . well, this calmed me down enormously . . . it seems that nothing else wants to come . . ." [standard termination].

*Case 21:* A 26-year-old hospital worker (reactive depression). The following passages are characteristic for a graduated thematic termination involving dynamics of transformation and progressive diminution.

"It's as if there were a couple of dancers behind the accordion . . . folklore dancers . . . they're far away and I can't really make them out . . . there's mostly some red, some white and some black in their costumes . . . and it seems to be a spirited tune because they're dancing swiftly . . . their movements are lively . . . the accordion is still playing on. . . . Now I no longer see the dancers . . . there's only the accordion . . . all stretched out . . . I now have the impression that it's all folded up . . . now it's just like a little ball of paper which seems to be placed on something that I don't want to see . . . as if it was just waiting to fall . . . it's as if the little ball of paper was on the edge of a window sill . . . the window of a gray stone house . . . at the foot of the window there's a little area where there's some grass . . . it's all wet because it's raining . . . it won't take long before nothing will remain of this little ball of paper . . . I see the small area of ground and the grass . . . I no longer see the little ball of paper . . ." [standard termination].

In other instances of cinerama-type dynamics the brain simply adapts the terminal development to the prevailing scene by producing a very calm and peaceful atmosphere, perhaps a beautiful sunset (see Case 22) or falling asleep in affectionate arms (see Case 23).

*Case 22:* A 40-year-old priest (anxiety reaction, ecclesiogenic syndrome, multiple phobic and psychophysiologic reactions). Toward the end of a very dynamic central phase of multithematic neutralization with emphasis on accumulated aggressive material, a brain-directed indication for termination is reached.

"These disagreeable teenagers disappear. . . . I go back again and lie down on the beach . . . and I observe a magnificent sunset . . . and there are the sounds of a harp . . . it is Ravel's concerto for harp . . . now I can hear it very clearly . . . I am still lying there . . ." [standard termination].

*Case 23:* A 34-year-old priest (anxiety reaction, ecclesiogenic syndrome, vocational conflicts). After a 45 min. autogenic abreaction which focussed on the neutralization of anxiety related to the father figure, Oedipal dynamics, confrontation with his dying mother and a prolonged period of ecclesiogenic material (damnation, tortures in hell, etc.), brain-designed termination occurred.

"I crush the devils . . . I crush the witches . . . I get rid of them . . . and I get out of hell. . . . And I am a huge road . . . and I don't know where to go . . . and I walk . . . I walk . . . I walk for a long time . . . and I arrive at a fountain and I drink water . . . and there's a young girl there who helps me drink . . . and who brings me along with her . . . it's Lucy . . . we're walking together . . . we walk together for a long time . . . and we sit under a big tree . . . and we kiss each other . . . and I fall asleep beside her under the big tree . . . all is quiet . . . I feel very comfortable . . ." [standard termination].

Certain interjected patterns of violent dynamics may abruptly shift to an interjected antithematic theme tending toward a soothingly comfortable situation (see Case 25). In other instances the brain emphasizes a maneuver of terminal readjustment in a particular desired direction (e.g., Case 14, p. 60: "I am now cannibal myself, tattooed in the wood, and *I have become a perfect man . . . quite suddenly I became myself again* . . . nothing . . . some drawing-like pattern on a dark background . . . that is all . . . I feel comfortable . . .").

*Case 24:* A 24-year-old male student (anxiety reaction). During the terminal phase, an increase of positively oriented elaborations occur before a relatively abrupt indication for termination is given.

"I see some crosses at night in a cemetery: it's a row of crosses . . . there are no names, only dates, there are many . . . a long row of crosses, it seems that it practically encircles the earth . . . I dig and at the bottom of each tomb, it's my damn fool of a nut with a computer, he has a cynical laugh . . . I open up all the tombs, he is still laughing, he's splitting his sides laughing. . . . I go to Holland, and I come back with flowers, and they all come out with flowers in their hands . . . they are like choirboys now . . . we build them cabins in the woods . . . now, they're being constructive, they build houses and homes, and they clear the land, they make bread, they like going for walks . . . they are happy and they are singing . . . they fill up the tombs, take out the computers, they fill up the tombs . . . and they use the crosses to make road signs. . . . I'm in an airplane now, and I see their colonies down there . . . I see gray . . . nothing new it is silvery gray . . ." [standard termination].

It often happens that patients who are sufficiently acquainted with termination requirements do indicate their wish to terminate at a certain point which appears to be favorable: "I think I could terminate here, I feel comfortable." Such an indication, when given by experienced patients, is often in good agreement with the brain-directed dynamics and the usual three-step termination procedure may be applied.

In certain patients, however, it might be advisable at times to verify whether or not the patient's indication is correct. Depending on the themes under neutralization, it may occur that such indications are manifestations of resistance, aiming at avoidance of dreaded or disagreeable confrontations (see Case 25).

*Case 25:* A 23-year-old male student (anxiety reaction). After 40 minutes of thematic neutralization focusing largely on sexual anxiety and aggression, the patient finds himself lying on a sunny beach. As he feels comfortable, he indicates "I could terminate here." The last three minutes preceding this indication and a following period of 14 minutes of "additional" neutralization are given below.

"I cut my penis and create a vagina . . . a big dark Negro appears with a big penis and he has intercourse with me . . . his penis is so long he is hurting me and I don't like it . . . I take an electrically sort of charged stick and press it against his abdomen and "bang" he sort of explodes. . . . Now I have become a baby again and I have a penis and I am laughing, running along a beach . . . there I meet a small girl . . . the girl is naked as I am and I take her by the hand and I kiss her, etc. . . . And now I see myself jumping into a swimming pool . . . I am about 20 years old, the water is nice and refreshing . . . and I go out and lie down in the sun and I feel fine . . . I could terminate here . . . [*Please continue to observe*] . . . A black bat appears and gets on my head . . . I am in hell and I have become a devil and there are many other devils, and the girl I met in the X hotel is there . . . and we are dancing around the fire and I throw vitriol at her and I am whipping her . . . I kill myself and I see myself in a coffin, in the funeral home, etc. . . . Now I see myself in my mother's womb, in the hospital and the doctor is cutting my umbilical cord and holds me up and is slapping my behind . . . and now I am in the water . . . and now in a sort of cradle, nice and warm . . . and suddenly I am growing up and I am in a coffin and they lower it into the hole . . . and I get out of there . . . walk out of the funeral home . . . and on my way to my parents home. I destroy everything . . . and I burn up the house with a flame thrower . . . and I let myself be eaten up by bears . . . I am sucking my mother's breast and I feel fine . . . now I am an adult and I am on a beach . . . and I fall asleep . . ." [standard termination].

Patterns dominated by intellectual elaborations usually enter the terminal phase with a significant increase of positively oriented elaborations which then may simply end with the patient stating, for example: "I have nothing more to say . . . my mind is blank . . . I feel comfortable . . . I could fall asleep. . . ."

TABLE 17. *Forms of Brain-directed Termination*

A. Progressive decrease of negative connotations followed by a phase of calm neutrality with positively oriented features (e.g., "And now I am lying on the beach . . . everything is peaceful . . . I feel comfortable . . . very comfortable . . . I am still lying here . . ."; see Case 22, p. 81)

B. Decrease of negatively loaded thematic elements and subsequent emphasis on positively oriented dynamics with indications of readjustment toward normality, which are followed by a cessation of differentiated thematically related elaborations (see Case 14, p. 60)

C. Thematically, positively oriented dynamics followed by cessation of differentiated elaborations, feelings of relaxation (warmth) and appearance of (a) light shades of uniform colors (e.g., light blue, turquoise blue, pale gray, silvery tones, light yellow; see Case 24, p. 81); (b) whiteness, blankness, "empty space" (see Case 16, p. 66; Case 26, p. 85); (c) "very strong light," "very bright light," "blinding light" (see Case 18, p. 79; Case 19, p. 79)

D. Brain-directed developments indicating by the nature of visual elaborations that the brain wishes to terminate before engaging in a thematic shift (e.g., sundown; see Case 27, p. 86)

E. Following a clearly positively oriented phase, onset of thematically incoherent elaborations which may be associated with elementary or significantly less differentiated phenomena of visual nature (see Case 27, p. 86)

F. Emphasis on neutral or positively oriented dynamics, agreeable feelings (e.g., relaxation, warmth, feeling clean, desire to sleep) and progressive cessation of differentiated visual elaborations which may be characterized by the following dynamics.
   (a) Distintegration, dissolution or progressive diminution of a given object or scene (see Case 21, p. 80)
   (b) Arrest of dynamic features of, for example, filmstrip or cinerama-type elaborations (e.g., "Now it looks like a postcard . . .") and subsequent "shrinking" or "progressive disappearance in the distance" (see Case 21, p. 80)
   (c) Loss of sharpness and clarity of visual elaborations which become progressively more "blurred" or "vague," and finally are replaced by light shades of colors (see Case 20, p. 80)
   (d) Processes in the course of which differentiated images are "folding up," "rolling up from the bottom" or "disappearing toward the top."

G. Relatively sudden cessation of brain-directed elaborations with terminal statements, for example: "Suddenly I am back here on the couch . . . I think it's all over . . . There is nothing to describe . . . I feel quite comfortable . . . ," or simply: "That's all. . . . My mind is blank. . . . I could sleep" (see Case 25, p. 82)

H. Slowing down of brain-directed productivity with sporadic incoherence of thematic neutralization, increase of silent intervals, and eventual onset of sleep (see Fig. 5, p. 55)

When the central phase features frequent and intensive discharges of a disagreeable nature (e.g., falling, spinning, pain, massive motor discharges, violent crying spells), these phenomena simply cease during the terminal phase, being replaced by agreeable feelings (e.g., relief, warmth, relaxation, calmness). Such terminal phases are frequently accompanied by slowly moving lighter shades of blue, gray, yellow, and silvery tones and other manifestations indicating a significant slowdown or cessation of brain-directed productivity. Sleepiness or sleep may or may not occur.

Studies of longer series of autogenic abreactions indicated that a given brain tends to indicate the end of its work in certain ways which are characteristic for its peculiar overall pattern of thematic neutralization.

### Delayed Termination

It is of practical and theoretical interest to know what happens when autogenic abreactions are not terminated in spite of positively oriented brain-directed elaborations signalling that the self-regulatory processes of neutralization have ended for the time. To find out how the brain reacts in such situations, various categories of autogenic abreactions, i.e., (A) Intellectual, (B) Motor and sensory, (C) Visual, (D) Mixed (see p. 49) were intentionally prolonged beyond brain-directed indications for termination. Under such circumstances a number of changes of brain-directed reactivity were noted.

When the central phases were of relatively short duration (e.g., less than 35 min.), it was frequently observed that certain dynamics which were characteristic for the central phase will reassert themselves. Thematic shifts may or may not occur at this point. However, even in cases of thematic shift, the level of productivity tends to be lower, and usually it will not take long and the brain will start to elaborate new indications for termination.

When autogenic abreactions were of relatively long duration (e.g., over 50 min.), the participating brain mechanisms appeared to be fatigued; and subsequent phases were unproductive with frequent indications for termination or the patient fell asleep, thus terminating the processes of autogenic neutralization in a natural manner. However, after several minutes of a sleep-like state, a patient may start describing again for a short while. In such instances previously dominating dynamics may continue or, and this is usually the case, the brain adopts a pattern of incoherent elaborations. Of particular interest in this connection are brain-directed changes as reflected by patterns of visual elaborations. When the dynamics of the central phase were largely restricted to elementary or intermediate stages of differentiation (e.g., I-V; see Table 33, p. 188), a very slow elaboration usually associated with functional regression to lower degrees of differentiation is noted. In many instances visual elaborations seem to stop, and the patient appears to be about to fall asleep (see Fig. 5, p. 55).

When reality-related cinerama-type elaborations dominated the central phase, intentionally delayed termination is usually followed by relatively incoherent and unproductive sequences of visual phenomena (see Case 26) with repeated brain-directed indications for termination (see Case 26; Case 27, p. 86). For brief periods more dynamic and more differentiated elaborations may reappear. However, such attempts at reengagement in thematic neutralization have been largely abortive.

When the central phase is composed of frequent motor or sensory discharges, the release of such phenomena simply ends, and the patient feels calm and relaxed. A similar development of reactivity has been noted when the central phase consisted largely of intellectual elaborations. The patient simply feels that for the time there is nothing more to say, that his brain seems to be empty and that he feels comfortable and would like to sleep.

*Case 26:* A 35-year-old businessman (anxiety reaction). In expectation of further development, termination was intentionally delayed. The terminal phase with the last sequences of reality-related material of this autogenic abreaction (68 min.) are given below (technically favorable possibilities for termination are indicated by *X*).

"Now I can see myself as a boy perhaps . . . yes, I can remember, the picture of me and my mother . . . I remember, it looked like that and somehow I see myself as that little boy in there . . . there is nothing there . . . it's blank . . . its sort of a whitish, sometimes irridescent sort of a round . . . I get the impression of a roundish face . . . now I can see my mother again . . . I am still trying to see myself in the dressing room. . . . Now I see sort of a yellowish copper ball . . . things are very dark now but I don't seem to see anything behind me, and its in front of me and I should be able to see in back of me, in all those mirrors reflecting back and forth but they're not . . . its blank . . . now I see sort of a triangle, it's sort of wisp of a yellowish thread dancing about . . . no it's not anything there. . . . (*X*) At first it looked perhaps like an embryo or like a clam on the half shell but that's about all I can. . . . That looks like water spilling across the floor . . . sort of grayish like . . . clouds rolling about . . . now it's still blank. . . . (*X*) There's nothing about with the odd slightly darker feature . . . I can't see anything at all. . . . (*X*) Blank . . . gray, medium gray, a little bit darker than mushroom gray. . . . (*X*) It's still the same . . . a bit of jet of slight color from the left to the right. . . . (*X*) I get the impression . . . like a snowball rolling toward me and sort of gathering up . . . it looks like its rolling . . . it is getting bigger . . . I can see the streaks

. . . possibly it could also be dough as it's being rolled up . . . there's dark things pushing up from the bottom of my vision . . . it seems to be like boiling up from the bottom . . . it's still doing it . . . little abstract yellowish golden rectangles. . . . (X) That looked like a pair of hands . . . for a moment I saw a dark slit, it looked most indefinite . . . sort of reddish abstract figure swirling about . . . sometimes it looks like legs . . . sort of a grayish yellow abstract . . . not abstract just blank . . ." [standard termination].

*Case 27:* A 35-year-old male technician (personality disorder, sexual deviation, ecclesiogenic syndrome). After 64 minutes of dominantly reality-related cinerama-type dynamics with active self-participation, the patient's brain mechanisms announce repeatedly that termination is indicated. In this case the application of the standard termination procedure was intentionally postponed, and the dynamics of visual elaborations were observed for another period of 23 minutes. In contrast to the reality-related pattern with active self-participation which characterized the first 64 minutes, the dynamics remained elementary, rather abstract and without possibility of further reality-related confrontations or thematic engagements. The passages given below start with the last reality-related elaborations: positively oriented masculine identification. This is followed by visual phenomena which approach the characteristics of a *Bright Light Phase*. As the brain is "forced" to continue, a series of similar brain-directed indications for technical termination (marked X) are elaborated.

"I now see Commander Trapp in his elegant uniform, and the image changes to become that of my brother-in-law, Joseph the doctor, it's his face with the commander's body, standing straight and impassive . . . he appears very determined . . . his face has suddenly changed to that of Prince Philip . . . and it's that of Robert that comes in now, smiling, and from far off behind this human figure rays of light are coming in . . . they're very clear and strong . . . and the man's image becomes vague, and I examine the flashes of light coming in from far off . . . they come and go . . . I see the earth's horizon, and I see something like a sunrise. . . . (X) There are still rays of light in the background . . . the colors intermingle and move from a bright yellow to a coppertoned red . . . but it's the sun in shape of a half-moon that predominates, very clear, it doesn't dazzle one's sight. . . . (X) The flashing of the rays of light is above the sun right now. . . . (X) The background is snow white, and the rays continue to vary the flashes coming from the infinite. . . . (X) I see something shaped like the tail of a prehistoric animal, this tail is wagging about like a kite in space, and it tapers off into many fine extremities, like fine stems . . . now I notice this animal's body which would come from the alligator family, the two front legs very big and long, the hind ones very short . . . its body in a somewhat elongated egg-like shape, its tail still floating about like a kite, and its head turned to the sky at which it's barking. . . . Always with the background and its colorful rays passing from yellow to coppertoned orange. . . . The image tends to become vague and nebulosities set in, and there are all sorts of very strange movements going on. . . . (X) I see a horizontal shape, narrow with little black squares . . . but projected, and it starts to move as if this projected shape was dancing . . . I see it in three dimensions, and this shape becomes a bit like the arc of a circle . . . a bunch of strange forms follow . . . all of them moving, and they're intermingling to form marbled patterns . . . and they're nondescript. . . . (X) Lights are exploding in the vagueness. . . . (X) A central point is coming into view quite clearly, but the strange forms continue to unfold around this center . . . this center seems to be a lit up hole with a sky-blue background, and the forms evolve around it as if they overlapped each other . . . these forms are like storm clouds in different tones ranging from pale gray to dark gray . . . this persists. . . ." (X) [standard termination].

## Premature Technical Termination

A premature termination, suggested by the therapist for technical reasons, is occasionally necessary in connection with the following circumstances:

(a) Repeated evidence of technical errors (e.g., intentional forms of resistance; see Vol. VI, Part I) which require a clarifying discussion to avoid an unproductive autogenic abreaction.

(b) After prolonged central phases when there is a reasonable probability that the brain can go on with the same pattern for a rather long, however unpredictable, time and the prevailing theme of neutralization is of such a nature that minimal or no particularly disturbing after-effects can be predicted.

(c) After prolonged central phases, when brain-directed termination is not likely to occur soon and the experienced patient is able to continue the current process of neutralization alone by performing autogenic abreactions at home.

(d) After successful neutralization of important material in the course of a relatively long central phase and there are indications that the brain prepares for a thematic shift aiming at engagement in neutralization of "new" material.

(e) Unforeseen and technically disturbing environmental changes (e.g., construction workers starting drilling on the floor above the office).

Whenever a premature termination for technical reasons is contemplated, it is therapeutically important to postpone the application of the standard termination procedure until the brain has reached a positively oriented, or at least a relatively neutral, phase of elaborations. In such instances it is necessary to indicate to the patient that a technical termination is intended by (a) asking: "Do you feel comfortable?" and, if the answer is affirmative, to continue with (b) "Well do you think we can terminate at this point?" If the patient agrees, the standard termination procedures follow. In case the patient indicates that he does not feel comfortable (e.g., frontal headache, chest pain, feels like crying, has the impression that something is about to come out), the technical termination must be postponed until the patient feels reasonably comfortable.

The adequate application of technical termination requires an understanding of the patient's particular pattern of neutralization and sufficient practical experience with autogenic abreaction. Generally it is advisable to wait for developments which resemble as closely as possible those phenomena which are frequently associated with terminal phases leading toward brain-directed termination (see Case 16; p. 66 ff.). As the therapist is familiar with the pattern of brain-directed termination in a given case, he will find it easier to determine a favorable point for the application of a technical termination. It is technically wrong to terminate at a point where the patient describes, for example: "Now I am really dead, I am lying in the coffin and everything is calm and dark. . . .;" or "The cars still keep rolling over me . . . and now I am flattened out on the pavement . . . like a piece of paper . . . I don't feel anything anymore." Such relatively calm phases are still too closely related to negatively loaded dynamics, and there is no evidence of engagement in "neutral" or "positively" oriented developments. A technically adequate but early termination which aims at a reduction of undesirable after-effects must await indications of relatively advanced neutralization and, if possible, be applied before a thematic shift occurs (see Case 28).

*Case 28:* The following passage is taken from a central phase (42-year-old housewife; anxiety reaction, depressive reaction) which largely focussed on neutralization of the general topic of death. A possibility for adequate premature technical termination is indicated by (X). Brain-directed positively oriented elaborations are in italics.

"I fall down . . . I scream . . . I fall on the middle of the highway. Cars keep going over me. The traffic just goes on and on. It is almost like robots . . . not cars driven by people . . . all of them are speeding straight ahead. They keep going over me until I am almost flat as the road itself . . . I am completely flat and then I break up to pieces. Some pieces roll into the ditch . . . some get stuck in the middle of the cars . . . some are just rubbed into the highway. The traffic just goes . . . goes and goes. It is still raining. *The rain is washing the road clean . . . there is no blood left . . . it just disappeared . . . now you can only see the cars going. . . ."* (X) (thematic shift).

After a technical termination has been applied it is helpful and instructive to explain to the patient why the autogenic abreaction was terminated at this particular point and why it would have been a technical error to terminate earlier. It is through such technically oriented postabreactive discussions that intelligent patients learn how to avoid technical errors when doing autogenic abreactions at home (see Vol. VI).

When premature termination is applied to a patient who has complained about disagreeable sensations or other disturbing phenomena, it is appropriate to use the following approach: "Well, I think we should terminate here and discuss the matter, and now you terminate in three steps, and you feel comfortable, and everything is working perfectly normally" (patient terminates in three-step fashion).

In other instances, when brain-directed developments have engaged the patient in situations which are in sharp contrast to the atmosphere of the therapist's office, unfavorable surprise reactions can be avoided by applying: "Well, now you return slowly here to the couch in my office. I think we are going to terminate here and discuss the matter, and now you terminate in three steps as usual, and you feel comfortable, and everything is working perfectly normally."

### Requested Premature Termination

Generally it is possible to distinguish three situations which may motivate a patient to request premature termination: (a) fatigue after long, unpleasant and relatively complicated central phases characterized by relatively frequent interferences from brain-antagonizing forms of resistance, (b) disagreeable experiences occurring in the beginning of treatment with autogenic abreaction (see Case 29, p. 91 ff.), (c) interference by forms of indirect psychophysiologic resistance (e.g., need to urinate; see Vol. VI, Part I).

Since any form of premature termination leaves the patient's brain in a mobilized state of semi-neutralization with subsequent risks of therapeutically undesirable psychodynamic and psychophysiologic reactions, it is clinically important to avoid premature termination as much as possible. In case premature termination cannot be avoided, attempts should be made to delay the requested termination until dynamically and thematically relatively neutral or positively oriented phases have been reached. However, there are instances where even this is not possible.

When a long central phase is loaded with unpleasant dynamics and, for example, prolonged phases dominated by accident-related pain, frequent crying spells, massive motor discharges, repeated episodes of vestibular elaborations (e.g., falling, spinning, dizziness) and other disagreeable confrontations (e.g., abortion, traumatic delivery, tortures in hell, accidents) which tend to elicit brain-antagonizing forms of resistance, it is natural that a stage will be reached where the patient feels exhausted.

Experienced patients know that it would be preferable to go on but they feel that it might be better to interrupt autogenic neutralization at a technically convenient point and to continue thematic neutralization later. Inexperienced patients who are still in the learning phase (see Table 16, p. 78) tend to be glad to terminate, not realizing yet that they are prone to experience difficulties within hours or two or three days. In such instances a very careful postabreactive discussion with clear instructions (see Case 29, p. 91 ff.; see p. 95 ff.) and case-adapted use of supportive medication is considered essential.

In about eight per cent of cases (see Table 4, p. 33) it happens that a patient's first autogenic abreaction is experienced as being outrightlly disagreeable and termination is requested and carried out within a few minutes after termination of the induction phase (see Case 29). Usually the second autogenic abreaction is more likely to be unpleasant; and most requests for early termination occur during the first 10 to 15 autogenic abreactions, when certain categories of patients are still in the learning phase and still have difficulties in maintaining passive acceptance. Such difficulties are encountered when very disturbing accident material or other severely traumatic situations are programmed for early neutralization. Onset of topographically rather specific (accident-related) pain, headaches, sudden onset of series of massive motor discharges and episodes of vomiting tend to be very disturbing for the inexperienced patient. Requests for early premature terminations were observed when brain-directed dynamics of thematic neutralization started to focus on particularly disturbing material usually accumulated by patients with a history of ECT, of traumatic abortions and deliveries, traumatic operations (e.g., inadequate anesthesia), severe accidents (e.g., plane crash, car collision, kicked in the head during football, falling down flight of stairs with loss of consciousness, accidents associated with alcohol intoxication, insulin reactions in diabetics). Often, when early termination is requested in relation to neutralization of such episodes, a skillful therapist should be able to persuade the patient to continue for a few minutes. As a few minutes are gained, the patient's brain usually comes to the therapist's help by engaging in a thematic shift toward antithematic dynamics with more neutral or agreeable phases, and the patient is more disposed to continue the autogenic abreaction. However, in other cases it might be therapeutically advisable to respect the patient's request and to apply standard termination without delay. During a subsequent discussion, the therapist has an opportunity to explain the medically favorable aspects of the brain-directed nature of relevant dynamics. After such clarifying explanations it is important to point out that it is in the patient's interest not to wait until the next appointment for another autogenic abreaction but to lie down again and to continue the interrupted processes of neutralization (i.e., standard induction procedure, etc.). When the patient refuses continuation during the same session, it is frequently advisable to facilitate the next autogenic abreaction by prescribing supportive medication (e.g., chlordiazepoxide, 10 mg. b.i.d.) for the interim period.

In patients who repeatedly show unusual difficulties and who are prone to request premature termination, it is advantageous to apply facilitating supportive medication for prophylactic reasons (e.g., chlordiazepoxide, 10 mg., 1 hr. before the beginning of autogenic abreaction).

*Case 29:* A 40-year-old nurse (anxiety reaction). The patient felt that there was something lacking in her, that she was not quite satisfied with herself concerning her planning and outlook for the future. She wondered if anything was wrong with her. Six years earlier, the patient was involved in a car crash which was fatal for three of her friends. The patient escaped death but suffered various fractures (pelvis, nine ribs, right patella), dislocation of the left acromioclavicular joint (screw and wire fixation required), and retrograde amnesia (6 mon. hospitalization).

The pattern of the patient's first autogenic abreaction (i.e., elementary visual elaborations, multiple sensory phenomena, disagreeable affffective components; see below) is characteristic for a relatively small group of those patients who have accumulated severely disturbing experiential material (e.g., accidents with loss of consciousness).

"Nothing . . . no meadow . . . it is all dark and on top there is a bit of brightness . . . it is dark on top and there is a bit of brightness and a little bit of slight flashing things like fire works . . . nothing . . . the same . . . nothing. . . . I have a slight headache all over my forehead . . . some tingling on my right foot and heel and a funny feeling on top of my feet and a feeling as if my toes are cramped . . . the headache is more on the right side . . . nothing . . . let's finish . . . [*Perhaps you can continue for a while*] . . . It is black and I see the same sort of clouds . . . no heaviness . . . right knee a bit of a strain . . . nothing . . . it is absolutely dark . . . nothing at all . . . some cloud formations . . . some brighter things are popping up, moving from right to left and from top to bottom . . . like moving clouds and they are getting together and disappear . . . the same thing again . . . it is getting a little yellowish, golden [8 min.] . . . they still come down and form a ball with a dark center . . . they are always coming down and are going into a dark center with a sort of golden rim . . . always going down and there is a sort of a black ball with a sort of golden sun around it . . . I still have a headache . . . it is not round anymore, is is elongated . . . and coming down . . . I think I have enough now, it is bothersome this black thing going up and down on the right side . . . now the golden thing is in the middle again . . . my left leg is twitching . . . now there is a golden ball in the center . . . without dark interior . . . the same . . . I really would like to stop now . . ." (12 min.; standard termination).

*Postabreactive discussion:* Asked why the patient wished to terminate the exercise at this point, she explained that "The whole thing bothered me. I felt frustrated. I did not see anything and I felt uncomfortable. I thought that all this was silly, a waste of time and just plain nonsense." and "The headache bothered me." During the following discussion, it was explained to the patient that her performance was indeed quite successful and that her brain had already taken the opportunity to discharge a number of things as, for example, tingling, twitches, certain feelings, various forms and colors. To illustrate this, the patient's verbal description of the abreactive period was read back to her, and it was explained how the elaborations of the brain started out in a very simple way and became progressively more dynamic and differentiated. The patient had not realized this while she was describing. She agreed that a certain progress was evident. The onset of headache was explained as a phenomenon which occurs occasionally in situations where the brain wants to elaborate or discharge something, but cannot do so for some reason and, that this might be a manifestation of resistance. Toward the end of the postabreactive discussion, the patient felt encouraged. She agreed to write down a detailed description of her autogenic abreaction as soon as possible, to reread her report at least once a day, to note down comments and dreams, to practice autogenic training regularly and to continue her protocol of training symptoms.

# 7. The Postabreactive Period

For practical reasons it appears useful to distinguish a postabreactive period, during which the patient is still in the therapist's office, from the interim period (see p. 120 ff.) which starts as the patient leaves the treatment room. The postabreactive period begins at the end of the standard termination procedure, with the immediate postabreactive phase, while the patient is still lying on the couch. Depending on the patient's postabreactive reactions (see p. 93 ff.), the second part of the postabreactive period which is largely devoted to a technically oriented postabreactive discussion (see p. 94) may follow after a few minutes. The duration of the postabreactive period is usually longer (e.g., 10-20 min.) for beginners who need a more detailed discussion of certain difficulties they experienced during the autogenic abreaction, and various aspects of their therapeutic program (e.g., homework, supportive medication, interim problems). Sufficiently experienced patients usually leave the office within ten minutes after termination of the autogenic abreaction (see Table 23, p. 148). Since adequate patient-adapted management of the immediate postabreactive period and the interim is of particular importance, a variety of therapeutic aspects will be discussed in the following two chapters.

## The Immediate Postabreactive Phase

With beginners the immediate postabreactive phase often starts with reminding the patient who is still lying on the couch to keep his eyes open, not to get up immediately, but stretch and to move the extremities for a while, and allow at least one minute for low-level motor activity before getting up slowly. As the patient's voluntary motor activity keeps him from falling asleep and helps to readjust circulatory and other functions (e.g., reflectory motor reactivity, transitory visual disturbances), there is a reduced probability that disagreeable after-effects will occur (e.g., dizziness after getting up) or persist (e.g., blurred vision, disturbance of motor coordination). During this period, the patient should be observed carefully. While many patients have no comment to make, others may express their impression spontaneously (see Table 18, p. 94). Occasionally when inexperienced beginners wrongly state that they felt comfortable to obtain termination (see p. 89 ff.), a crying spell may start, frontal or occipital headache is noted or there are other manifestations (e.g., pain in topographically specific areas, feeling of nausea) which indicate that the termination was premature. In some of these instances

TABLE 18.  *Spontaneously Mentioned After-effects Directly after Termination of the First and the Second Autogenic Abreaction*
(100 Psychosomatic and Neurotic Patients)

| Autogenic Abreactions After-effects Noted within Three Minutes after Termination | AA 1 (N = 100) | AA 2 (N = 96) |
|---|---|---|
| (a) Feeling relaxed, refreshed, better, less nervous, rested, as after a good sleep | 21 | 9 |
| (b) Feeling tired, wishing to sleep | 13 | 10 |
| (c) Transitory disturbed vision | 2 | — |
| (d) Dizziness | 4 | 1 |
| (e) Headache | | |
| 1. Disappeared | 3 | — |
| 2. Less | 1 | — |
| 3. Same | 6 | 1 |
| 4. Feeling of pressure in forehead area | 2 | — |
| (f) Various aches | 1 | 1 |
| (g) Residual feeling of heaviness | 5 | 2 |
| (h) Feeling of stiffness | 1 | 1 |
| (i) Feeling of warmth | 2 | 2 |
| (j) Feeling depressed, crying | 1 | 1 |
| (k) No comments | 46 | 73 |

it is advisable to aim at continuation of the interrupted processes of neutralization by simply stating: "I think it is better for you to continue for a few minutes, please assume the training posture again." [Patient assumes training posture] "My right arm is heavy . . . My right arm is heavy . . ." etc., until the patient starts describing again. In other instances it may be preferable to discuss the patient's resistance before suggesting that it would be to his advantage if the brain could be given an opportunity to continue neutralization for a few minutes.

POSTABREACTIVE DISCUSSION

Initial parts of the postabreactive discussion are usually related to the nature of the autogenic abreaction and specific difficulties which the patient has encountered during certain processes of thematic neutralization. Of particular concern are patients who have frequent difficulties in remaining passive and giving *carte blanche* to their brain. As various forms of brain-antagonizing resistance may interfere very unfavorably with the brain's own program of thematic dynamics and adequate level of neutralization with brain-directed termination cannot be reached, the brain remains in an undesirable state of mobilization. In instances where early application of premature technical termination was applied and in other cases of premature patient-directed termination, the postabreactive discussion aims at understanding and clarification of the patient's resistance. After a sufficient level of technical understanding on the part of the patient has become evident, it is therapeutically desirable that the prematurely interrupted brain dynamics are given immediate opportunity to arrive at more satisfactory levels of neutralization by starting another autogenic abreaction.

Inexperienced patients who terminate their autogenic abreactions prematurely and others whose pattern of the central phase show unusually frequent occurrence of brain-antagonizing forms of resistance (see Vol. VI, Part I) and who did not agree to continue autogenic neutralization after a clarifying discussion tend to experience a variety of difficulties (see Case 30) during early phases of the *interim period* (see p. 120 ff.).

*Case 30:* A 42-year-old housewife (anxiety reaction, moderate depression). During the initial phase of the patient's sixth autogenic abreaction, her brain focussed on dynamics aiming at neutralization of very disturbing material related to the general topic of death. Frequent *thematic evasion, abortive engagement,* and other forms of brain-antagonizing resistance kept interfering with the brain's program of thematic neutralization. To avoid continuation of such functionally unfavorable patterns, premature technical termination was applied at a relatively favorable point. As the patient was glad to terminate, she was not particularly interested in the postabreactive discussion and rejected the therapist's proposal to continue. She evidently wanted to get out of the office as quickly as possible.

Four hours later, at 9:30 P.M., she called the therapist, stating that she felt utterly miserable, panicky, confused, that she had had a fight with her husband, and that she wondered if she could see the therapist as soon as possible. Autogenic neutralization was continued half an hour later in the therapist's office. Having learned her lesson, she maintained an adequate level of passive acceptance this time, and gave her brain a good chance to follow its own program of neutralization. After about 45 minutes, brain-directed termination occurred, she felt calm, comfortable and relaxed. Her sleep was undisturbed and there were no further difficulties at home. The following week the patient stated that she had felt particularly well and had been in good spirits during the interim.

Whenever there is a probability that premature termination may be followed by disturbing emotional or psychophysiologic reactions because adequate levels of neutralization of severely disturbing material could not be reached, it is therapeutically important to explain the reasons (e.g., resistance, unusually great need for neutralization), to warn the patient, to invite him to call the therapist at any time when he does not feel well and emphasize that it would be wrong to wait in a state of distress until the next appointment.

One of the most frequently observed manifestations occurring after premature terminations are disturbances of sleep and the experience of disagreeable dreams, which are considered as brain-directed abortive attempts to deal with semi-neutralized and mobilized material during sleep. In such instances the poorly rested patients tend to wake up in the morning with a headache which may last for many hours. To facilitate quick neutralization of the disturbing material by scheduling an early appointment, the patient should be told about the significance of such disturbing phenomena, which are an indication for calling the therapist.

In situations where prompt communication and flexible arrangements for an early appointment are not possible, the transitory use of supportive medication (e.g., chlordiazepoxide, meprobamate, chlorpromazine) may be considered. When supportive medication is acceptable to the patient (i.e., stat., interim period), it is helpful to explain the reasons and answer all relevant questions during the postabreactive period.

Occasionally a patient's pattern of thematic neutralization conveys an unusual load of aggressive, self-destructive material which may require a series of autogenic abreactions until adequate levels of neutralization are reached. In such cases it must be explained to the patient that his brain dynamics make him accident prone, and that it would be in his interest not to drive his car for a while, or at least to reduce driving to a minimum, and to be particularly careful. While intelligent patients understand this readily, others should be warned that the brain-disturbing effects resulting from, for example, car accidents add very undesirable functional complications to his brain which may require a high number of additional autogenic abreactions. As these patients respect the highly uneconomic brain-disturbing consequences of car accidents, more readily than other forms of reasoning, there is a good probability that they will be careful and follow the therapist's suggestion. Such advice during the postabreactive period is particularly important for diabetic patients (see Vol. II, p. 107ff.) who as a group are known to have a higher accident rate than others. Similar explanations and warnings are indicated for patients with known difficulties in controlling their consumption of alcohol.

## THERAPEUTIC HOMEWORK

A large proportion of the postabreactive period is usually taken up by discussions focussing on the nature of the patient's therapeutic homework. As it is therapeutically important to adapt the patient's program of therapeutic homework to his capacity, to his environmental and professional circumstances, to the particular exigencies which are closely related to the nature of his autogenic abreactions, and to his practical experience with the method, there are considerable variations of the therapeutic activities carried out during the interim period (see Table 19, p. 97; Table 20, p. 108). The following paragraphs are only an example of a therapeutic program which may be applicable under very favorable circumstances (i.e., tape recorder, own room, good motivation, reliable collaboration, sufficient time, sufficient intelligence).

Since no detailed information about the specific nature of the patient's homework has been given before his first autogenic abreaction, the patient expects relevant explanations and suggestions after getting up from the couch. Depending on the nature of the first autogenic abreaction and the patient's possiblity in engaging in therapeutic homework, one, several or all of the following tasks may be suggested:

1. To transcribe the autogenic abreaction or make a summary.
2. To reread the transcript aloud.
3. To make a thematic commentary.
4. To practice autogenic standard exercises regularly and keep a training protocol.
5. To make notes on dreams.
6. To make drawings (e.g., diagram of accident, certain sequences of images).

TABLE 19. *Therapeutic Homework carried out during Interim Periods: Transcript, Rereading, Commentary*
(120 Psychosomatic and Neurotic Patients)

| Homework of patients | Transcript or Summary of Autogenic Abreaction | | |
|---|---|---|---|
| | Rarely or none (%) | Occasionally (%) | Regularly (%) |
| Male (N = 60) | 18 | 13 | 69 |
| Female (N = 60) | 25 | 30 | 45 |
| | *Rereading Aloud of Transcript or Summary* | | |
| Male (N = 60) | 20 | 38 | 42 |
| Female (N = 60) | 40 | 42 | 18 |
| | *Written Commentary* | | |
| Male (N = 60) | 21 | 27 | 52 |
| Female (N = 60) | 52 | 38 | 10 |

These suggestions for therapeutic homework (particularly 1, 2, 3 and 6) are designed to copy as closely as possible those self-curative elements which the brain itself uses during autogenic neutralization: feedback of complex stimuli which originated from brain-directed self-curative elaborations with thematic confrontation, thematic repetition and motor (vocal, graphic) reexpression. Of therapeutic value is the psychophysiologically important fact that these tasks are carried out during a normal state of conscious control, thus helping to mobilize desirable integrative functions which facilitate the treatment process.

### 1. *Transcript of autogenic abreaction.*

A really fruitful discussion of the dynamics and various forms of brain-antagonizing resistance is very difficult or in many instances almost impossible without a transcript. As such technical discussions are particularly important in the beginning when the patient needs to learn about the dynamics of his brain and his technical errors, it is to the patient's advantage to accept the few hours of homework which are needed for the transcription. Associated with the task of transcribing the autogenic abreaction is an acoustic self-confrontation with informative stimuli which were generated by the patient's brain during the autogenic abreaction. From relevant studies it is known that a patient's confrontation with his own acoustic image enhances realistic self-perception, promotes expansion of awareness and mobilizes other mental functions which are generally considered as helpful in accelerating the psychotherapeutic process.

To make the verbalized material more readily available for an accurate assessment of the brain-directed dynamics, it is suggested that the tape-recorded autogenic abreaction be transcribed word for word, to indicate intervals of silence by three dots (e.g., . . .), and to use six dots or more (e.g., . . . . . . . . .) when exceptionally long intervals of silence occur. In this connection it is helpful to explain that the transcript of intervals is technically necessary to distinguish intervening forms of resistance more readily. Furthermore, copies are needed (one for the therapist, one for the patient) to facilitate therapeutic work together prior to the next autogenic abreaction.

The best time to transcribe the autogenic abreaction is as soon as possible after the patient arrives at home. Where the transcription is postponed for several days (delayed feedback), stronger emotional and psychophysiologic side-effects resulting from self-confrontation and premature mobilization of related material tend to occur. Since the next appointment may still be several days away and the inexperienced patient cannot readily neutralize the mobilized dynamics, he may feel disturbed until the next autogenic abreaction is carried out in the therapist's office. The emotional and psychophysiologic reactions are usually less intensive and of a more transitory nature when the transcript is made right after the therapeutic session while the patient's brain is still in a state of relative neutralization. To maintain a low level of unfavorable reactivity, the patient should be encouraged to follow the next suggestion (see 2).

*Case 31:* A 40-year-old architect (personality disorder, sexual deviation, psychophysiologic reaction; gastrointestinal system).

"Every time I type these reports, or express my thoughts, I am constantly drinking something and constantly smoking. I am writing this report a week after 'experiencing' it. My stomach improved progressively after the session but with disturbing recurrences daily."

*Case 32:* A 33-year-old housewife (anxiety reaction, moderate depression). In the following passages (AA 9, see below), the dynamics of neutralization focus on disturbing material (e.g., feeling of guilt, incomprehension of certain aspects of a specific situation) related to an episode which happened while the patient worked as a nurse. Of particular interest is the patient's comprehensive insight which occurred *while she was transcribing* AA 9. She noted: "At the time, and also during the trip,° I did not realize why I actually felt that the supervising nun was unfair, and why I felt that I should have been punished instead of the other nurse. Now I think I felt that way, because the supervisor acted largely on behalf of her own emotional reaction resulting from the fact that the other nurse did not obey her, while actually the patient's well-being should have been considered first. In that respect I did not take my responsibility correctly, by somehow avoiding the catheterization which I did not like to do anyway. I felt guilty because of that, and also because the other nurse got punished." The example illustrates the therapeutically advantageous implications of a reconfrontation in a normal state of conscious control with material described during autogenic abreaction.

*From AA 9:* "In order to become more independent, I have decided to enter into a nurses training program . . . I am in the hospital, I pass my examinations, and there . . . I see myself performing a catheterization . . . I always thought that my aseptic technique was not perfect . . . I always had the feeling that I did not take enough precautions when I needed sterile things, I was afraid of contaminating them . . . I was never sure that what I did was really done perfectly . . . I always had feelings of guilt . . . once I was on night shift, and I was supposed to catheterize somebody, and I did not do it because there

---

° Non-technical expression for autogenic abreaction.

was no catheter on the floor . . . I went to another floor and they didn't have
one, so I told myself I am not going to do it . . . I went to bed, and in the
morning the nun woke me up . . . no it wasn't the nun, it was a nurse I think . . .
the nun had asked another nurse to do the catheterization during the morning
shift . . . that nurse had refused to do it, and she had been suspended for six
months . . . I had not done the catheterization, it was really my fault, and I
didn't get anything . . . I think I went to see the nun later . . . and she told
me that she suspended the other nurse because she had refused to obey me . . .
but I had the impression that I should have been punished also, because I
should have looked for the catheter more thoroughly or I should have called the
supervising nun . . . I think the nun was unfair . . . quite often I was protected like this . . . the others got punished, when I should have been punished
. . . : I think they always treated me differently than the others . . . I don't
know why. . . ."

*Case 33:* A 24-year-old male student (personality disorder, sexual deviation,
ecclesiogenic syndrome, hypothyroidism) who delayed transcribing his autogenic abreaction for four days (delayed playback).

"I found it very difficult to finish typing the last AA. I experience quite a
bit of anxiety. I just had to stop a number of times, before I managed to
finish this."

Without having been asked to do so, many patients prefer to listen
once or several times to their descriptions before they start transcribing
the tape-recorded material (see Case 34, Case 35, p. 101). As has been
observed by other investigators who used similar techniques of feedback of self-generated acoustic stimuli, these patients tend to commit
that, while only listening to themselves (without transcribing) they became aware of essential elements, were more readily able to establish
thematic interconnections and thus arrived at certain new perspectives
or conclusions (see Case 34; Case 43, p. 109). It is of particular interest,
however, that on many occasions still other therapeutically important
information was "discovered" only later while going with the patient
through his homework during the *preabreactive period* (see p. 147),
prior to the next autogenic abreaction. From the patient's remarks it
became evident that the pattern of reactivity while just listening to the
tape-recorded material is not the same as the reactivity which occurs
during the transcript period (see Case 35). Many patients find it particularly difficult and painful to reexpress through writing what they have
described relatively easily during the autogenic abreaction (see Case
33; Case 35, p. 101). Observations in this area indicate that variable
degrees of dissociation which are characteristic for brain-directed processes of autogenic neutralization are significantly reduced during the

normal state of conscious control, and that the acoustic self-confrontation with its undeniable facets of reality contributes effectively to promote therapeutically desirable integrative processes between different levels of awareness and variable degrees of dissociation.

*Case 34:* A 30-year-old priest (obsessive-compulsive reaction, sexual deviation, multiple psychophysiologic reactions, ecclesiogenic syndrome).

"While I was listening to my last trip, three times in a row I became aware of a number of things. Incredible but true, for the first time I noticed a fact: the link between my weakness of concentration and my psychologic problem is quite clear. I am so preoccupied, or obsessed by my problem, that I continually avoid reality and thus I don't need to face it. This seems to be a sort of a gimmick or a safety valve fabricated by the subconscious mind, which permits me to take evasive action. Concentration has something to do with this. I also think that my constant feeling of tiredness is to a large extent also caused by my problem."

*Case 35:* A 32-year-old housewife (depressive reaction, anxiety reaction, multiple psychophysiologic reactions). Before starting to reread her transcript of AA 5 in the therapist's office, the patient commented on the difficulties she experienced while transcribing the autogenic abreaction.

"Oh, it really was quite difficult to type all that, but once it was done I felt relieved. I felt sick enough to my stomach to start vomiting, but afterward I felt unburdened, really relieved, and the sick feeling was gone. I listened to the trip once before transcribing it, and at that time the whole thing left me rather cool, I had no emotional reaction. But that started during the transcript, to write all that, that's what is really tough, particularly the passages where I kill and slaughter my mother, I felt like crying again, and I had to stop several times. I felt that all this was very sad. I did the transcript in small sections. Afterward I felt really relieved. I also noticed that I was much less aggressive and my attitude toward my children has changed. With my husband things are going much better than before."

*Remarks:* The patient's comments reflect significant differences of reactions, experienced merely during listening to her descriptions and while re-expressing her material during the various phases of transcription. In keeping with observations made by many other patients, a marked change toward normal re-activity and a feeling of relief is noted, after a re-integrative confrontation and re-experience of emotional reactions has occurred in a normal state of conscious control.

## 2. Rereading the transcript aloud.

In contrast to a passive acoustic self-confrontation while listening to the tape-recorded autogenic abreaction, and complementary to the graphic re-expression of the verbalized material, this part of the therapeutic homework aims at active vocal re-expression of brain-elaborated disturbing material. It constitutes a repetition (and feed-back) of the original brain-directed process of verbalization, how-ever at a normal state of conscious control. As vocalized reading of the transcript is carried out repeatedly throughout the interim period, the initially mobilizing effect on affective dynamics decreases (see Case 37). Generally it has been observed that reading the tran-script aloud twice per day helps decisively to keep the patient's mobilized psychophysiologic reactivity at a desirably low level.

A number of patients find it very difficult to go through this pro-cess of self-confrontation and re-expression. However, the task be-comes easier when emotional and psychophysiologic reactions sub-side as the number of repetitions increase (see Case 37). In case a regular practice of rereading the transcript repeatedly *aloud* is not observed for several days after the autogenic abreaction (de-layed feedback), the patients tend to experience an amplified effect of mobilization with more disturbing emotional and psychophysio-logic reactions (e.g., headaches, crying spells, gastric discomfort, palpitations, sweating).

In many instances, while rereading their transcript, patients dis-cover "new perspectives," "interesting interrelations," "new ideas" or realize the significance of certain brain-directed elaborations which they did not notice while transcribing the tape-recorded material. It is in this connection that it may be suggested that a few notes should be made during or after rereading the transcript. Such notes are of preparatory value for the next task (see 3.).

*Case 36:* A 33-year-old housewife (anxiety reaction) commented on her homework.

"This trip left me confused, I read it 10 or 15 times and I could not see any continuity or link, all loose ends. I sat there, thinking it over, going over the symbols, checking the previous trips. I did some exercises and went back. Then on Tuesday night, I thought of a sort of a line where things would fit on one after the other: my listening to mother, not marrying Dick because of her, and then later my decision to marry Bob, etc. Yesterday during the transcript of my notes I started crying again."

*Case 37:* A 33-year-old housewife, nurse, three children (anxiety reaction, moderate depression).

"I find it quite depressing to transcribe these trips and particularly to have to read them repeatedly. In the beginning when I just listened to the trip, I started to cry, and I started again to cry when I transcribed the trip. But later, after reading the trip several times, I felt more relaxed, the whole story appeared to be farther away, and I felt less depressed."

3. *Thematic commentary.*

Based on the assumption that the patient's brain knows the answers to its own elaborations much better than the therapist ever can, the patient is invited to try to make a commentary on the possible significance of the various brain-directed elaborations. The type of commentary a therapist may suggest depends largely on the pattern of neutralization, the patient's interest, and the time he has. What is essential is that the patient occupies himself with the content of his autogenic abreaction (self-confrontation, feedback, broadening of awareness) and tries to understand the language and messages delivered by his brain. Commentaries are less necessary in those cases in which the brain has adopted a very clear reality-related pattern of elaborations (e.g., affective and sexual activities in patients suffering from sexual deprivation; patterns dominated by intellectual elaborations). In other instances commentaries may vary from a few scribbled notes which serve as a base for a discussion during the preabreactive phase of the next appointment, to very systematically elaborated step by step interpretations and drawings. Generally it has been found helpful to suggest to the patient that he elaborates his commentaries by trying to answer the following questions:

(a) What does my brain want to tell me by producing this and this in such and such a manner?

(b) What does this have to do with certain situations in my past?

(c) What does this have to do with my present situation?

(d) What are the possible relationships between the past and the present situation?

Inexperienced patients need to be repeatedly assured that only their brain knows the correct answers, that often many answers are possible and that it actually does not matter whether their answers are correct or not. It is more important that the patient try to understand the language of his brain in order to advance his own treatment by mobilizing and facilitating more efficient brain-directed processes of neutralization.

When the brain-directed processes of neutralization are slow and restricted to, for example, elementary and intermediate stages of visual elaborations, a detailed step by step commentary appears to be particularly helpful in facilitating and widening the range of brain-directed elaborations (see Case 39). When such commentaries are worked out carefully, patients tend to become aware of the progress their brain has made during the same autogenic abreaction;

and also that in the course of an entire series while being engaged in working out comments, or typing of the commentary, a variety of emotional and psychophysiologic reactions may occur (see Case 38). When such reactions occur, the patient should be encouraged to find out by himself whether a particular topic or problem may have triggered these.

*Case 38:* A 35-year-old saleman (moderate depressive reaction). While typing the following passage of his commentary, which refers to the beginning of a hopeless love affair, localized headache occurred.

"I guess the really overt incident occurred when Jos went to Bermuda in June '63 and I dropped over there on the way back from the States. It was about 10, and it led to the kiss on the couch and much kissing that evening; am sure possibly that we had had an alcoholic drink or two. There was not any bodily caressing. (*I seem to be getting a headache at the back of the head, this time over the right ear, but about two inches farther back*). . . ."

*Case 39:* A 36-year-old priest (personality distorder, homosexuality, ecclesiogenic syndrome). The following short sequence of thematic analogies (i.e., penis, tip of breast) are associated with antithematic elements (i.e., masculine, feminine).

| **Passages from AA 7** | **The patient's comments (homework)** |
| --- | --- |
| "I see a penis, the tip is uncovered . . . again I see a woman's breast, especially the tip which is darker . . . it's as if I saw the exterior of a building lit up, but it's rather just a circle of light . . . I see the tip of an uncovered and shiny penis. . . ." | "There is certainly a link between the tip of the penis and the tip of the breast as mentioned here. These two paragraphs express the desire to touch or to suck a woman's breast, but because this desire cannot be satisfied actually it transformed itself into a desire to touch or to suck a man's penis. Regardless of my hidden desire to see and to caress a woman's breasts, it is certain that I have always experienced a sort of fear in doing so. I even experience a certain fear in looking at a woman's breasts. This circle of light on a building probably signifies that the penis and the breasts constitute for me two precise sexual attractions." |

*Case 40:* In the following commentary on cinerama-type processes of neutralization, the patient (Case 16, 66 ff.) attempts to interpret a number of items which she has described in AA 10 (see p. 66 ff.). Initially her comments are relatively restricted, avoiding a number of rather obvious possibilities of interpretation. However, as the commentary continues (i.e., guided by brain-directed elaborations) her initial tendency toward thematic avoidance appears to decrease.

| Items described in AA 10 | The patient's commentary worked out at home |
|---|---|
| 1. Bloodshot eye. | "My father had bloodshot eyes. So did my brother (when drinking) and Jean. |
| 2. Dead eyes. | Reminding me of the dead eyes I first saw in AA 3. I actually saw them on the screen and the sight stayed with me. |
| 3. Peeling potatoes. | This goes back to AA 7: there is half a skeleton and there is a man with a knife. Short pointed one . . . the kind you use for peeling potatoes . . . (see p. 53). This could mean that one has to peel layers of skin (or peels) to find oneself— one has to go to the bones or to the eye of the potato. Or is it aggression? |
| 4. Bucket. | When you have an abortion there is in fact a kind of 'bucket' underneath where all the blood drips. |
| 5. Sharp knife. | Probably I need a knife later in the trip, so my mind provides me with one. |
| 6. Eye. | Eye of a potato. |
| 7. Eye in triangle. | 'God's eyes see everything,' My past indoctrination. Draw and memorize . . . ad infinitum. |
| 8. Bleeding heart of Jesus. | Also mentioned in AA 7: 'blazing heart . . . little flames come out of the heart.' |
| 9. Red heart. | Still refers to Jesus' heart plus fear of death. When one's heart is taken out, one is dead. Heart is life, but stupid life. It is the center of emotions (goodness, badness). |
| 10. Taking the brain out. | Without the brain 'I can't see.' Not in the physical sense obviously. What I mean is 'I can't think,' i.e., 'I can't see myself.' Fear of madness (referring to AA 9: quiet mad woman, a friend who is in the hospital now). |
| 11. Waking up after operation. | Theme of death comes up again. |
| 12. Bottom of a well. | 'Bottom of a deep hole' is introduced (death). The brain also goes back briefly to AA 9: fear of being buried alive; people throwing earth on you. |
| 13. Big red eye seen from the bottom of the hole. | Seeing eyes from below, looking upward into eyes (see 14). |

| Items described in AA 10 | The patient's commentary worked out at home |
|---|---|
| 14. Climbing up a wall that is crumbling. | Age 8-10. We lived at a place where there was a hill. The wall of it was almost vertical: sand, clay and some soft stones. We used to have races with the boys (I always played with boys) who can get up to the top faster. Those who were close to the top tried to push the ones below back down. I was often scared and often slid all the way back. Got punished for torn clothes. I would have liked to hit (kill) the boy on top, but did not dare. I was the only girl, and the youngest in the group. My mind is elaborating on this now to neutralize (a) fear of death, (b) some unpleasant sexual episodes and (c) aggression. |
| 15. White liquid—it is spraying on me. | The same day when I went to the exhibition at Victoria Place on St. Denis street, in a shop window, I saw a sign saying 'SPERM BANK.' I only noticed it at the time, but after a few minutes—by the time I was on Notre Dame—the thought came back, and I was wondering what it could have meant. So: both the red eye and 'SPERM BANK' were flashed at me the same day. |
| 16. Sperm in mouth. | I never objected, actually used to enjoy this form of sexual experience. As far as I can remember, it became unpleasant twice: (a) during a casual affair, many years ago, (b) when I was pregnant with Yves, I gagged and nearly got sick in my stomach. After that I found that putting any object in my mouth while my hands are occupied (e.g., pencil, card, button) makes me gag. |
| 17. It just fills up—then it is quiet—whiteness, coolness. | It seems that by now the thought of death is less frightening. Coolness, whiteness, altogether not important images. |
| 18. Wrinkled red eyelids— long eyelashes. | These images gradually introduce the next point which will be the eye turning into a penis (foreskin). |
| 19. I want to stay quiet so it would reach up quicker and would be finished. | I want the stuff to cover me *quickly*. Still fear of *slow* death (like drowning). This points back to previous trip when I made sure that *court-martial team kills immediately*. |

| Items described in AA 10 | The patient's commentary worked out at home |
|---|---|
| 20. Kill the eye. | Violence: I stab the eye harder, I want to *kill* the eye. Only in reality I want to kill the boy on top of the sand pit, or I want to kill the penis—or rather the man to whom it belongs. If this is so, it must be Jean. |
| 21. I have such a quantity in my mouth. | The 'great quantity' of sperm also refers to Jean. This is one reason of my disliking intercourse with him. I feel so *messy* afterward. AA 7 is referring repeatedly to messiness, which could have been an indication of this. |
| 22. My throat is sore. | Introduction for taking the penis into my mouth. Again I remember gagging. I do not understand why I did not use my potato-knife on the penis. Why dare I kill the eye and not dare to kill the penis. I probably do not want to. Or I do not want to in this general fashion as I enjoy love-making. I wanted to kill only a particular one, that reminded me of Jean. |
| 23. I feel relaxed and peaceful. | Here, death becomes 'rest.' I feel 'relaxed and peaceful.' Probably my mind had enough death and violence for one trip." |

4. *Autogenic training.*

It is important to explain to the patient that the practice of autogenic abreactions cannot substitute for the psychophysiologically beneficial effects resulting from autogenic standard exercises. The methods complement each other, and autogenic training provides the psychophysiologic base for effective work with autogenic abreaction. Therefore the patient is encouraged to continue practicing autogenic standard exercises regularly and to continue writing his training protocol. In this connection it is of particular importance to emphasize that the patient should not permit his brain to engage in autogenic abreaction. To avoid the spontaneous onset of brain-directed dynamics aiming at complex processes of autogenic neutralization, it is essential that a continuity of passive concentration on autogenic formulas is maintained during the practice of autogenic training.[19,20,174,2221] As formula-related passive concentration is kept at a functionally adequate level, a mental shift toward passive acceptance with onset of dynamics characteristic for autogenic abreactions can be avoided. Furthermore, it must be emphasized to patients who have not yet acquired technically sufficient knowledge to be able to engage successfully in unsupervised autogenic abreac-

TABLE 20.   *Therapeutic Homework Carried out during Interim Periods: Autogenic*
*Standard Exercises, Training Protocols and Notes on Dreams*
(120 Psychosomatic and Neurotic Patients)

| Homework of patients | Autogenic Standard Exercises | | |
|---|---|---|---|
| | Very irregular pattern (%) | Irregular pattern (%) | Regular pattern (%) |
| Male (N = 60) | 2 | 17 | 81 |
| Female (N = 60) | 5 | 28 | 66 |

| Homework of patients | Training Protocols | | |
|---|---|---|---|
| | Rarely or none (%) | Occasionally (%) | Regularly (%) |
| Male (N = 60) | 10 | 15 | 75 |
| Female (N = 60) | 26 | 39 | 35 |

| Homework of patients | Notes on Dreams | | |
|---|---|---|---|
| | None (%) | Occasionally (%) | Frequently (%) |
| Male (N = 60) | 27 | 63 | 10 |
| Female (N = 60) | 40 | 58 | 2 |

tions, that they terminate autogenic exercises as soon as they have
the impression that brain-directed dynamics try to push toward
dynamics of autogenic abreaction (see Case 50, p. 125). When
brain-directed pressure in this direction leads to frequent interferences in formula-related passive concentration, it is advisable to
practice a series of *very brief* (e.g., 10-30 sec.) autogenic standard
exercises, and to terminate each exercise correctly in the usual three-
step manner before starting another very short exercise. As the
autogenic standard exercises are kept very brief, it is easier to maintain a continuity of formula-related passive concentration. When
these technical suggestions are observed, no particular difficulties
related to spontaneous conversion into dynamics of autogenic abreaction are encountered. However, when these technical requirements
are not observed, very disturbing experiences may occasionally
occur.[1356,2128,2129,2390] Technically inexperienced patients may find
themselves confronted with anxiety-producing brain-directed elaborations; and in their technically inadequate brain-antagonizing efforts
to suppress the forceful dynamics, they are prone to work themselves into states of confusion and panic.[1016] Other patients who
already have gained some technical experience with autogenic
abreactions know at least that when spontaneous conversions to
complex processes of autogenic neutralization takes place, it is a

basic requirement to maintain an attitude of passive acceptance, and not to antagonize the brain, but to go along with the brain-directed elaborations until these end.

*Case 41:* A 42-year-old housewife (anxiety reaction, multiple psychophysiologic reaction) who already had advanced experience with autogenic abreactions, reported an incidence of conversion into complex dynamics of autogenic neutralization which occurred while she was practicing autogenic standard exercises.

*Transcript of the patient's report:* "Endless tears, well seemingly so, feeling of choking. See my mother, she is holding her head looking down at me. I am a baby nine months old, I am lying naked on a table . . . she is looking down at me saying: 'shut up, shut up, why for God's sake don't you shut up, you've had your bottle, SHUT UP. . . .' This is repeated several times as she is getting nearer and nearer to me . . . suddenly I black out. My mother is now sitting on a chair and she is crying bitterly: 'What have I done, oh Christ what have I done?' As my mother is saying this she is putting her mouth on mine, blowing into my mouth . . . I am naked and the tears are falling all over me . . . she is rocking back and forth. I as a baby am experiencing all sorts of sensations, the feeling of no breath, tension from throat dissolving . . . I am very cold and the tears are still falling over me . . . I am now wrapped in a brown blanket, warm being rocked by my mother."

*Case 42:* A 26-year-old male student who complained about tiredness, unpleasant dreams, difficulty of concentration, bothersome homosexual phantasies, periods of palpitations, disturbing tensions, periods of diffuse anxiety, aquaphobia, feeling of constriction around his head, headaches, cold hands and feet, feeling of isolation in groups, buzzing in ears.

"During one of my exercises, I see again the young soldier whom I liked and I start to masturbate him. This takes some time. Then I press him against me from behind and very gradually he dissolves and it is myself whom I masturbate. After a few moments I experience a violent urge to suck. All the muscles of my mouth are active, and it is just as if I suck a breast in reality. To my knowledge it is the first time that I ever experienced such movements with my mouth. The whole thing functioned completely automatically. At the same time I experience a feeling of unusual pleasure in my mouth, my tongue, in my whole abdomen and including my penis. This is as if the pleasure is absorbed by my mouth and runs out of my penis. Then I become aware that I suck my mother's breast and the sexual excitement becomes quite intensive. At the same time I see my mother embracing me and happily I let her do so. Then my mother starts masturbating me while I suck her breast and while this is going on my sexual excitement gets more and more intense until a real ejaculation is produced. During the days which followed this spontaneous trip, I experience an intense and real feeling of liberation."

*Case 43:* A 30-year-old priest (anxiety reaction, obsessive-compulsive manifestations, vocational conflicts, ecclesiogenic syndrome). Three days after the twelfth autogenic abreaction, the patient's training protocol mentions a number of distractions which reflect his preoccupation with certain vocational problems. The nature of these "distractions" is closely related to the dynamics of neutralization of the preceding (AA 12) and the following AA 13.

| Formula | Reports on the effects of the exercises |
|---|---|
| SE I-VI | (a) "Medium heaviness in right arm and left leg toward the end, some numbness. Heaviness starting in right leg at the end. Heart about normal. Few reactions. Well relaxed. Concentration weak. Distractions: My summer course program. It would be possible, quite possible to start in philosophy. I already have two years of university studies in this area. Thought of a nice girl, my wife, and intercourse with her. |
| " | (b) Right arm and left leg heavy toward the end. Both legs are a little numb. On two occasions some slight pain in the left temporal area. Heart all right. Well relaxed. Concentration disturbed: the tape recorder and particularly the summer course (finances, living quarters, clothing, etc.). |
| " | (c) Right arm and left leg numb, medium heaviness. Heart okay. In the beginning there was quite a strong pressure-like sensation over the left temple. Concentration disturbed: new insight. I asked myself how come that now, several years after my ordination, everything, my whole life is in question. As I listened to my last trip, the answer came like a flash: it's because, when I committed myself with two vows, and the ordination, I was not mature enough to know what I did, to appreciate the importance of my commitment. This actually means that I did not commit myself in the real sense, I did not give myself. Therefore this pledge did not have a real value. And that is why everything is now questionable. Before the Lord, I think it's logic, and I can start a new life. But this time with lucidity, either by remaining in the order or by going into another profession. It seems to me that this conclusion deserves to be considered. This reasoning appears to be so simple, and still it's only now that I grasp its real significance." |

After the beginning of treatment with autogenic abreactions a number of patients tend to notice (during AT) the occurrence of brain-directed phenomena which appear to be closely linked to the dynamics of the preceding autogenic abreaction or which may indicate the nature of the material which is going to dominate the central phase of the next autogenic abreaction. Such training-related phenomena may be of intellectual nature (see Case 43), may consist of brief episodes of visual elaborations (which the patient is supposed to interrupt as early as possible by terminating the autogenic exercise), phasic onset of vestibular discharges (e.g., accident-related) or other topographically rather specific sensory (e.g., pain, pressure) or motor discharges (e.g., twitching of right foot, related to a ski accident). When the patient's training protocol reflects massive or increasing phenomena which thematically are related to the patient's pattern of autogenic abreactions, this is usually an indication for giving more adequate opportunity to the brain to neutralize the mobilized material. In case this indication is not respected, it may not take long until more forceful brain-directed elaborations start to interfere (e.g., many distractions, restlessness, headaches) unfavorably with the regular practice of autogenic training.

5. *Notes on dreams.*

In various respects the patient's dreams are of particular interest during treatment with autogenic abreaction. Generally it may be helpful to explain to the patient that it is not intended to spend time on the interpretation of dreams, because it has become evident that such interpretations are of relatively limited therapeutic value when compared with the efficiency of processes of brain-directed neutralization during autogenic abreaction. Therefore, it is therapeutically of greater practical value to use the available time for autogenic abreactions instead of time-consuming dream interpretations.[837] In this connection, particularly when patients have been under psychoanalytic treatment before, it may be mentioned that the brain takes its opportunity to repeat dreams, or parts of them, during autogenic abreaction in order to neutralize the disturbing potency of the underlying material.

Since dreams may be regarded as relatively abortive attempts at neutralization of accumulated disturbing material, the dream content may serve as a valuable source of information.

Firstly, the dream content may indicate material and specific dynamics which have not occurred during autogenic abreaction. In such instances it may be suspected that brain-antagonizing forms of resistance (e.g., thematic avoidance; see Vol. VI, Part I) are exerting inhibitory effects during autogenic abreaction, and a relevant technically oriented and thematically related discussion is indicated.

Secondly, the dream content may serve as an indicator of the level of thematic neutralization. Relevant studies have shown that particularly massive and disturbing material tends to be thematically repeated during dreams, when it was technically impossible to arrive at adequate levels of neutralization (e.g., after premature termination). When dreams occur repeatedly and are closely related thematically to dynamics observed during autogenic abreaction, it is advisable to give the brain better opportunities for autogenic neutralization (i.e., prolongation of future AAs, increase of office visits, increase of AA at home for experienced patients).

Thirdly, dream content may forecast essential topics which will be taken up for more detailed neutralization during the central phase of the following autogenic abreaction. Such advance knowledge is usually helpful for the therapist in his evaluation of the brain-directed pattern and subsequent indications for technical support to help the brain to overcome brain-anatagonizing forms of resistance (see Vol. VI, Part I).

*Case 44:* A 48-year-old male patient (anxiety reaction, personality disorder, homosexuality, obsessive-compulsive reactions, ecclesiogenic syndrome) reported the following dream which indicates that the brain needs more opportunity to neutralize anxiety material related to feelings of guilt, death, fear of punishment by God and suffering in hell.

"I had terrible dreams in the course of the night: I saw myself in a colony of lepers who were taking diabolical delight in imprisoning me along with themselves. It's as if I was seeing myself in hell. I felt I was being punished, and well punished for my offenses against my superiors, my colleagues, my plans to leave the order, my arrogance, my desire to show off, my stubbornness in resisting superiors and colleagues. When I awoke, I tried in vain to get my mind off it and to fall back asleep, but no, all this terrible business came back to me so I preferred staying awake; and God knows how sleepy I was. I felt unhappy and guilty; and in the dream and even when awake, I had the terrible fear that things would always remain as such in my mind; because even when awake, I thought as in the dream."

*Remark:* The central phase of the following autogenic abreaction was dominated by processes of neutralization which focussed almost exclusively on dynamics indicated by the dream.

*Case 45:* A 49-year-old priest (anxiety reaction, obsessive-compulsive manifestations, vocational conflicts, ecclesiogenic syndrome). Following an initial seven-minute period of elementary visual elaborations (stages I-II), the visualization of the devil's face led to a repetition of essential elements which occurred during a dream the patient had had the night before. Brain-directed indications for termination follow after adequate levels of neutralization have been reached.

"A devil's face on a blue background, a blue that somewhat nears purple . . . a devil's face with oblique eyes and a muzzle, a large and round aquiline nose . . . I saw a devil last night . . . it was a television commercial . . . putting us on guard against the devil . . . damn catechism. . . . Later I had a dream . . . the devil was at a short distance, as if in a field beside a bunch of flames coming out of the ground . . . a warning, a recalling that it could suddenly come . . . the earth opening up . . . a nun's story in catechism . . . sudden death . . . the devil who could appear unexpectedly . . . it, it profoundly marked me . . . it caused great anxiety in me for years . . . like it is said, in a state of mortal sin . . . the fear . . . the quaking . . . the devil . . . we'll go there . . . I go down into hell by way of Vesuvius, right to the bottom of the abyss . . . there we are tortured: the traitor, the hypocrite, the sacrilegious, all like me . . . into the burning sulfur . . . torches of fire. . . . In the midst of devils pricking me with pitchforks, snakes, reptiles, octopuses, giant spiders scratching me, stinging me, sucking me. . . . The background turns orange, red a beautiful red, there's orange, some yellow . . . now it's blue, a beautiful blue . . . there's a paler blue with a pinkish tone mixed into it . . . a clear blue, a beautiful blue, a clear blue . . . clearer than navy blue . . . I was in hell . . . for quite a while with some monsters . . . in the fire forever . . . some green . . . ah yes, lots of it . . . it's like green streaks . . . there's a little bit of orange in there, not clean . . . well yes, some orange, some green, a clear enough pale green . . . clear blue . . . it's all a bit dirty, a little bit in the gray tones . . . it's blue . . . oh, a beautiful blue with yellow going through it, a clear yellow . . . before that, it was of a slightly purplish magenta tone . . . clear blue, a large enough face in the background . . . get out you devils . . . all sorts of colors in the background . . . there aren't too many . . . now some blue, some blue tones . . . there's a pale blue, a darker blue . . . all sorts of blue shades, and it all oscillates like sheets in the wind, it moves like the surface of water . . ." (40 min.; standard termination).

*Case 46:* A 37-year-old businessman (anxiety reaction). During cinerama-type elaborations with active self-participation, mainly involving themes related to childhood material (fear of death, horror stories told by a maid), the brain focusses upon reconfrontation with a nightmare which the patient had at the age of six or seven.

"Ah! I am seeing all sorts of things from these tapestries or what have you . . . yes, exaggerated, goblins, witches or what have you, yes I'm sort of seeing that dream I had that night . . . more about rolling down the hill . . . about rolling the heads down the hill, from a cemetery, I remember that scared the hell out of me when I had this nightmare when I was a kid. . . . And the screaming rabbit. . . . Yes, it's all there . . . I don't know where the heck I got that nightmare from, its stuck with me a long time . . . oh, its sort of a spooky cemetery on a hill . . . all these witches were rolling the heads of dead people down the hill, and it just scared the life out of me . . . the hill and the heads rolling down, they were not skulls, they were heads, and it was pretty weird seeing all these witches doing that . . . then I remember seeing a rabbit that was screaming and so I started screaming and I woke up in the middle of the night . . . and my parents came over, to see what the heck was the matter with me . . . it was pretty . . . I'll always remember that nightmare, because it was one of my very first impressive . . . why I saw it, what made me see it I don't know . . . well I'm still seeing this hill with this churchyard . . . partly it's a graveyard running from the top to the bottom . . . it seems to me sort of a church or chapel at the top . . . I don't know what there is at the bottom . . . a wall or a moat or something . . . heads all bouncing down, very strange . . . well there are graves, a couple of open ones there, and a lot of tombstones . . . what gets me, how these heads all keep rolling down without stopping . . . they are hitting some of the tombstones . . . I can see these heads and they are rolling down, all sorts of pirates and bandits and regular people . . . and now I am getting this striped effect again [*elementary visual elaborations indicating a thematic change*]. . . . The tiger, the yellow and black, yes, I'm seeing a tiger sort of stalking through the underbush . . . now he is jumping . . . I sort of caught him in mid-air . . . [*anticipatory resistance*] . . . he's going to jump at me, and sort of tears me apart. . . ."

*Case 47:* A 49-year-old lay brother (anxiety reaction, personality disorder, sexual deviation, obsessive-compulsive and phobic reactions, ecclesiogenic syndrome) who had wished to become a priest for many years, but who hesitated to ask permission to do so. During an autogenic abreaction carried out at home, the patient's dream of the previous night was spontaneously repeated during the central phase.

"I see myself in a clergyman suit . . . I'm a priest . . . and I see myself among missionaries with a fellow priest, newly ordained as I . . . we're very happy, very relaxed . . . we're experiencing the plenitude of the priesthood and of being missionaries . . . we feel wholesome, void of complexes, lighthearted, satisfied, fully happy that we're priests . . . and we're there to help . . . we're studying the language, we're looking through books that will help us adjust our ministry to that particular corner of the world . . . we're preparing ourselves with much joy and ease in this work . . . on the veranda, I see . . ." (thematic shift).

## 6. Sketches and drawings.

When central phases are dominated by a mixed pattern of accident-related sensory, vestibular and motor discharges, and the accompanying visual elaborations remain vague or incomplete, it has been helpful to ask the patient to try to reconstruct the accident by making a sketch of its location and dynamics. While doing this, or soon afterward these patients tend to remember details which are of importance for the understanding of certain brain-programmed elaborations, the significance of which remained obscure during the autogenic abreaction.

Series of drawings are also of therapeutic value when central phases are dominated by descriptions of elementary stages (i.e., I-III; Table 33, p. 188) of visual elaborations which show slow progress to higher degrees of differentiation (see Fig. 18, p. 304). The step by step execution of colored drawings according to the transcript of the apparently uninteresting autogenic abreaction reveals to the patient more clearly that very complex elaborations of structural, chromatic and dynamic nature have actually occurred, and that the sequences of simple forms of objects show a progressive trend toward higher degrees of differentiation. Patients are normally encouraged by such "discoveries," and their comments on the largely symbolic elaborations tend to become easier and more sophisticated (see Case 88, p. 208 ff.). As these patients continue to draw the sequences of their autogenic abreactions, a supportive brain-facilitating effect toward a speedier development to more differentiated stages of visual elaborations appears to occur. The therapist's suggestion to make such drawings would be misunderstood, however, if the patient is left with the impression that visual elaborations are more important than other kinds. It should be emphasized repeatedly that it is essential to remain open-minded toward any kind of brain-directed elaborations, and that it would be a technical error to restrict the brain by overemphasizing the value or description of phenomena in the visual field.

## 7. Other tasks and recommendations.

As the treatment with autogenic abreaction pursues its brain-directed course, a variety of specific suggestions closely related to prevailing themes of autogenic neutralization may be appropriate to widen and to verify the patient's awareness. For example, it may be helpful to obtain more information about a certain childhood accident, about certain traumatic family situations, or about certain aspects which are related to the patient's professional activity or occupational orientation.

In many instances, when autogenic abreactions emphasize neutralization of anxiety material related to death as, for example, witnessing relatives dying in the hospital, traumatic funeral episodes, participation in shootings and other life-threatening situations of violence, a thematically adapted discussion is indicated; since the brain-directed elaborations which occurred during the autogenic abreaction have clearly shown that the patient's brain is still disturbed by "long forgotten," but severely disturbing events. In such cases it is therapeutically desirable that the brain be given a favorable opportunity to continue its original program of neutralization and that undesirable thematically related confrontations during the patient's daily life are avoided, reduced and if possible eliminated. As long as adequate levels of thematic neutralization have not been reached, further confrontations with, for example, dying relatives or closely related situations are known to result in a reinforcement of negatively oriented dynamics with undue mobilization of still existing insufficiently neutralized, underlying disturbing material. To avoid such thematically undesirable and complicating brain reactions, additional loading of already overloaded systems should be avoided as much as possible. This leads to practical recommendations, such as not to visit severely sick persons, not to visit funeral homes or participate in burial ceremonies. However though these patients tend to agree in principle with such recommendations, they are usually worried about the reactions of other persons who would not readily accept the patient's "heartless," "unsocial" behavior (e.g., not attending a funeral). As social practices must be respected up to a certain point to avoid new sources of disturbances, it is advisable to make efforts to find a compromise solution with the aim of reducing the negative consequences of premature confrontations to a minimum. In many instances it should be explained to the patient that his own health is more important than social practice, and for medical reasons it is necessary to avoid such activities or confrontations for the time.

Recommendations of a similar nature may be necessary when relatively high levels of anxiety are repeatedly associated with various kinds of violent and morbid themes of autogenic neutralization. The undeniable fact that the brain is attempting to reduce the disturbing potency of already accumulated material makes it easier for the patient to understand that additional loading by material of similar nature is not to his advantage. Patients belonging to this category tend to agree readily that further watching of tension and anxiety promoting films (e.g., *The Birds, The Snake Pit*), exciting television stories, scenes of violence, or reading of literature with morbid themes (e.g., E. A. Poe, F. Kafka, violent thrillers) are therapeutically contraindicated. The emphasis should be on neutral and positively oriented brain input. While listening to such explanations and recommendations, a relatively large number of patients tend to be somewhat surprised, because they have felt particularly attracted to exactly this category of thrilling film, to precisely this type of literature, or they find themselves compelled to look at a messy accident scene or a devastating fire. To these patients it must be explained that relevant studies have indicated that their particular attraction or interest appears to be actually an attempt on the part of their brain to neutralize disturbing material through confrontation. However, since adequate neutralization requires many repetitions of the same stimulus within a certain period of time to obtain a response decrement to levels which permit the development of enhanced adaptation at various functional levels, quantitatively and qualitatively inadequate number of confrontations tend to act rather as negatively oriented reinforcements associated with undesirable additional loading, without reaching brain-desired levels of adequate neutralization. Furthermore, evidence indicates that in such abortive attempts at neutralization through confrontation with reality (e.g., scenes, films, pictures, literature, comic strips) there results an even greater brain-desired need for neutralization, thus creating a self-reinforcing vicious circle with the probability of increasing functional disturbances in the brain. In this context it may be appropriate to mention that it may be of therapeutic interest at a later point, after technically adequate levels of neutralization have been achieved, to test the patient's reactivity by permitting "experimental confrontations" with previously disturbing reality material.

Recommendations of a similar nature are indicated in the area of sports. For example, when flying, skiing, water skiing, diving or acrobatics are found to be associated with severely brain-disturbing material, it is preferable to reduce or eliminate such activities during the treatment period for two reasons: (a) to avoid additional loading and (b) to avoid the risk that brain-directed dynamics (e.g., self-destruction) are given a chance to project into reality what should be neutralized during autogenic abreaction. In certain instances it is in the patient's interest to reduce or to stop driving his car for a certain period to avoid the increased probability of getting involved in accidents.

Homosexual patients who have already had the opportunity to see that their brain is continuously aiming at progressive heterosexualization, with neutralization of brain-disturbing dynamics which promote brain-undesirable homosexual activities, usually realize themselves that continuation of brain-antagonizing homosexual activities are not to their advantage. As this invariable observation (see Vol. VI, Part III) indicates the brain's natural efforts to promote a development toward heterosexual activities, it is therapeutically justified to recommend during early phases of treatment with autogenic abreaction a reduction of brain-antagonizing homosexual activities.

Other recommendations such as keeping the transcriptions under lock at all times, the patient's temporary removal from a neurotogenic household, or therapeutically desirable occupational adjustments are usually discussed after the interim period has been reviewed and before engaging in preparatory work for the next autogenic abreaction (see p. 120 ff.).

### Schedule of Appointments

Toward the end of the postabreactive period the patient is invited to discuss the date of the next appointment. In the course of such a conversation it may be explained to the inexperienced patient that the scheddule of appointments must be adapted to the need of unloading as indicated by his brain, and for this reason it is a therapeutic disadvantage to adopt a predetermined fixed program of appointments (e.g., every Wednesday at 3 p.m.). As an instructive example, the brain's need to unload and the consequences which tend to result in cases where the brain's functional state is not respected may be compared with the functional state of the bladder which is slowly filling up. As one responds in a natural manner to the prompting of the bladder by emptying it on time, disturbed periods and embarrassing episodes are avoided. However, in case one has no opportunity to void, increasing disturbances of concentration, discomfort, increasing apprehension and anxiety are usually noted. These disturbing phenomena subside promptly as one finds an opportunity to urinate. Analogous changes of reactivity are noted in patients who do not permit their brain to unload when the need to do so is not respected. Depending on the nature of the material involved, one may notice various kinds of psychophysiologic reactions (e.g., gastric discomfort, headaches, sleep disturbances, crying spells, palpitations, feelings of impatience, aggression, experience of episodes of anxiety, more use of alcohol than usual, difficulties for oneself and others, difficulties of concentration, loss of creative productivity and perhaps regrettable mistakes in judgment and inadequate decisions). To avoid such therapeutically undesirable effects which tend to be associated with mobilized but unneutralized material, it is essential to adapt the program of appointments to the patient's need. Only later, when the patient has gained enough technical experience to carry out unsupervised autogenic abreactions at home in accordance with the needs as indicated by his brain, is it possible to adopt a more regular schedule of appointments (e.g., once every two weeks). In the beginning, during the learning phase, most patients are seen within ten days (see Table 21). Only in exceptional circumstances is a patient seen twice a week. Since it is difficult to determine in advance a patient's need for the next autogenic abreaction it is advisable to adopt a flexible approach. The patient should feel that he can call at any time when he does not feel well and that efforts will be made to accommodate him when necessary. Emphasis on such a flexible policy is of particular importance to those inhibited patients who initially show difficulties in maintaining passive acceptance during initial autogenic abreactions and who are prone to experience disagreeable reactions during the interim. Generally, it is recommended to begin with appointments spaced at about one-week intervals. When unforeseen intervening variables (e.g., intercurrent diseases, prolonged absence) make it impossible to carry out the next autogenic abreaction within about ten days, the transitory use of supportive medication may be considered.

TABLE 21. *Intervals between the First and the Second Autogenic Abreaction*

| Autogenic Abreaction | Interval in Days | | | | | | | | | |
|---|---|---|---|---|---|---|---|---|---|---|
| | Same Day or Session | 1 | 2 | 3–4 | 5–6 | 7 | 8–14 | 15–21 | 22–28 | Over | M |
| 96 psycho-somatic and neurotic patients | 5 | | 2 | 12 | 10 | 14 | 20 | 20 | 7 | 3 | 3 | 9.5 |

# 8. The Interim Period

The interim peroid covers the time between the patient's departure from the therapist's office and his next appointment in the office. Generally it is possible to distinguish three major interim phases: (a) the initial interim phase, (b) the central interim phase and (c) the pre-appointment phase. Each of these interim phases is characterized by certain features of psychophysiologic reactivity which are in many respects related to the disturbing nature of the material undergoing autogenic neutralization, the program of therapeutic homework and the patient's reactivity to variables which may intervene during the interim period (e.g., death of mother, fight with husband, accident, hospitalization, confusion resulting from discussions with other patients who are also treated with AA).

Since a variety of therapeutically important problems may occur during the interim period and a patient-adapted management in relevant situations is considered essential, some of the more frequently encountered observations and variables will be presented in the following chapters.

Of general interest are postabreactive improvements and difficulties which have been reported by patients after their first and second autogenic abreaction (see Table 22).

## THE INITIAL INTERIM PHASE

The initial interim phase comprises a six- to eight-hour period which starts after the patient leaves the therapist's office. If possible, it is advisable that patients use this postabreactive period of relative neutralization for transcribing their autogenic abreaction. In most instances patients tend to feel relieved, certain bothersome symptoms disappear (see Table 22, p. 121) and no particular problems are encountered. Only a relatively small number of patients, who are usually still in the learning phase, tend to experience difficulties which require the therapist's immediate attention. Usually it can be predicted that undesirable emotional and psychophysiologic reactions will occur during the initial interim phase, when the pattern of the autogenic abreaction has involved frequent occurrence of various forms of brain-antagonizing resistance (see Vol. VI, Part I), and adequate levels of neutralization could not be reached (see Case 30, p. 95). Premature patient-directed terminations, early technical terminations and refusal of the patient to continue the interrupted processes of neutralization

during the same appointment, or an unusually massive load of thematically specific material (e.g., neutralization of hell, severe car accidents)
are the most frequent reasons why unsufficiently neutralized material
produces postabreactive difficulties. Inexperienced patients are usually
glad to leave the therapist's office, and they hope that everything will
be satisfactory until the next appointment (see Case 48, p. 122). However, as the hours pass they tend to feel more and more uncomfortable.

TABLE 22.   *Changes Noted by Psychosomatic and Neurotic Patients
during Intervals between AA 1, AA 2, and AA 2 and AA 3*

| Changes Reported after Autogenic Abreactions | Intervals between Autogenic Abreactions | |
|---|---|---|
| | Between AA 1 and AA 2 (%; N = 100) | Between AA 2 and AA 3 (%; N = 96) |
| **A.** *General* | | |
| (a) Feeling better generally | 40.0 | 50.0 |
| (b) Improvement of specific complaints or disorders | 7.0 | 6.2 |
| (c) No improvement of feeling badly | 22.0 | 20.8 |
| (d) More disturbed by specific disorders | 6.0 | 10.4 |
| (e) No changes reported | 25.0 | 12.5 |
| **B.** *Specific improvements* | | |
| (f) More relaxed, less nervous, less anxiety, less depressed, less irritable | 19.0 | 18.7 |
| (g) Improved social contact | 7.0 | 13.5 |
| (h) More efficient at work, better concentration | 8.0 | 9.4 |
| (i) Better appetite, gain of weight | 6.0 | 6.2 |
| (j) Improvement or normal sleep | 7.0 | 7.3 |
| (k) Improvement or normal gastrointestinal functions | 2.0 | 1.0 |
| (l) Improvement or disappearance of headaches or dizziness | 5.0 | 4.2 |
| (m) Other specific improvements | 9.0 | 20.8 |
| **C.** *Specific difficulties and complaints* | | |
| (n) Periods of tension, nervousness, restlessness, depressive feelings | 11.0 | 16.6 |
| (o) Less appetite, nausea | 1.0 | 1.0 |
| (p) Social contact more difficult | 1.0 | — |
| (q) Work concentration more difficult | — | 1.0 |
| (r) Poor sleep | 3.0 | 3.1 |
| (s) Gastrointestinal complaints | 2.0 | 2.0 |
| (t) Headaches and dizziness | 6.0 | 8.3 |
| (u) Other specific complaints | 6.0 | 10.4 |

They may decide to go to bed early, and while practicing autogenic exercises, their brain uses the opportunity to press for neutralization of the mobilized material. Technically inexperienced patients then attempt to antagonize their brain; consequently they feel increasingly uncomfortable, bothered by restlessness, diffuse anxiety and even states of panic. If they do manage to fall asleep, disturbing dreams, frequent waking up, crying spells and despair may interrupt the night. In other instances the insufficiently neutralized material may project its dynamics onto family members (see Case 48), and very disturbing episodes tend to result (see Case 30, p. 95).

To reduce the negative consequences of such reactions, it is absolutely necessary to warn these patients and to ask them to call the therapist as early as possible when they notice that disturbing manifestations persist after arriving at home. Prophylactic application of supportive medication (e.g., chlordiazepoxide, meprobamate) is always helpful, but therapeutically it is more desirable to invite the patient to return to the therapist's office and to neutralize the disturbing material by another autogenic abreaction. Such episodes, when taken care of without delay, are quite instructive for the patient and help to improve his collaboration (e.g., less brain-antagonizing resistance). For these patients it is important to realize that attempts to be wiser than one's own brain mechanisms are never successful (see Case 48).

*Case 48:* A 38-year-old businessman (anxiety reaction, obsessive-compulsive manifestations, ecclesiogenic syndrome) began his fourth autogenic abreaction with an unusually long latent period. The subsequent pattern of his descriptions was particularly slow, with frequent intervals of silence and appeared rather to be a well-formulated speech than a description of brain-directed processes of neutralization. The thematic content kept revolving around pleasant memories of his adolescent years. After 23 minutes the patient expressed that he felt comfortable and wished to terminate. During the immediate postabreactive phase he admitted: "I have the impression this was not a real trip." The therapist agreed and in the course of the postabreactive discussion invited him to call anytime in case he did not feel well.

Three days later, around 9 A.M. on Sunday morning he called and asked for an appointment because he had some difficulties and felt he could not allow them to continue because a particularly heavy load of important work was planned for the coming week.

When the patient was seen two hours later he stated that he had felt badly for the last two or three days, that he had been more aggressive toward his wife and his children, that generally his reactions were more violent, that he felt somewhat confused, with periods of disturbing inner tension and diffuse anxiety. No dreams were remembered, but he had tried to keep himself very busy and had no time to practice his exercises or to finish typing his last autogenic abreaction. He also admitted freely that he thought the therapist was

joking when he invited him to call at anytime, simply because the last autogenic abreaction had not gone well. A little later he remarked that he knew
why he felt badly and that he kept thinking of certain things he had visualized
during AA 4 but which he did not wish to describe (i.e., *intentional resistance*,
see Vol. VI, Part I).

AA 5 was started, and a 56-minute period of brain-directed processes of
neutralization focussed on exactly those themes which the patient did not want
to mention during AA 4. Afterward he felt relieved and in good spirits. No
further difficulties were encountered.

## THE CENTRAL INTERIM PHASE

The central interim phase usually comprises a variable number of
days (see Table 21, p. 119) ending about 24 hours before the next
appointment. Patients who have obtained adequate levels of thematic
neutralization during the preceding autogenic abreaction tend to feel
unburdened and they notice certain positively oriented changes in their
behavior and during work. However in many instances such changes
last only for about two to four days. Then certain difficulties may reappear, or "old complaints" seem to become more prominent again.
Such manifestations usually indicate that relevant brain mechanisms
have mobilized program-related thematic material which starts pressing
for unloading and neutralization. In case the next appointment is only
a few days away and the functional disturbances are not too bothersome, the patient may wait and maintain himself by practicing series
of *very brief* (e.g., 10-20 sec.) autogenic standard exercises more frequently. However, when the patient feels more acutely disturbed, he
should feel free to call the therapist and ask for an earlier appointment.
Experienced patients who are permitted to carry out autogenic abreactions at home can help themselves effectively by performing autogenic
abreactions as they feel the need to do so (see Vol. VI, Part I). In this
connection it may be mentioned that disagreeable dreams occurring
during the morning hours and subsequent onset of frontal or occipital
headaches belong to those categories of symptoms which usually indicate the brain's need for neutralization. When these phenomena occur
during the night or during early morning hours, it is particularly helpful to neutralize the underlying dynamics before getting up (see Case
50; Case 52, p. 145). Otherwise the patient is prone to experience more
difficulties during working hours.

Of particular diagnostic and therapeutic concern are patients with a
history of cardiac disorders (e.g., paroxysmal tachycardia, see Case
23, p. 67/II), iatrogenic reactions and other forms of psychoreactive
cardiac complaints. More frequently than other groups of patients,

these cases are prone to experience subjectively very disturbing heart sensation, episodes of tachycardia, palpitation and oppressive feelings (see p. 126 ff.). As these reactions are usually closely related to specific themes which are under neutralization, a feeling of acute anxiety, with fear of heart attack and sudden death tend to be associated. For these patients it is particularly important to communicate with the therapist during the interim period and to undergo a reassuring differential diagnostic evaluation without delay. Only after the physical examination has ruled out cardiac lesions can the treatment with autogenic abreactions continue (see Case 49).

Case 49: A 46-year-old priest (anxiety reaction, iatrogenic reaction, ecclesiogenic syndrome). During a physical examination shortly after the patient entered a religious order, the examining physician remarked that his heart was weak and that probably he would not live much longer than the early thirties. Repeated electrocardiographic studies carried out later did not reveal any abnormalities.

During a treatment period which focussed on thematic neutralization of his father's death (which the patient had witnessed) and anxiety dynamics related to damnation in hell, the patient repeatedly complained about discomfort in his heart, menacing palpitations, tachycardia, a "racing irregular heartbeat," and fear of sudden death.

A physical examination carried out during the interim period shortly after he called the therapist's office revealed a normal heart condition (P. 72 reg., B. P. 132/84).

During treatment phases which are devoted to brain-directed neutralization of certain accidents (e.g., with shock, brief loss of consciousness, near drowning), acute episodes of gastric discomfort and feeling of nausea may occur during the interim. After other causes have been ruled out, and as the thematically related pattern of reactivity becomes known, it is appropriate to encourage these patients to permit vomiting as often as they feel nauseated. In case this suggestion is not followed, or the frequency of vomiting is inadequate, the patient is prone to suffer from gastric discomfort, nausea and anorexia for longer periods.

Diabetic patients should be advised to test daily their urinary glucose levels during the interim and to adjust their insulin dosage in such a way that slight spilling of sugar provides reassuring evidence against the fear of sudden insulin reactions (see Case 40, p. 108 ff./II). Clinically oriented observations have indicated that adequate levels of thematic neutralization over series of autogenic abreactions may require a progressive reduction of insulin dosage. Inversely, during treatment periods characterized by frequent interferences from brain-antagonizing forms of resistance, when the brain is not permitted to reach and to maintain adequate levels of neutralization, it may be necessary to increase the number of insulin units (see Fig. 19, p. 109/II).

*Case 50:* A 27-year-old housewife (anxiety reaction, allergic reactions, sleep disorder, multiple phobic reactions, multiple psychophysiologic reactions, ecclesiogenic syndrome). The patient started feeling progressively more uncomfortable and tense after transcribing her autogenic abreaction (AA 5, Monday) which was largely dominated by aggressive dynamics against family members, the therapist and herself. Anxiety material related to comic strip-like childhood literature (e.g., being devoured by tigers, bears, lions, monsters) came up briefly, but appeared to have been evaded (*thematic evasion,* see Vol. VI, Part I). The patient's evasion of neutralization of the brain-programmed topics during AA 5 led to brain-directed interferences during autogenic standard exercises (see below) and are also reflected by thematically related elaborations during a dream.

An early appointment was indicated, and the patient was told to continue practicing *very brief* exercises in the meantime. While she practiced these brief exercises no particular problems were encountered (see: c, d, e, f).

Particularly instructive are the brain-directed dynamics of AA 6 which include several interjected phases of bright monochromatic colors (see AA 6 below). As potent anxiety material (e.g., films, stories, car accident, religious education) underwent neutralization in AA 6, the patient did not experience any of the previous difficulties (see a) during subsequent practice of autogenic training. No further nightmares were reported.

| Formula | Reports on the effects of the exercises |
|---|---|
| SE I-IV | (a) *Tuesday,* 8:10 P.M. |

"As I start thinking of my formulas, many of these small monsters are coming up. Now since they have been awakened during the last trip, they keep dancing around, and they don't want to go away. I also see these nightmare landscapes. Then a terrible face of a witch grimacing at me. She puts me into a huge pot, she cooks me and I am disintegrating and die. Then there was a giant gluey octopus on top of me, squeezing me with its cold and slimy tentacles; she suffocates me, and I literally felt her weight crushing down on my chest, and I died. Right after this, a huge black hairy tarantula came toward me, stinging me right into my heart, sucking all my blood [third death]. During all this I tried to keep my formulas going and just let myself die. I was quite afraid. I cry and shiver when I think of the night ahead, my teeth are chattering and I have a headache on the left upper side.

**Formula**                              **Reports on the effects of the exercises**

*P.S.* Each of these episodes of death are related to a story or a film which I saw when I
was a child. I realize this now. But is it not
always possible that one terrible thing links
up with the next one, and that most of this
goes actually back to childhood experiences?

"

(b) *Tuesday,* 11:45 P.M.

Since my last exercise I felt like calling you,
but I managed to do the exercise without
aggressive elements. That is encouraging for
the night ahead. I only see sort of curdled
milk or some clotted liquid substance, like
during experiments in chemistry. Some twitching of muscles of my right upper lip and in
my neck. Some pain in my chest, left shoulder
and in my heart.

"

*Wednesday,* 5:20 A.M.

I had a nightmare and woke up. A bulldog bit
somebody in the chest and legs. And this
somebody became me. All my extremities are
sore as if I had been under great tension. This
makes me think of other nightmares when I
had similar sensations.

Then there was a pool of dismembered
corpses, all in pieces, stinking, and all
around me, and on top, everywhere. I let this
go into my mouth and nose, and finally I
suffocate and die. All the little monsters came
back again surrounding me, they dance and
laugh. I order them to go away, but they don't
want to and cry: 'We will kill you, kill you,'
and I let them go ahead—crying.

I would like to get up, but I am afraid of
the darkness, and I am afraid just as I was
during my childhood. I just could not go down
into the basement to call you. What I am most
afraid of is that I could not take all these
gimmicks of my brain, and that I am going to
go crazy. Did a thing like that already happen
during treatment? Are these hallucinations
going to last for a long time to come?

Called Dr. *L.* at 7:00 A.M. Was told to do
many very brief exercises and to come to his
office at 3:00 P.M.

| Formula | Reports on the effects of the exercises |
|---|---|
| SE I-VI (very brief) | (c) *Wednesday*, 7:10 A.M. |

I succeeded in doing the exercises in one stretch, I kept them very short. I had many distractions, but they did not bother me very much. Stinging pain in left upper leg. Pressure at both temples. Pain in left fingers. Heaviness in arms and legs.

| SE I-VI (very brief) | (d) *Wednesday*, 9:15 A.M. |
|---|---|

Some shivering over left temple, pain in right upper arm, itchiness on forehead. I see light yellow, and I see myself sitting at a table with a towel around my neck and I have to eat a big bowl of shit. Tension and heaviness in both arms. Tingling and excitation in both breasts. Some distractions.

" (e) *Wednesday*, 11:15 A.M.

I see yellow and orange-red. Some pain in fingers and both hands. Some muscular pulling on top of my head, and it is warm at the same time, as if it were bleeding and something is going into my skull. Visualized a big white man, made of smoke or as if in the clouds, he was not disagreeable. I think I am going to kill my husband during the next trip, put an ax into his face. Pain coming up the left upper arm. Relaxed, some distractions.

" (f) *Wednesday*, 1:30 P.M.

Sharp localized pain on upper right side, and some pressure on upper part of the back of my head. Many distractions: fast sequences of strange images which I could not really identify. I feel sleepy. There was a dragon, immobile like on a Japanese print, and the tarantula from yesterday, the octopus, the witch, etc. After the exercise I slept for an hour, but I did not feel rested afterward.

| RAH, LAH, BAH, RLH, LLH, BLH, ALH. (Induction, AA 6) | (g) *Wednesday*, 3:15 P.M. (AA 6 in the therapist's office; 58 min.) |
|---|---|

At the moment I can only think of my . . . the monsters of yesterday . . . of last night . . . and I . . . I see again . . . I . . . I . . . see again the . . . the . . . the huge tarantula . . .

## Transcript of AA 6

which . . . which came down on top of me . . .
I find this funny because . . . well, as I
said . . . there . . . there . . . is always a link
with . . . with something which made me
afraid when . . . in these type of images . . .
the tarantula was . . . I was perhaps nine or
ten years old, and it was . . . I was in school
and they had shown a film about the . . . the
small animals in the desert, the . . . the animals
which managed to keep alive in the desert . . .
there was . . . three were tarantulas, and
scorpions, and there were . . . there were
snakes . . . I was quite impressed . . . by that
film . . . probably that's where the . . . the
tarantula comes from . . . I never saw this
thing elsewhere . . . perhaps much later . . .
but that was really . . . that . . . I . . . I was
really . . . really impressed by this thing . . .
it's . . . it's as if it really happened . . . I saw
her, and then she put her sting into me . . .
right into my heart . . . and then I saw myself
like a dried up fly in a spider's net . . . I saw
her . . . she was terrible, she was all hairy . . .
it was terryfying like . . . like . . . like . . .
quite an experience . . . there I . . . I see her
again, but she doesn't . . . she doesn't make
me afraid as before . . . I don't know if I
should . . . ah . . . ah . . . no she does not
come closer . . . the octopus, that was a
story, a . . . a . . . a story I read . . . which
was read to me . . . and there was . . . there
was a small . . . a small mermaid, who was
living on the bottom of the sea . . . well . . .
and then, the witch made her . . . well, she
had to pass between rocks full of octopus to
come to the witch's place . . . then she had to
take a potion . . . to become a real girl
again . . . and in exchange for that she had to
give her tongue . . . and after she had drunk
the potion she could not talk anymore . . .
and, she had to charm the prince in other
ways . . . she became a cloud . . . the . . .
the . . . these images . . . I must have been
about the same age when . . . when I read
this story . . . perhaps . . . well, that's funny,

### Transcript of AA 6

because I think at the time . . . I don't think
that I only thought of that . . . that that was
a story which I liked very well . . . a story
which . . . which I really liked . . . I . . . I
. . . now it comes back as if this was not
digested properly . . . as if . . . I wonder . . . I
wonder if it was so terrifying, in any case, the
octopus was terrible . . . she was also full of
tentacles, she was all slimy and she fell on
me . . . and she started squeezing me . . .
she squeezed me . . . I was completely
crushed . . . well, she is still on top of me . . .
still on top of me . . . she is still there, but . . .
I am much less afraid now . . . well . . . she
has green eyes . . . green with flames . . . red
flames . . . she . . . she has suction cups along
the arms . . . and she has them all over on me,
all over . . . it feels cold, cold everywhere . . .
she is squeezing . . . well . . . at the same
time . . . she has a mouth, which she puts
on me . . . and she is sucking . . . it . . . it
. . . it squeezes more and more . . . slowly . . .
my bones start cracking . . . well, it's as if all
the . . . the . . . as if it is going to burst . . .
because all my . . . my circulation is stopped
. . . all the blood has stopped . . . a very tight
squeeze . . . and . . . she takes me to her
cavern on the bottom of the sea . . . I . . .
I . . . I don't know what to do . . . well . . .
the witch is there also . . . she . . . she
succeeded . . . she got there because she has
a magic stick . . . the place is full . . . full, full
of octopus, all over the rocks . . . ah . . .
everywhere . . . they are everywhere . . .
they move . . . and there is one making ink
clouds . . . but . . . there . . . there are two
who are . . . fighting each other . . . they
are . . . I am . . . I am like dead in the
back of the cavern, that's all, but I can see
them anyway . . . preparing . . . something
. . . in her big pot . . . that's all . . . she is
not interested in the octopus . . . she is
making . . . she puts frogs and, then . . . I
don't know what . . . poisonous mushrooms . . .
she is very ugly . . . she has a big wart on

**Transcript of AA 6**

her nose . . . and the hair are all gray . . .
they are sort of sticking out . . . crooked
fingers . . . she has, well she has just two
teeth . . . now I am not afraid of her . . . I
don't know, she is not really ridiculous . . .
she is somewhat ridiculous, she is not . . . she
is not so frightening as before . . . now she is
getting bigger and bigger, and still bigger . . .
she has become enormous and . . . that's it,
she puts me into her pot . . . that was funny
the other time [*see: a*] when I started to melt
in the pot . . . I . . . I . . . I dissolve . . .
as she keeps stirring . . . I . . . I . . . I melted
. . . she keeps stirring . . . it is very hot, I am
cooking, it is cooking, I am boiling . . . it is
terrifying, and it smells bad, this pot . . .
that's all . . . now she has . . . sort of dragons
with her . . . that's . . . they are . . . that's . . .
the other . . . that makes me think of the
other image . . . the pool with the corpses
which piled up on me . . . they were all . . .
all in pieces . . . there are arms . . . and legs,
and heads . . . half decomposed . . . that's . . .
that was this part of the nightmare . . . I . . .
that makes me think . . . that's . . . I don't
know where this comes from, but in any
case, there was . . . once . . . when we came
back from a trip we took . . . we . . . we were
. . . we took a ferry . . . and we had traveled
all along the other side on the northern coast
of the St. Lawrence river . . . and at one
point . . . we were with the children . . . and
we had stopped . . . on the roadside . . . we
saw a small dirt road going off . . . and we
decided . . . we are going to stop there and
eat something . . . and we parked in this dirt
road, and we took our things out to eat
something . . . and occasionally there was . . .
it smelled very badly, it . . . it . . . there was a
funny odor . . . and Frank said there must be
a garbage dump around but I . . . that was
not what I thought, that made me think of a
putrefying corpse . . . in decomposition . . .
well . . . I did not mention this . . . but just

### Transcript of AA 6

before we went on, I said to Frank, I told him
that's not . . that does not smell like garbage,
that does not smell like a dump . . . it just
came with a wind, and then it was not there
all the time . . . I said it smells like decaying
carcass . . . and . . . well, I had just said a
few words to Frank, and Frank said . . . that
he did not say that he had no intention to
go and look to see what it was, but he said
one . . . one should perhaps notify . . . the
police . . . the Provincial Police or something
. . . to find out where this comes from . . .
and . . . I . . . I . . . that's . . . I got terribly
afraid that he would go himself to find out
what it was . . . what smelled so badly . . .
I . . . I wanted to leave the place as fast as
possible . . . that's . . . I could not forget
that . . . that's . . . I thought often about it
. . . well, it's not . . . it's not so long ago, but
. . . that's a thing . . . I wanted to express . . .
my fear . . . during the trips, and . . . in any
case [*Can you go into the woods and find out
what it is?*] . . . well, that's it . . . that's it . . .
I thought I should go and find out . . . I
don't know if that . . . if that is really
necessary for me . . . to do that . . . he is
there, there . . . he is a terrible sight . . . he is
half decayed . . . and there must have been
animals which started . . . to gnaw . . . his
clothes are mouldy . . . it is . . . it is a man in
his fifties . . . perhaps a . . . that's . . . that's
. . . I see a . . . hole in his head . . . he got
killed . . . he got killed . . . I don't know . . .
who . . . [*Can you describe the face?*] . . . the
face is . . . it is full of worms . . . the eyes are
gone, there is . . . the skin is . . . decaying . . .
one can see the bones, the nose . . . the mouth
. . . there is no tongue anymore . . . only the
teeth . . . [*Can you look into the eyes?*] . . .
There is nothing it is just black, there are
worms . . uh, that makes me feel sick . . .
that's difficult, because I never saw, let's say,
as I . . . as I imagine this . . . I don't see this
very clearly, but I imagine this . . . and there

### Transcript of AA 6

it is full of worms inside . . . he . . . the hair
. . . I don't touch anything, the hair fell out
. . . I know that the hair is coming off when
. . . the hair becomes longer, after death, and
the hair can fall off just like that, when touching them . . . that's all . . . I don't know how
that . . . it is all soft . . I don't know anymore,
what shall I do? Shall I . . go away or shall
I stay there? I don't know . . . now, I am . . .
I am sort of very low again . . . it . . it starts
exactly as before . . . I am . . . I am at the
bottom of my grave . . . and above it's an
open hole . . . and I let things go . . . and I
let them throw the earth on top, and I am
burried alive . . . they are filling it up . . . I
am on the bottom of the grave . . . on the bottom of the pit . . . I have difficulty to breathe,
there is earth in my nose . . . but why is this
always slanted, that's what I don't understand . . . a grave is not slanted . . . now I
feel like . . . like in a V . . . I don't really
touch the bottom . . . my arms are resting on
the . . . on the sides of the V . . . it's still the
same thing . . . I am all buried, on the bottom
. . . that's . . . ah now I am dead, there is
nothing more to do in there . . . I don't feel
anything in particular . . . but I don't understand why . . . I am in this V, like that . . . I
have the impression it is getting deeper, the
V . . . I see . . . I see red-orange, it is all
fire . . . ah . . . ah . . . I see all kinds of small
devils, jumping around . . . and they have the
long spears . . . and they hit with their forks
in . . . to . . . make sure that everybody
burns well, that they are fried well . . . and
they scream . . . and cry . . . they . . . they . . .
I see one who just got caught by the flames
. . . he is going up in flames . . . that's . . .
well that makes me think of those Buddhist
monks . . . who burned themselves alive
. . . in India . . . he is engulfed in flames,
he, he . . . he is burning up . . . he is screaming, and . . . that's it he cannot burn himself
because . . . he is still there, there forever . . .
but he is all . . . ah, it is cracking, crackling,

### Transcript of AA 6

it's terrifying . . . it's not . . . I don't see
anything else . . . [*Can you keep describing?*]
. . . Now there are many little dragons, and
they are all red, and they have horns . . . and
they have a split tail like . . . like they are
shown in children books . . . they grunt and
they are full of energy . . . and they jump on
everybody . . . and they push them back into
the flames . . . that makes me think of a
picture . . . of a picture I saw in one of these
story books, *Hérauts,** I don't know which
saint, but in any case there was a saint who
was at the edge of a, of a . . . of a precipice
. . . and on one side one could see the con-
demned who were caught in the flames . . .
it's . . . it was really stupid as a representa-
tion . . . and there was one who asked for
help to get out of there . . . that's, that's . . .
what is funny, for example, it was quite hot
down there . . . very hot, and . . . it's not
uncomfortable, I want to say . . . it is supposed to be very hot . . . but it is a representa-
tion which . . . which makes me feel, which
impresses me not so much as another thing . . .
I . . . I . . . I don't know, but I think that I
never had any fear of hell, of that kind of
hell . . . it's, it's like . . . the only thing I could
use as a comparison, that's the big furnace of
the . . . like they have on the big ships . . .
with the enormous fire of I don't know how
many degrees . . . a glowing furnace . . . it
screams, that's all . . . and . . . there are
people screaming, but I don't know anybody
. . I knew . . .the flames are red with . . .
with yellow sparks, and it is turning, and it,
it . . . it crackles . . . it's going up and . . .
there are some . . . some which appeared to be
detached . . . and there in the dust which . . .
but dust but pieces which . . . in the mounting
flames . . . because there is a current of air
which makes them rise, which is pushing all
this up into the air . . . and then it all falls
back. . . . But I see again this person in the

---

* *Hérauts. Le trésor des belles aventures.* Fides, Montreal, Vol. 6, 1949.

**Transcript of AA 6**

forest who is decaying . . . that reminds me
of . . . it's just that what I am seeing at this
moment . . . that makes me sick I have a
feeling I would like to touch it . . . to see if
. . . the joints are really stiff . . . if one still can
bend them . . . I . . . I touch the arms, and
it breaks, very easily as if . . it's very dry . . .
that's . . . the bones . . . there are no joints
anymore . . . ah I feel very tense, my legs
are very tense . . . now I see . . . yellow almost
white . . . it is very clear, very bright . . . very
very light pale . . . I sit down near the corpse,
and I wait . . . I don't know what . . . I am
sitting at the side of the corpse, and I stay
there . . . nothing else is happening . . . I
don't know what . . . I see red with purple
mixed to it . . . suddenly the corpse sits up
and starts talking, well . . . he looks terrible
. . . one side of his face is . . . is all . . .
there is no skin anymore . . . there is skin on
the other side . . . and he is talking, that's,
that's, that's . . . that's terrible, how it smells
that makes me also think of certain types of
cancer which . . . or it is perhaps rather like
. . . a decay during life . . . there are some
which look like that . . . or it is like leper, or
. . . it smells, it smells terrible . . . now I see
lepers in Africa . . . they are all . . . it's just,
there are some who have no hands anymore,
they have just a stump . . . they have no
fingers anymore . . . there are, that's that's . . .
it's down to the bones, all the skin is gone . . .
completely gone. . . . They make me think of
the people of Pompei . . . when one visits
the ruins and the museum of Pompei there are
people who are . . . who are there . . . real
people who are in lava . . . in certain places
they have scratched the lava, and one can
see the bones . . . that is terrible to see, it's
. . . there is one who is sitting and . . . he is
holding his head, another is . . . who is . . .
almost . . . who is like . . . as if he fell while
trying to run . . . there is also a dog . . . all
twisted, really terrible . . . that must have been

### Transcript of AA 6

a terrible ordeal . . . I see the location of
Pompei . . . and Herculaneum . . . and that
makes me think of the trip . . . in Italty . . .
summer . . . winter . . . last fall . . . last . . .
it was really interesting to visit Herculaneum
. . . well, I don't know whether I shall continue
with this . . . there is no aggression in this . . .
I don't know . . . I just see Herculaneum . . .
it was . . . I read at that time . . . a sort of
pamphlet which . . . which reconstructed the
scene of the moment when the . . . the volcano
erupted, and the lava was . . . it was not lava
actually it was . . . at Her . . . Herculaneum it
was a sort of mud which covered the city and
which became a solid mass . . . that's why . . .
that's why it's better conserved than at Pompei
. . . he described a bit how the people were
living at that time when . . . when that occurred . . . when this sort of gigantic mud
wave arrived . . . because the journal exactly
. . . the tables were set and the bread was
baking and a blacksmith who was about to
finish . . . to repair furniture . . . that's . . .
I found that . . . that is . . . I found that . . .
very moving to read . . . that was real . . .
real life . . . that was not just a big great
story which actually does not touch us . . .
these were the little small facts of daily life
which were described in . . . at the moment of
the big tragedy . . . and I think of the eruption
of Mount Pelée on Martinique, we visited the
ruins of St. Pierre . . . and this . . . it was full
of things which were . . . all twisted by the
heat . . . pieces of glass, completely deformed,
and clocks, and . . . all these small objects of
daily life . . . it was quite saddening to look
at all this . . . it was . . . it was painful to
look at this. . . . I don't know what to say . . .
I keep seeing yellow, light yellow, now . . .
*very bright . . . it's whitish.* . . . I think . . . I
think I am supposed to visit a funeral home,
well . . . it's it's . . . I invented quite a story
to . . . to free myself today . . . a friend of
mine took the children . . . took my children

### Transcript of AA 6

out to their cottage . . . actually . . . I didn't
want to . . . but she offered to do this . . .
we are supposed to see some family member
who died and . . now I am about to go over
my aunts, in the funeral home and . . . the
old aunts one hardly knows . . . and I can see
them, I see them, I don't know these women
but . . . I imagine them . . . well it's still, it's
still in the funeral home . . . and they are
talking all kinds of things and . . . for a
long time they did not see each other . . .
they are . . . are . . . they are old and ugly, I
don't even know them . . . so what's the use
of going there . . . I went there just to
vis . . . to bring the . . . the other aunts . . . to
meet them . . . it's something which I find . . .
which I find particularly difficult . . . to meet
these, these . . . old aunts . . . they are sort of
sour sweet, they are, they are . . . tiring, they
keep repeating the same old stories . . . I see
them, they annoy me . . . I take them and
I . . . I smack . . . I hit them in the face . . . I
push them . . . I . . . I . . . I tear their hats
off, I undo their hair . . . I find them ugly . . .
I wish they would be dead, all of them . . . I
don't even know them . . . I . . . I don't
know . . . I give them . . . I pump bullets into
their heads . . . real gun bullets . . . so there
are more dead people in the funeral home . . .
at least I did not come for nothing . . . several
of them are there . . . they are dead . . . I kill
everybody. . . . That makes me . . . that reminds me of a film . . . called *If* . . . that was
a story in a British college and . . . that was
about violence . . . to show the contrast between the methods used in, in . . . in the
English colleges . . . the high-class ones and
. . . which are for the, the . . . all the elegance
and all the subtleness of the methods of
education . . . and on the other hand the
revolting youngsters who are full of . . . aggression, well . . . and one of the youngsters
discovers a hidden place full of old weapons
in the college . . . and he goes up to the top

**Transcript of AA 6**

of the college during a distribution of re-
wards . . . and he forces the people to leave
the hall . . . by throwing tear gas bombs and
. . . . he guns down everybody . . . with a
machine gun . . . and . . . well . . . the title
of the film, I find . . . it's fantastic . . . this
*If* . . . and the actor . . . that's, that's really . . .
I find this film extraordinary . . . it's full of,
of . . . full of aggression, full of life, this actor
. . . in case he would have had a chance I
don't know I . . . a chance of a better education, I mean if the education would have been
less superficial and . . . almost medieval he certainly . . . he certainly would have been able
to achieve something . . . and all he does in
the college makes him bitter and he ends up
like that . . . he kills everybody . . . I think
that's regrettable . . . I think . . . I think that's
. . . a good example for . . . for understanding
our actual period. . . . I also think, the strike
of the police . . . the day before yesterday . . .
that's quite something . . . I don't agree at all
with them . . . but I find it's somehow significant for, for . . . for . . . it characterizes our
. . . the time in which we live . . . the aggression, it's everywhere, everywhere, everywhere . . . I don't know . . . I don't know if
that makes sense to talk about all that, I
don't know if all this has something to do
with me . . . or what should I say . . . I see
just all that, anyway these manifestations,
these, these . . . these guys who fight in the
streets . . . the policeman who got killed. . . .
That makes me also think of . . . it looked as
if these . . . these guys who are trained in . . .
South America or in Latin America . . . to
make guerilla warfare, these . . . these agitators . . . these professional agitators who
seemed to be around . . . who were doing
their thing . . . I don't know if it's true but
. . . I don't know, I just see . . . they are
about to break all the show windows and . . .
going at it with guns . . . that's what I am
thinking of . . . *I see nothing but white* . . .

## Transcript of AA 6

my eyes are fluttering a bit . . . I don't know
what to say . . . I think . . . ah, I am thinking of the police, that reminds me of the film
I saw . . . on safety day, the one which was
shown by the police in New York, the film
about the car accidents. . . . I thought also . . .
it was myself who was one of these, these . . .
these road victims . . . and he was all in
pieces, like that, it was . . . it was terrible to
see these films . . . I . . . I have . . . I see
again the pieces of of . . . all is bloody . . .
there were no extremities anymore . . . just
the body with the legs, and the arms were all
cut off, and no head . . . and there was one . . .
his head was like red jelly . . . no face anymore, that's that's . . . I don't know . . . they
tried to get him out of there . . . and it was
going like Jello, it . . . just the bloody skin . . .
that makes me think of . . . of . . . you talked
about the possibility that anxiety can take all
kinds of forms . . of the fear of having a car
accident, but I have that fear already . . . I
mentioned that before . . . I am not able to
take the car without . . . without thinking of
the accidents . . . that does not stop me to
drive very fast, but I am thinking of it anyway
. . . but now I do that less often . . . I don't
know what to say. *I see blue, a little . . . a
little blue . . . pale blue . . .* I have . . . my
eyebrows are all tense . . . I see again these
accident scenes . . . it's, I don't know, it's . . .
always the same thing . . . and . . . the police
arrive . . . the cars are completely finished . . .
they are a heap of scrap . . .the doors are
torn off . . . the seats . . . all the springs are
sticking out . . . I don't know . . . last Sunday
we went up North, and there was . . . I don't
know if it was only to remind the people to
drive carefully . . . or if this really happend . . .
but there was a car which was like that . . .
near St Jérôme . . . it was completely . . .
completely smashed up . . . and on it was
written, be careful, drive safely . . . the life
you are saving is perhaps your own . . . and
there was this smashed up car . . . all scrap

### Transcript of AA 6

. . . I . . . I see it again, when we went up North, we stopped there, it was all . . . we ate there . . . we went with my mother. . . . And that makes me think of my mother . . . and I am also afraid of . . . when I am afraid of, of . . . of loosing my senses like that, that's . . . that . . . and now I see my mother standing there . . . it's just . . . it . . . it will only take a few years and . . . I am going to be like her . . . she is terrible . . . she . . . she has no, she has absolutely no reality sense . . . she is living in her own world . . . on that Sunday when we went up North . . . Frank asked her to wait at the corner of . . . of the boulevard and . . . the metro station . . . and she, she understood it was at the X metro station, and she went there waiting there . . . she does things like that . . . she does these things very often . . . she does not understand anything, she understands everything wrong . . . when you call by phone at home, she understood it was Dr. X who had phoned . . . and she started wondering whether I was sick or what, I don't know . . . I . . . it's, it's let's say I am afraid of the worst . . . to become like that . . . I don't know . . . I have the impression she transmitted a good deal of her . . . of her anxiety on to me, because she must have . . . a lot of anxiety, and what I am afraid of, I have . . . I have . . . I have the impression I am also . . . I am also transmitting this onto my children . . . I don't know when. Recently, Bobby talked to me about monsters . . . I don't know if that . . . he asked me if that exists . . . I told him no, and that this was just, just sort of . . . imaginations . . . and that things like that did not exist . . . anyway, he . . . I don't know if . . . I think that's not sufficient and I have the impression he is in a better position than me, because he . . . he is talking about this, I did not talk about this often . . . he asked me what it was . . . it was dark in his room and he asked me what it was . . . the lights moving on the wall, and I was exactly like that when I was small . . . I told

## Transcript of AA 6

him that these were lights coming from outside, I explained to him that . . . there are
lights outside, and lights were reflected on the
wall, and then I left his door wider open than
I usually do . . . I put more lights on . . . but
I wonder . . . I . . . I . . . I really don't
know if . . . if he is about to develop the same
system. . . . Now I start seeing red again
with yellow-orange . . . my knees are all
tense . . . I don't know, I see red with purple
. . . I think again of my mother . . . I find
that really . . . tragic I don't know . . . that is
something which really bothers me because
. . . it . . . that's terrible, I don't know, perhaps it's myself who has messed up my life,
she, she . . . she was not aware of all that . . .
she is really lucky that she is not concern of all
this . . . I find it really tragic, her case . . .
[crying] . . . something I could scream when I
see her . . . it hurts me . . . [crying] . . . [*Can
you describe?*] . . . I don't know how old
she is, she looks about 66 . . . [crying] . . .
luckily she is not aware of this, it would be
more difficult for her . . . [crying] . . . and I
cannot be nice to her . . . I just cannot . . . I
just cannot do anything for her . . . [crying]
. . . I see her . . . I don't know . . . she is like
a prisoner, it's terrible . . . it will not take
long . . . and she cannot go out alone anymore . . . she has all kinds of things . . . she
has neuralgia . . . she is often sick . . . she
could travel . . . she has money, she could . . .
she could live an interesting life, but she does
nothing, nothing . . . I think that's terrible . . .
her . . . and her . . . her only satisfaction is
when I manage to do something . . . when she
sees the children . . . during that . . . and not
even the . . . [crying] . . . it's terrible such a
messed up life, it's sickening . . . [crying] . . .
I don't want to become like that . . . [crying]
. . . I don't know what to talk about, nothing
is coming up . . . I only see her when she . . .
when she is with the children . . . then she is
really happy . . . but in case . . . in case my
father would die . . . I don't know what is
going to happen to her, I wouldn't be able to

### Transcript of AA 6

live with her . . . I couldn't have her around
all the time . . . when I have seen her . . .
two days, and I can't see her anymore for at
least a week . . . I know she is at least partly
responsible for all that, and . . . myself, I
don't know, it does not only depend on my
father, but I cannot think of all that without . . . without thinking it's all his fault . . . I
keep telling myself that it is not fair because
actually . . . in case she would have . . . she
would have been quite stable, she would not
have chosen a man like him . . . probably . . .
and actually that they are completing each
other, but they functioned together, that's why
they decided to . . . to get married . . . but it's
because . . . that's what makes me feel too
aggressive against him, it's . . . I think he
managed to get the better part of it, he managed to . . . he had his profession, he, he
managed all right, he was always away from
home . . . she, she did not have a nice life
. . . that's exactly why . . . that's why I am so
aggressive against my father, I suppose . . . I
am going to kill him . . . I hit him with a
hammer on the head and . . . I bury him . . .
I kill him . . . I hate him because he did . . .
he is responsible for my mother being like
that, I don't know why, I keep hitting his
head with an ax . . . I don't know what to
say. . . . *It's blue . . . I see blue with yellow.* . . . I think of Frank . . . yesterday . . .
we . . . we talked . . . it's funny . . . he
said he noticed that I am changing . . .
that I was less . . . less insecure, and . . . that
I was less . . . after him . . . I . . . I was
more self-reliant, more independent, that's
what he he said . . . as I kept talking . . . I
asked him if . . . I asked him if he ever
thought of the possibility to be separated . . .
to separate . . . that is . . . that would according to him what could happen, how, how would
one do that . . . he said that . . . in case that
would happen . . . that would be less difficult
for both . . . than before . . . now, before . . .
according to him that was a possibility which
was less important now than before because

### Transcript of AA 6

. . . we have been making progress . . . each
of us . . . I . . . I . . . I don't know . . . I did
not ask for that . . . I just asked, I was just
curious, I wanted to know . . . I know it's
crazy to ask that, I wanted to know . . . how
he would react to that if . . . if we would get
separated . . . I asked him if . . . if he would
forget me easily, I don't know . . . I don't
know, that again must have been one of those
manifestations of . . . anxiety . . . of fear . . . I
have some pain in my knees . . . that's like . . .
like . . . like a sort of paralysis, I don't know
. . . it really hurts inside of both knees . . .
I don't know what to say . . . I just see *light
blue* . . . ah I think that's enough . . . that's
really enough . . . well . . . I don't know . . .
now . . . I think of living alone . . . I keep the
children naturally . . . I don't know if . . .
I certainly would not do all what I want to
do . . . I would have to find something . . .
a job . . . and since I don't know much . . . I
would not do very much . . . that would not
be an interesting job . . . I would find it quite
hard . . . I know that . . . often . . . when,
when I think of that possibility, in case Frank
would die or something like that, that's all
right, because at that moment I have the
insurance, and that would give me some time
to go back . . . I don't know, to take a course
of something which would give me a better
salary . . . to do more interesting things, but
. . . just being separated from Frank, that
seems . . . that would be easy . . . I don't
know, I . . . I would return to university,
but . . . I would have difficulties . . . to get
along . . . I think . . . well to live . . . it
would be quite tight . . . I don't see anything
well, there is something which disturbs me,
that's . . . the children are going to come back,
and I have to be at home on time, I don't
want to . . . I cannot think of anything else, I
think it's already quite a while that I am here
. . . and . . . they are going to arrive before
me, that's what is crossing my mind . . . I
cannot think of anything else. . . .

**Formula**

**Reports on the effects of the exercises**

*The patient's comments:* I find the trips are getting more and more interesting. For example, I find it most interesting to see how the situation with my corpse unfolded gradually via the lepers, Pompeii, Herculaneum and Mont Pelée; and how through the car accidents I was finally brought to talk about mother who causes me a lot of worries. I now think that the topics which on first sight do not appear to be of immediate interest, are necessary to come to the point by serving to bring about a transition to other areas of anxiety.

*Remarks:* Toward the end of the postabreactive discussion, it was suggested that the patient make colored drawings of the monsters, practice autogenic exercises regularly, and call the therapist at anytime. No further difficulties were encountered and the patient's subsequent training protocol (see h, i, j) indicate that the potency of acutely disturbing material had been significantly reduced by AA 6.

**SE I-IV**

(h) *Wednesday,* 11:30 P.M.

Slight headache in the back of my head, left side, and left eye. Itchiness over both temples. Occasional muscular twitches on top of the head. Some pain above the right eye, in right knee, some burning upper right leg. Some distractions, I thought of the drawings of the monsters which I did and I see some as I did them in my drawings.

"

*Thursday,* 9:00 A.M.

My head feels heavy. Some ache on the left side, pain in left eye, pain left ribs, pain left shoulder. Distractions: I think again of the paintings of the monsters, which I did last night, the tarantula, the trips, and I see them again and remain very calm, there is really nothing to be afraid about.

"

*Friday,* 12:00 P.M.

I see again the dragon, I remember there was one like this on a vase at home, when I was a small girl. I feel tired and almost fell asleep during the exercise.

## THE PREAPPOINTMENT PHASE

The last 24 hours before the next appointment are often experienced as more difficult than the initial and the central phase of the interim. Various emotional and psychophysiologic reactions (e.g., crying spells, headaches, abdominal discomfort, hostile reactions, sleep disturbances, nightmares, diffuse anxiety, tension, increased consumption of alcohol, difficulties at work) are reported to be more marked than before. Such changes in reactivity are considered to be partly due to inadequately programmed homework. For example, postponement of transcript until the day before the appointment (delayed feedback), avoidance of regularly reading the transcript aloud during the interim and the subsequent preparation of a commentary are potent stimuli which easily lead to a mobilization of psychoreactive dynamics and disturbing psychophysiologic reactions. Furthermore, it must be considered that even when the patients have followed the recommended pattern of therapeutic homework correctly, it is therapeutically normal that new material mobilized during the interim starts pressing more forcefully for unloading. Therefore it is not surprising that the preappointment phase of the interim is also associated with variable degrees of apprehension, ambivalent attitudes toward the therapist and the treatment, and other manifestations characteristic for the activation of defense mechanisms (see Case 51).

*Case 51:* A 37-year-old female office worker (anxiety reaction, moderate depression) remarked at the beginning of her appointment: "Yesterday was a real hectic day, I worked until 6 P.M. and was quite exhausted. I felt tired, got a headache, I looked pretty awful and I could not eat. I went to bed quite early. This sort of a thing seems to be a pattern, it happens almost everytime the day before I have an appointment. I really accumulate pressure, and I think all that proves to me that I have to come to see you because I am not feeling well. Actually I am making myself sick, and it sort of proves to me that I can work in case I really want to."

Generally it is recommended that the patient try to organize his activities during the preappointment phase in such a manner that he is relatively well rested. This recommendation is based on the observation that a tired brain prefers to sleep, and that autogenic abreactions carried out in a state of fatigue tend to remain relatively unproductive (see Vol. VI, Part I) or the patient falls asleep. Similarly, brain-disturbing interferences (*indirect psychophysiologic resistance*) are also observed in patients who have had no time to eat and who start autogenic abreactions in a state of hunger. In these instances brain-directed dynamics tend to interject elaborations referring to the patient's need to eat. To avoid the phenomena of *indirect psychophysiologic resistance,* some patients need to be reminded to eat properly during the preappointment phase.

As in other instances when brain-disturbing material is pressing for neutralization, disturbances of sleep and periods of dream activity involving material which is identical with or closely related to patterns of current trends of thematic neutralization tend to occur more frequently during the preappointment phase (see Case 45). In consequence, certain patients tend to feel less rested on the day of the appointment, and they also tend to complain about persisting headaches after waking up in the morning. Such headaches, which are usually well localized (e.g., temporal, occipital, frontal), appear to be similar to the types of headaches which are encountered after premature termination of autogenic abreactions, or which may start during autogenic abreaction when brain-antagonizing forms of resistance do not permit brain-desired processes of thematic neutralization (see Case 52).

*Case 52:* A 44-year-old housewife (anxiety reaction, moderate depression, multiple psychophysiologic reactions). One week after AA 10, the patient had a dream (see below) which was followed by a migraine-type headache, starting in the occipital area and progressively involving the entire left side. The dream focused on material, certain parts of which already had been subject of brain-directed neutralization during previous autogenic abreactions.

"In this dream I was kind of an outside observer and did not really take part in it myself. There was a group of people, as one sees them arriving at airports or meetings. The men were apparently scientists or medical doctors, and most of the ladies present were in fur coats. It was somewhere outside, in winter time, with leafless trees, a pale sun and a bluish sky. Then there was WL coming into the picture from the right, and a man from the left eagerly stepped up to him and said, wasn't he WL, and that he always had wanted to meet him and how glad he was to meet him. Meanwhile I was looking at the ladies and thought that I would fit in there rather well in my mink coat (which I inherited brand new from M). And then I thought how those ladies were kind of sunning themselves in the importance of their husbands and how I would never be able to sun myself in the importance of K (who in reality is once again in a period of trying to withdraw from the world more than ever), since he doesn't understand 'it' referring to my having to be here so long and that he does not really know what goes on. And then I awoke with kind of a slight left-sided headache. I knew I wouldn't go to sleep again, worked for two hours on a journal (in the bathtub) and went back to sleep for another three hours. The headache was still present when I woke up, and stayed with me up to this appointment."

Other phenomena of resistance which are related to the dynamics of the preappointment phase involve "forgetting" the homework material at home, or more often, the tape recorder, or even "having an accident" with the tape recorder are not unusual (see Case 53, Case 54, Case 55).

*Case 53:* A 39-year-old priest (personality disorder, ecclesiogenic syndrome, sexual deviation, obsessive-compulsive reactions).

Since his initial psychosomatic evaluation four years earlier, this patient had shown a pattern of massive resistance which had hampered and interrupted his therapeutic progress in many ways. He spaced his appointments at relatively long intervals. Against recommendations, he assumed more professional responsibilities, thus being "forced" to cut down his time for treatment purposes. With sophistication he carefully planned professional obligations which would "force" him to be out of town for long periods. While he was in town, he came irregularly, his therapeutic homework was carried out in such a manner that efficient technical control was very difficult. After a long period of procrastination, he finally bought a tape recorder. However, he bought a model which was inadequate for treatment purposes. Realizing this, he finally bought the right machine and had it repaired three times before ever coming with it to the office. When he finally arrived with it at the office, he proceeded to lie down for the autogenic abreaction leaving the tape recorder untouched as he brought it. Then, when he was asked to prepare and use the tape recorder, he at last discovered that he had left the microphone at home. Confronted with this, he kept insisting that he had not done this on purpose, and that he believed it to be a coincidence. Upon the therapist's remark that this was merely another manifestation of resistance, he laughed and remarked: "But what do you want me to do about this?"

*Case 54:* A 24-year-old male student (personality disorder, anxiety reaction). After forgetting to bring his tape reels a number of times, the patient decided to leave a complete set of reels in the therapist's office. From there on he never again forgot to bring his reels.

*Case 55:* A 22-year-old male student (personality disorder, depressive compulsive manifestations, hypothyroidism). Aware of certain aspects of his pattern of resistance, the patient appeared for the appointment with the broken pieces of his expensive tape recorder. He excused himself profusely, explaining that he had fallen in front of the building, and that this had absolutely nothing to do with resistance.

*Case 56:* A 36-year-old housewife (anxiety reaction). During her first ten autogenic abreactions it occurred on three occasions that the patient appeared without the transcript of her autogenic abreactions. Each time she explained that the machine did not record properly, that she could not hear anything, and that this was definitely not her fault. When asked if this might perhaps have something to do with her dislike for reading the transcript, she flatly rejected such a possibility. However, after this she did not report any further difficulties with her tape recorder.

# 9. The Therapeutic Session: Preparatory Period

During treatment with autogenic abreaction it has been found useful to observe a certain sequence of therapeutic procedures which is closely related to the nature of the method and the therapeutic homework carried out by the patient. Generally a pattern of three major periods called the *preparatory period,* the *abreactive period* and the *postabreactive period* are distinguished. Each period evolves through various phases which are characterized by relatively specific therapeutic tasks and dynamics. Since the structure and dynamics of the *abreactive period* and the *interim period* have been presented in the preceding sections of this book, the reader now may find it easier to understand a variety of technical implications and problems of therapeutic management which are associated with the *preparatory period.* The preparatory period usually comprises four phases: the initial *general discussion phase,* the *autogenic training phase,* the *thematic mobilization phase,* and the *immediate preabreactive phase.* The therapeutic dynamics of each phase directly or indirectly emphasize certain aspects which are considered to be of facilitating value for the brain-directed dynamics of autogenic neutralization. For this reason the first part of the therapeutic session may be considered as a preparatory period for the therapeutically fruitful application of autogenic abreaction during the second part of the appointment.

An adequate case-adapted management of therapeutic dynamics and a variety of technical problems encountered during the four phases of the preabreactive preparatory period depends largely on the therapist's understanding of (a) various elements, patterns and dynamics of autogenic neutralization (see Part III and IV; Part I, Vol. VI), (b) the particular profile of postabreactive emotional and psychophysiologic reactivity as related to the patient's history and actual clinical condition, (c) the nature of the patient's homework (see p. 96 ff.) and (d) the clinical significance and psychophysiologic repercussions of certain medical and non-medical events which may have occurred during the interim period.

## THE GENERAL DISCUSSION PHASE

At the time when treatment with autogenic abreaction is started, the patient already knows that technically oriented discussions related to autogenic training are usually postponed until after the therapist has had an opportunity to review the patient's training protocol (see

TABLE 23.  *Variations of Time Devoted to Different Areas of Therapeutic Work in the Therapist's Office*
(Psychosomatic and Neurotic Patients)

| Patients | General Discussion Phase (min.) | Autogenic Training Phase (min.) | Thematic Mobilization Phase (min.) | Immediate Preabreactive Phase (min.) | Abreactive Period (min.) | Post-abreactive Phase (min.) | Therapeutic Session; Total Time (min.) | Treatment Level |
|---|---|---|---|---|---|---|---|---|
| M. D. (m) | 5 | 1 | 18 | 1 | 123 | 12 | 160 | Advanced, control |
| A. B. (f) | 4 | 2 | 49 | 2 | 32 | 11 | 100 | Intermediate, AA 19 |
| M. L. (f) | 10 | 10 | 51 | 2 | 49 | 13 | 135 | Intermediate, AA 21 |
| J. D. (m) | 33 | 4 | 42 | 1 | 136 | 13 | 229 | Advanced, control |
| G. T. (m) | 6 | 1 | 4 | 3 | 13 | 9 | 36 | Advanced, control |
| M. G. (f) | 6 | 1 | 5 | 1 | 15 | 8 | 36 | Advanced, control |
| P. L. (m) | 2 | 5 | 36 | 2 | 27 | 5 | 77 | Intermediate, AA 18 |
| M. T. (f) | 2 | 2 | 2 | 1 | 32 | 4 | 43 | Advanced, control |
| C. L. (f) | 4 | 4 | 8 | 3 | 26 | 24 | 69 | Learning phase, AA 2 |
| W. C. (m) | 6 | 4 | 12 | 2 | 22 | 18 | 64 | Learning phase, AA 1 |
| M. L. (f) | 14 | 6 | 12 | 2 | 15 | 13 | 62 | Learning phase, AA 1 |
| C. D. (m) | 39 | 4 | 6 | 2 | 62 | 23 | 136 | Advanced, control |
| P. L. (m) | 28 | 5 | 2 | 2 | 26 | 23 | 86 | Intermediate, AA 22 |
| H. R. (f) | 8 | 4 | 19 | 2 | 36 | 11 | 80 | Learning, AA 11 |
| J. T. (f) | 19 | 2 | 38 | — | — | — | 59 | Advanced, control |

p. 107 ff.). Similarly, it is preferable to discuss questions or certain therapeutic aspects which are related to autogenic abreaction during or after a review of the transcript(s) and commentary of his last autogenic abreaction(s) (see p. 103 ff.). Therefore it is generally preferable to begin the therapeutic session with discussions of a more general nature. Usually there are a number of events, developments, observations, and specific problems which have occurred during the interim period, and the patient would like to discuss these items before entering the more technically oriented phases which emphasize matters related to the patient's therapeutic homework.

The duration of such general discussions may vary considerably (see Table 23, p. 148). During advanced treatment phases, usually less than ten minutes are required, unless particular developments require a more detailed evaluation and exchange of views. Patients who are passing through a terminal treatment phase and who are seen after longer interim periods (e.g., 3-6 wks.) usually have a prepared agenda of items of general nature. In these cases the general discussion phase may take 30 minutes or longer.

The patient-adapted dynamics of such discussions do not follow any prearranged patterns, but are kept as flexible as possible to allow the problem-adapted use of those psychotherapeutic elements which, regardless of their origin, appear to be of supportive, constructive or otherwise helpful nature concerning the patient's specific problem or situation. However, in distinction from other forms of psychotherapy, such discussions are conducted with reference to the case-specific nature of brain-directed dynamics and the information which has evolved from the patient's autogenic abreactions. It is in this connection that special consideration is given to a number of psychophysiologic dynamics which appear to be also of interest for other forms of psychotherapy.

In the field of autogenic therapy and particularly when methods of autogenic neutralization are used, patients usually start considering the importance of understanding and insight. For example, during the general discussion phase, many patients, and particularly those who have undergone psychoanalytically oriented forms of treatment before they started autogenic therapy, eventually tend to direct the conversation toward topics which are related to questions involving the therapeutic significance of understanding and insight, the role of dreams, the usefulness of interpretations, and occasionally about the therapist's view on the phenomena of transference. When such topics are raised, it is therapeutically important to clarify them.

From his experience with autogenic training the patient already knows that certain improvements occur without any evident participation of insight and without, for example, engagement in dream interpretations. Such therapeutic experience may have led to the erroneous conclusion that understanding and insight are of no particular importance during autogenic therapy. In such instances it is advisable to point out that understanding and insight are certainly very helpful therapeutic elements particularly as far as they can contribute to improved adaptational functions and can assist in reducing or eliminating certain psychogically disturbing situations or developments. However, understanding and insight *cannot* neutralize, undo or erase brain-disturbing material which has been recorded and accumulated in the past. Patients who have experience with autogenic abreactions can see this without difficulty and readily agree that desired improvements have a better chance to come about by giving due consideration to at least two therapeutic requirements: (a) to use one's understanding, insight and intelligence to reduce possibilities of negatively oriented reinforcement of already existing disturbances by avoiding or eliminating exposure to, and additional accumulation of, material which is thematically related to the disturbing material already existing in the brain and (b) to attempt to reduce the pathofunctional potency of already accumulated disturbing material through autogenic neutralization in combination with autogenic training. In other words it is therapeutically essential to realize that it does not make sense to put more tension-producing material into a system which has indicated that it is already under too much tension. As the patient progresses through an increasing number of autogenic abreactions, his brain provides him continuously with information about the nature of the disturbing material he has already accumulated and thus keeps the patient informed about the nature of the stimuli (e.g., activities, situations) he should avoid as long as brain-desired levels of thematic neutralization have not been reached. It is in this connection that the therapist may point out that methods of autogenic neutralization cannot erase disturbing material from the brain. Even in instances when previously existing disorders seem to have disappeared for longer periods, it is not believed that the originally recorded disturbing material has disappeared. However, it is assumed that processes of brain-directed neutralization significantly help to reduce the disturbing potency of such material.

As patients realize that the processes of neutralization follow their own program of self-curative action whether thematic understanding or insight exists or not, they also agree more readily that it is to their advantage not to spend valuable office time with matters which do not advance the neutralization of brain-disturbing material (e.g., interpretation of dreams).

In respecting the psychophysiologic implications of naturally given brain dynamics, it is one of the therapist's responsibilities to help the patient to recognize and to reduce or eliminate those categories of stimuli (activities, situations) which are known to reinforce, amplify or complicate already existing disturbances. While pointing out and explaining why, for example, certain anxiety-promoting confrontations (e.g., looking at messy accident scenes, watching violent TV films, reading murder stories, visiting severely sick persons, participating in funerals) are to the disadvantage of the patient at this point of his treatment, it must be clearly understood that the therapist has no intention of making decisions for the patient. However, patients who decide not to follow such technical advice will eventually discover during thematically related autogenic abreactions that they have done a disservice to their brain for which they have to pay. In this connection it is also the therapist's responsibility to give due consideration to the fact that treatment phases during which brain-directed processes focus on neutralization of specific material (e.g., witnessing father's death in hospital, disturbing identification) are associated with a psychophysiologic state of increased susceptibility and proneness to overreactions in thematically related areas of stimulation. In practical terms this means that exposure to stimuli (activities, situations) which are related to topics which are actually undergoing neutralization is more disturbing than before or after neutralization. Once adequate levels of thematic neutralization have been reached, intentional exposure to previously harmful stimuli may become a part of therapeutically desirable reality testing and verification of adjustments in reactivity.

As a practical consequence of such psychophysiologically oriented therapeutic perspectives, the general discussion phase may emphasize certain technically oriented aspects of the patient's behavior during and after specific interim events. It is of therapeutic interest to know how the patient has managed to avoid known areas of disturbing stimuli, what difficulties he encountered while avoiding them or certain negatively oriented dynamics (e.g., self-punishment) which help to promote exposure to stimuli (situations, activities) which he knows are to his disadvantage. From such discussions a variety of case-specific self-protective suggestions may evolve. For example, a patient who has already had three car accidents in six weeks and who has had another one during the interim, may be asked to stop driving for a while or, in other instances when it is obvious that the patient's homosexual activities are quite disturbing to his brain, it is of therapeutic importance to find means to reduce the frequency of such brain-disturbing engagements. In this connection it must be clear from the start that it is always up to the patient to reject, modify or contribute his efforts in going along with the therapist's recommendations, and thus accelerate his treatment progress.

Of particular brain-disturbing consequences are unexpected confrontations with potent stimuli (situations, activities), the nature of which is very closely related to disturbing thematic elements which are known but which have not become the central topic of brain-directed neutralization. When such situations occur during the interim period, the phenomenon of *premature overamplification* with exaggerated reactions results. This therapeutically unfavorable development is usually associated with a disturbance of the brain-designed order of thematic priorities and may cause additional functional complications which are reflected by alterations of the habitual pattern of thematic neutralization. To save the patient from such unfavorable time-consuming and uneconomic complications it is the therapist's responsibility to explain, to warn and to suggest to the patient that he stay away from areas of stimuli which are likely to produce undesirable thematic over-amplification. In certain therapeutic situations this may, for example, mean that the patient is asked to move out of a neurotogenic family setting for a temporary period. For others this may imply the evaluation of the possibility of a temporary change in professional activity (e.g., nurses, surgeons, priests, teachers, aircraft pilots).

As the patient's experience with autogenic abreaction advances and he has had repeated opportunity to study the significance of thematically specific elaborations provided by his own brain, he tends to agree more readily with recommendations which aim at a reduction or elimination of those categories of stimuli which may reinforce already existing brain-disturbing dynamics (see Case 57, Case 58, Case 59, Case 60).

*Case 57:* A 39-year-old engineer (anxiety reaction, mild depressive reaction). During his initial psychosomatic evaluation the patient stated that his hobby was flying and that there was nothing more exciting and enjoyable than traveling in his airplane. After several autogenic abreactions, when his brain had repeatedly engaged in neutralization of anxiety related to certain hazardous flying episodes (e.g., possibilities of crashing, fear of death, fatal accidents of pilots he knew), he decided himself that it might be better to stop flying for a while.

*Case 58:* A 44-year-old priest (anxiety reaction, multiple phobic and gastrointestinal reactions, ecclesiogenic syndrome) had noticed increasing difficulties in celebrating mass, during other ceremonies and while giving various courses in the general area of religious education. During these functions he experienced tension, headaches, diffuse anxiety, onset of palpitations and profuse sweating. As his brain kept emphasizing neutralization of anxiety material related to his own religious education, he concluded that he could no longer accept many of those things which he was taught and which he felt obliged to teach others Since the circumstances did not permit him to express his own views, he realized that he felt like a liar, and that this was probably one of the reasons why he experienced progressively greater difficulties during the functions he was assigned to perform. Realizing this, he decided to ask his superiors to change his duties to administrative tasks where he was not obliged to say or to do things in which he did not believe anymore.

*Case 59:* A 28-year-old nurse (anxiety reaction, moderate depression) who, because of her efficiency in the operating room, was highly appreciated by all surgeons of the hospital in which she had been working for several years. Of late she had become more irritable, felt progressively more depressed and wondered why this was so. After her brain confronted her for long series of autogenic abreactions with various scenes related to her activities in the operating room, she arrived at the conclusion that this was not good for her health and she decided to give up nursing.

*Case 60:* A 29-year-old female teacher (anxiety reaction, moderate depression, multiple phobic and psychophysiologic reactions). During neutralization it became evident that she had accumulated considerable quantities of aggression, which to a large extent appeared to be continuously reinforced by her teaching activities ("I actually like teaching and I have no difficulties in controlling myself"). After several months of treatment with autogenic abreaction, she decided to go back to the university and prepare herself for another professional career which appeared to agree better with her personality dynamics.

Occasionally it has happened that the patient uses the general discussion phase as a welcome opportunity to unload himself. When such spontaneous non-autogenic processes of verbal unloading fall into already known patterns of thematic neutralization as observed during previous autogenic abreactions, it is therapeutically favorable to invite the patient at the earliest convenience to continue his verbalization on the couch as an initial part of an autogenic abreaction.

Sometimes the general discussion phase is used by a patient to gain enough time to avoid the scheduled autogenic abreaction. Such manifestations of resistance are more often encountered in patients with hysterical dynamics. As the therapist is aware of this possibility, it is in certain instances justified to interrupt the patient's time gaining maneuvers, to postpone the reading of the last autogenic abreaction until the next appointment, and to move directly to the *immediate preabreactive phase* (see p. 162) with preparation for autogenic abreaction. Such technically indicated interruption of an unduly prolonged general discussion phase may be followed by manifestations of brain-antagonizing resistance during the *initial abreactive phase*, when the patient may feel blocked by certain ideas or items which he has had no chance to discuss (see Case 61).

*Case 61:* A 36-year-old housewife (hysterical personality, anxiety reaction, multiple psychophysiologic reactions). To forestall the patient's known tendency to gain time by engaging in long drawn-out sophisticated tirades, the general discussion was intentionally cut short, and the patient was invited to get ready for autogenic abreaction. This technically indicated interruption was followed by initial blocking (see below) as related to subjects the patient was not given an opportunity to discuss prior to the beginning of autogenic abreaction.

"I see absolutely nothing . . . there is nothing . . . neither visual nor 'sensitory' . . . I think this is resistance . . . I wanted to discuss two points before we were starting . . . I think that's what is blocking now . . . [*Can you mention these two points now?*] Well, the first one has something to do with my will which I have changed . . . but I did not sign it . . . and the second concerns the proposed trip with M. P. . . ."

The management of displacement of affect onto the therapist largely depends on the nature of the prevailing pattern of autogenic neutralization. In patients who have reached a wide scope of flexibility with cinerama-type visual elaborations, positively and negatively oriented dynamics of transference may receive instant gratification while permitted to undergo autogenic neutralization (e.g., attacking the therapist and hacking him to pieces; making love; see Vol. VI). Such therapeutic possibilities greatly facilitate the therapist's task, help decisively in reducing undesirable interferences, and promote the treatment process in general. When patterns of autogenic neutralization are still restricted (e.g., elementary stages of visual elaborations) and the emphasis is, for example, on intellectual elaborations, it is technically indicated to encourage the patient to include the therapist in whatever topic his brain wishes to engage.

To avoid undesirable interruptions of the preparatory dynamics associated with the following *thematic mobilization phase*, it is suggested that the patient's medication be discussed as well as clinical appointments and other matters which are not related to autogenic training or autogenic abreaction in the course of the general discussion phase. Psychologic tests and physical examinations are usually carried out before entering the preparatory mobilization phase (see p. 158). Notes on dreams are often a part of the patient's training protocol and are usually discussed briefly in connection with certain training symptoms or thematically related processes of autogenic neutralization.

## THE AUTOGENIC TRAINING PHASE

After the general discussion phase has ended, the emphasis shifts to the patient's practice of autogenic standard exercises. The time devoted to this part of the preparatory period varies considerably, depending on (a) whether the patient already practices all six standard exercises or not, (b) the complementary use of organ-specific or intentional formulas, and (c) the nature of certain topics of neutralization and their particular clinical significance for the therapeutic process (see Table 23, p. 148).

Patients who have already practiced all six standard exercises for many weeks or months are usually advised to limit their training protocols to notes on training phenomena which appear to be unusual or which seem to be of particular interest in connection with current patterns of autogenic neutralization or dreams. Of further interest are these patients' difficulties with autogenic training which may or may not have occurred before (e.g., periods of restlessness during AT at night). Training difficulties and various new or unusual modalities of autogenic discharges may be related to certain events which have happened during the interim period. For example, different kinds of accidents (e.g., sports, traffic, household), certain medical procedures (e.g., abortion, insertion of intrauterine device, dental or other operations), changes of reactivity related to pregnancy, intoxications, epileptic seizures and other traumatic episodes (e.g., father's death) may modify the patient's reactivity during autogenic training (and autogenic abreaction). As such training difficulties and unusual training symptoms are important for the patient, case-adapted explanatory and technically oriented information must be given (see Vols. I-VI).

While uneventful training protocols with a pattern of largely formula-related training phenomena require little ground for discussion, more time is required when the profile of training symptoms repeatedly contains elements which point toward specific problems. For example, frequent occurrence of falling asleep during autogenic exercises usually indicates a persistent sleep deficiency. Frequent occurrence of frontal headaches is often related to a need for crying. Whenever a patient finds it difficult to cry, a problem-focussed discussion may help the patient to better understand the medically valuable nature of crying and thus help him to change his attitude toward crying. When the crying mechanisms appear to be blocked by self-imposed inhibitions, it may be necessary to emphasize that it would be most helpful for the patient to relearn how to cry (e.g., to imagine himself as an actor supposed to produce a crying spell in a play). In case the biologic crying mechanism remains blocked, difficulties during autogenic abreactions and slowing down of the treatment process may be expected. In this connection it is in certain cases essential to explain that crying is a very complex process of discharge involving not only a production of tears, but also the release of motor impulses (e.g., face, shoulders, chest, respiratory), and that these different functional components may be dissociated (i.e., motor discharges without tears, tears without motor discharges). It usually is therapeutically very encouraging once a patient who has not cried for many years finally reports that he has had a good crying spell. Generally the crying mechanisms appear to be facilitated during and after autogenic exercises and during autogenic abreaction.

Of further interest are certain types of autogenic discharges which in the past have had a specific significance in connection with autogenic neutralization. For example, heart pain may be associated with accumulated aggression toward close relatives (e.g., husband, parents, children) or against oneself. Repeatedly in these cases various forms of brain-antagonizing resistance interfered during autogenic abreaction with brain-programmed neutralization of accumulated aggressive impulses, and problem-focussed discussions aiming at a reduction or elimination of such forms of resistance are indicated. Similarly repeated ocurrence of pain in topographically specific areas and vestibular discharges as they are frequently encountered in trainees with a history of severe accidents may point toward inadequately neutralized areas of brain-disturbing material (i.e., thematic evasion, thematic avoidance, abortive engagement, repetition resistance; see Vol. VI, Part I).

When treatment with autogenic abreaction is started before the patient has learned to practice all six standard exercises (see Table 3, p. 19), a part of this phase of the preparatory period is devoted to the introduction and supervised practice of progressively added new standard formulas (see Vol. I).

In relatively rare instances, when treatment with autogenic abreaction has been started before the third standard exercise was introduced, and disagreeable sensations in the left chest (e.g., oppression, cramp-like sensation, pain) were experienced during autogenic abreactions, it is advisable to postpone the heart exercise until symptom-related thematic material (e.g., aggression against oneself, mother's heart attack) has been neutralized or the patient is technically far enough advanced to engage in autogenic abreactions without supervision.

When autogenic abreactions are associated with gastric complaints, nausea or vomiting, the practice of the fifth standard exercise is not indicated until after these thematically related dynamics (e.g., accident, near drowning) have reached adequate levels of neutralization.

So far no particular difficulties have been encountered with the application of the fourth and sixth standard formulas. The application of organ-specific formulas is guided by the same principles as outlined in Volumes I, II and III.

In certain cases it has been found helpful to make additional use of Intentional Formulas once the trainee has learned all six standard exercises. During the discussion of the content and structure of a patient-adapted intentional formula, due consideration should be given to relevant pattern of brain-directed dynamics as elaborated during the trainee's autogenic abreaction.

The simultaneous use of autogenic verbalization (see Vol. VI; Vol. I/209) is usually reserved for patients who have shown reliable collaboration and who are permitted to perform unsupervised autogenic abreactions. In case this precaution is not observed, it may easily occur that the dynamics of autogenic verbalization convert spontaneously into more complex processes of autogenic neutralization, and the technically inexperienced patient finds himself in a precarious situation which may be followed by an increase of anxiety and disturbing psychophysiologic reactions.

Patients who practice autogenic verbalization are usually required to make thematic summaries of their verbalizations. These are read and discussed toward the end of the autogenic training phase and before the therapeutic work concentrates on the patient's preceding autogenic abreaction.

Generally, few training difficulties are encountered in experienced trainees during simultaneous treatment with autogenic abreaction. Difficulties of concentration, intruding thoughts, spontaneous visual elaborations and periods of restlessness usually indicate that thematically related material presses for more adequate neutralization. In these cases it is particularly technically helpful to instruct the patient to practice long series of very brief exercise (see Case 50, p. 125). As the patient finds it easier to maintain more adequate levels of formula-related passive concentration, for brief periods (e.g., 10-20 sec.) the brain has less opportunity to interject other technically undesirable elaborations; and the patient finds it easier to maintain an encouraging level of calmness and relaxation (see Case 50, p. 125).

## THE MOBILIZATION PHASE

This part of the preparatory period is devoted to more specific therapeutic work focussing on the patient's last supervised autogenic abreaction and, in sufficiently advanced cases, on autogenic abreactions the patient may have carried out at home (see Vol. VI, Part I). Because rereading of the transcript is done in the presence of the therapist, thematically related discussions and technically oriented explanations (e.g., brain-antagonizing resistance; see Vol. VI, Part I) may be considered as preparatory procedures which are associated with mobilizing effects on thematically related psychodynamic and psychophysiologic functions, this period is distinguished as the *mobilization phase*.

Usually the mobilization phase begins with inviting the patient to start reading his transcript aloud, and it is at this point that certain patients begin to apologize for having forgotten to make two copies or that they forgot to bring the transcript. Such manifestations of resistance which are closely related to the nature of the therapeutic work (e.g., self-confrontation, feedback, re-experience of emotional reactions, broadening of awareness) require technically oriented discussions aiming at a reduction and elimination of resistance (see Case 62, Case 63).

*Case 62:* A 24-year-old student (personality disorder, sexual deviation, ecclesiogenic syndrome, hypothyroidism) who repeatedly complained about his difficulties in transcribing his autogenic abreactions, stated at the beginning of the mobilization phase: "I am very sorry, but I did not make a copy, I cannot read the transcript, I didn't have any carbon paper."

*Case 63:* A 26-year-old female patient (personality disorder, anxiety reaction, multiple phobic and psychophysiologic reactions, ecclesiogenic syndrome). Repeatedly this patient had indicated her difficulty in reading her transcript in the presence of the therapist. This difficulty and other relevant dynamics were viewed by the patient as exerting an obstructive influence on her behavior in general and her attitude during autogenic abreaction. Related directed and indirect forms of brain-antagonizing resistance tended to interfere with giving *carte blanche* to her brain and hampered a free, uncensored verbal description of brain-directed elaborations. Problem-focussed discussions helped the patient to increase her feeling of security and to reduce the unfavorable consequences resulting from the brain-antagonizing forms of resistance. The patient's elaborations (see below) convey her views quite acurately.

"I think it is quite natural that I have a certain dislike to read aloud, to verbalize those things which come from the deepest part of myself, which are the most secret of me. In a certain way I think this is a reflex of natural shyness.

"I really hate to read an autogenic abreaction, it really demands quite an effort of concentration from me, and I feel the same dislike to read any literature aloud. I feel uneasy, unstable and my mind keeps wandering off the subject by, for example, having the impression that I need to sleep or by all kinds of other thoughts. I think this problem is not limited to reading before the therapist, who represents my father, my mother, a man I would like to seduce; and I want to present myself to his eyes in the best possible perspectives. I am afraid that when I uncover what I am really, one would be disgusted as I am disgusted with myself.

"When I read aloud or when I hear myself, I feel uneasy, ridiculous and feel that I fight against the material, in order not to recognize that it is actually my own. This is more or less a rejection of myself, a fight not to accept myself. In case this reflex would not exist, I would not be under treatment, because I would accept myself as I am. All the way, while I am reading I have only one idea, to do my very best in pretending that this material does not affect me, that it leaves me indifferent, and to read in a detached voice. In other words, I am very much afraid of this material, I don't take my autogenic abreactions as manifestations of my brain elaborations, but rather as sort of oracles which are going to determine the decision I have to take in real life. For example, at this moment, I am very reluctant to talk about my adventures in Rio, not only because there is a certain feeling of guilt, but also because I am afraid that the therapist may say that I should go back down there. I have the impression that I did not profit enough from the experiences, more are needed, and that all that has nothing to do with my new preoccupations and my life here in Montreal.

"I particularly believe that my rejection to read aloud is a refusal of admitting that the material is my own, even as I am forced to recognize that it was me who produced this material; I don't want to admit that this is true. It's very nice to explain to me that this is a technical procedure to overcome a certain resistance, but I think my brain is closing itself at any explanation. I think there is a neurotic aspect in this resistance, it is of the same order as my refusal to live happily, of my mechanism of self-punishment. I refuse to read in the same manner as I refuse to recognize myself being a woman."

While the patient is reading the transcript, the therapist has an opportunity to review the content and pattern of the autogenic abreaction and to make notes on specific points (e.g., technical errors, resistance, thematically related confrontations) which are to be considered during the subsequent discussion. The manner in which the patient reads his transcript often conveys therapeutically, particularly important areas of reactivity. Hesitancy, stuttering, crying spells or reading in a very low voice, coughing spells, laughing, inability to continue reading or aggressive reactions may indicate that (a) the patient's homework requires readjustment (e.g., increase of frequency of reading the transcript aloud at home), (b) inadequate levels of neutralization, and (c) brain-antagonizing forms of resistance (see Vol. VI, Part I). Explanatory discussions of these points usually follow after the reading is terminated or during therapeutic work related to the patient's commentary.

When a tape recorder is not used, the patient's homework usually consists of writing his autogenic abreaction down from what he remembers, and reading this material. In these cases note what the patient forgets or does not mention. In other instances, when the brain-directed elaborations are initially restricted to visual elaborations of largely elementary or intermediate stages (see Table 33, p. 188), no particular reading difficulties are encountered, and it may be preferable to replace the reading task by a step by step description and discussion of the patient's drawings and the comments he likes to make (or avoids making).

During advanced treatment phases, when sufficiently experienced patients are encouraged to carry out autogenic abreactions at home (see Vol. VI, Part I), the reading and discussion of the patient's homework may become the most important part of the therapeutic session. Occasionally when processes of neutralization engage in long series of almost monotonous thematic repetitions as, for example, encountered in obsessive-compulsive reactions, it is advisable to replace the transcript by a thematic summary and to limit a detailed transcript to passages which contain new material.

Occasionally it happens that a patient interrupts the reading of his transcript and makes certain remarks which appear to be out of context. Such interjected out of context remarks or patient-directed discussions which may also occur during the *general discussion phase,* and more often during the *immediate preabreactive phase,* are of particular interest. Often these out of context remarks (questions, conversations) are containing elements which become of focal importance during the following autogenic abreaction (see Case 64, Case 65, Case 68, p. 163). It is for this reason that it is considered technically more favorable not to engage in time-consuming discussions of the patient's out of context remarks, but to manage the situation in such a manner that more time can be devoted to autogenic neutralization of thematically related areas of mobilized material.

*Case 64:* A 28-year-old male postgraduate student (anxiety reaction, obsessive-compulsive reactions, habit disorders, multiple psychophysiologic reactions, ecclesiogenic syndrome). About ten minutes before starting his next autogenic abreaction, while the patient was reading the last page of his previous AA, he suddenly interrupted his reading and started recounting theme-related stories of drowning incidents involving others and himself. After relating several drowning incidents of which his mother told him when he was a young boy, he associated a bicycle accident which had not been mentioned before. He recalled that at the age of 11 or 12, he left the garage, speeding. He did not watch out, his eyes fixing the pavement and thus he suddenly crashed head first into the rear of a parked truck. He remembered hitting his head, losing his breath and hurting his hands badly. A few minutes later, the initial abreactive phase began with this particular accident.

"I see myself as I crash with my head against the truck. . . ."

*Case 65:* A 40-year-old housewife (hysterical personality, anxiety reaction, moderate depressive reaction). Toward the end of a technically oriented discussion of brain-antagonizing forms of resistance encountered in her last autogenic abreaction, the patient unexpectedly remarked that the treatment is like a bulldozer, flattening her out completely, and "I have to be flattened out before I can get up again, I feel sort of flat now." A few minutes later, during autogenic abreaction, the dynamics of neutralization focussed on neutralization of suicidal dynamics, in the course of which she got flattened out on a highway by a seemingly endless series of cars passing over her body.

Although studies of longer series of autogenic abreactions have shown that the brain follows its own particular program of neutralization with sophisticated logic, it is in many instances difficult to predict correctly what the next autogenic abreaction will be about. For example, neutralization of severely traumatic accidents tends to begin in a rather unexpected manner (see Case 66) and can be predicted more easily once a particular pattern of neutralization has already started. During treatment periods which are temporarily restricted to an emphasis on visual elaborations of elementary nature (see Table 33, p. 188, it can be expected that the same pattern will continue in a slow however progressively more differentiated manner. In these cases the nature and content of the general discussion phase and technically oriented explanations during the mobilization phase appear to remain without obvious effects on the prevailing pattern.

*Case 66:* A 35-year-old nurse (anxiety reaction, multiple psychophysiologic and phobic reactions, moderate depression). In obvious contrast to the apprehensiveness she conveyed before the beginning of earlier autogenic abreactions which emphasized progressive neutralization of a severe car accident (i.e., multiple fractures, prolonged loss of consciousness, six weeks hospitalization), the patient remarked repeatedly in a rather casual tone that she felt fine, more like herself, almost as before the accident, and that she had no complaints during the interim. Shortly before commencing the next autogenic abreaction, she also remarked "Oh, I don't think that this trip is going to be anything." A few minutes later, the brain engaged in neutralization of various phases related to a fall when she fractured her nose and lost consciousness. However, the dynamics were much less disagreeable than during previous car accident-related dynamics of neutralization (e.g., no headaches, only slight transitory discomfort, no brain-antagonizing resistance).

The neutralization of obsessive-compulsive dynamics usually follows a program of long series of autogenic abreactions revolving around the same themes. However, as the brain is given ample opportunity to repeat relevant dynamics, a slowly progressing trend toward normalizing can be recognized. When aggressive and depressive feelings have been coloring the general discussion and the mobilization phase, corresponding topics of mono- or multithematic neutralization (e.g., destruction of others and self) tend to follow. In sufficiently advanced patients the habitual pattern of multithematic neutralization may be characterized by new dynamics which are related to certain traumatic events which occurred during the interim period (e.g., death of mother, severe accident, near accident, traumatic medical procedures, significantly disturbing events in the patient's occupational sphere). However, in all these instances, it has not been observed that the brain mechanisms engaged in monothematic patterns which are exclusively devoted to the interim event. As a rule, the neutralization of disturbing interim events appears as a new addition to more complex and thematic material which is closely related.

## The Immediate Preabreactive Phase

This phase which covers the short period (see Table 23, p. 148) between the moment the patient and the therapist agree to get ready for the next autogenic abreaction and the beginning of the induction phase of the abreactive period usually comprises the routine of setting up the tape recorder, testing it and lying down on the couch. With advanced and experienced patients this phase usually passes in an uneventful manner. However, certain difficulties which are largely related to various forms of resistance (see Vol. VI, Part I) are encountered during initial treatment periods with autogenic abreaction. Dynamics of resistance may involve tape recorder (see p. 100 ff.), forgetting to visit the bathroom, or difficulty in finding a comfortable horizontal training posture on the couch. Depending on the nature of the patient's resistance it may or may not be advisable to engage in a clarifying confrontation and discussion before entering the induction phase. When manifestations of massive resistance are evident it is generally preferable to delay or postpone the planned autogenic abreaction until the patient has reached an adequate level of understanding and his collaboration appears to have become adequate.

Out of context remarks of thematically related or of paradoxic nature (see Case 67) occur more frequently during this part of the preparatory period than during the general discussion or mobilization phase. Occasionally patients indicate onset of frontal headaches while setting up and testing their tape recorder. In instances of crying, vestibular or motor discharges may start as soon as the patient has assumed the habitual horizontal training posture, and the standard induction procedure must be delayed until the patient has calmed down or is able to relax adequately.

*Case 67:* A 48-year-old housewife (anxiety reaction, multiple phobic reactions, moderate depressive reaction) who several years earlier went through a traumatic delivery and lost her baby a few hours later. The patient reported that the interim period had been very difficult. She had been crying a lot, her sleep was poor and several times when she practiced her standard exercises, crying spells had started again. While preparing to lie down for the next autogenic abreaction, she remarked: "I know what's going to come, I have been thinking of my baby all week." Several minutes later the dynamics of neutralization focussed on traumatic delivery, the delivery (inadequate anesthesia), the hours of tension which followed, and the circumstances under which she was told her baby had died.

*Case 68:* A 44-year-old housewife (anxiety reaction, moderate depressive reaction, multiple psychophysiologic reactions). During the mobilization phase, the patient had made two remarks, which appeared out of context: (a) the patient suddenly interrupted herself by interjecting that she had forgotten to tell the therapist that over many years she had been dreaming repeatedly of being sick, and (b) while preparing her tape recorder for the planned autogenic abreaction, she suddenly wanted to know if Dr. Lindemann (see Vol. III, p. 184) had published other articles about autogenic training, apart from his report on using it while crossing the Atlantic in a kayak-type boat.[841-844,1416,2392]

Both subjects were discussed briefly and no allusions were made to the fact that these items were taken as cues forecasting items of neutralization of thematically associated material. The dynamics of the central abreactive phase of the following AA focussed largely on disturbing material related to a series of past sicknesses, various accidents and certain other traumatic events. One of these involved capsizing with a kayak-type boat (like Dr. Lindemann's) and fear of drowning while being sucked down by a strong whirling current.

*Case 69:* A 28-year-old female teacher (anxiety reaction, multiple phobic reactions, moderate depression). While setting up her tape recorder, the patient mentioned that for the last ten days she had felt like crying and that occasionally this feeling has been overwhelming. When asked if she did cry, she explained that with one abortive exception, circumstances had not permitted her to cry because she was staying with relatives. Three minutes later during the induction phase, the patient interrupted the therapist at LLH with "I feel like crying" and then a prolonged crying spell followed.

# PART III. PSYCHOPHYSIOLOGIC MODALITIES OF AUTOGENIC NEUTRALIZATION

## 10. Introduction

The diversity of autogenic discharges and other training phenomena which occur during autogenic standard exercises suggests that a variety of cortical and subcortical systems may patriciate in centrally coordinated brain-directed functions which are facilitated or triggered by psychophysiologic changes resulting from the regular practice of passive concentration on autogenic formulas. The functionally relatively restricted nature of brief episodes of thematically dissociated discharge activity during autogenic training involve essentially the same modalities as those encountered during autogenic abreaction. However, since the processes of autogenic neutralization are significantly more complex and functionally more differentiated, there is a wider range of combinations of modalities and a greater diversity of thematically determined variations within each group of modalities (e.g., motor, vestibular, visual, olfactory). To provide an opportunity of general orientation in the vast area of psychophysiologic phenomena of autogenic neutralization, it may be helpful to discuss essential aspects of each of the more important modalities. In an attempt to remain brief, a variety of interesting but, for purposes of general orientation, less important observations have not been mentioned. The highly differentiated area of sensory modalities requires detailed consideration after completion of further studies. A separate book on the variety of brain-directed dynamics involving the body image, which goes into greater detail in the area of visual elaborations may be indicated. Furthermore it was decided to refrain for the time being from a space-consuming discussion of affective, ideational and intellectual modalities of autogenic neutralization.

# 11. Auditory Phenomena

The variety of auditory sensations which occur for brief periods during the practice of autogenic standard exercises (see Table 13, p. 41[887,888]; Fig. 3, p. 142,[886]) are also encountered during autogenic abreaction. Here, however, auditory phenomena tend to be of longer duration and of a more complex nature. They range from thematically associated modalities which are actually void of auditory sensations (not included in Tables) and which *may* appear to play merely an illustrative role in the patient's description of certain phases of neutralization to auditory sensations which may be as clear and as complex as life experience itself.

Initially, during the first and the second autogenic abreaction, auditory elaborations are still relatively restricted and occur only in about 12 to 15 per cent of psychosomatic and neurotic patients (see Table 24). Later when the dynamics of brain-directed neutralization have gained more flexibility, auditory sensations are more frequently a thematic element of multithematic processes of neutralization in about 35 per cent (N=150) of psychosomatic and neurotic patients.

Relatively undifferentiated auditory sensations, such as buzzing, humming, hissing and pure tones, which are localized in or near Heschl's gyrus, occur less frequently during autogenic abreactions (see Table 24) than during the first standard exercise of autogenic training (see Table 13, p. 41[887,888]). In the course of multithematic neutralization there is a clear emphasis on more complex phenomena which are usually classified as psychic hallucinations. These are about equally distributed between auditory sensations of human nature (e.g., speech, singing, crying, groaning, laughing) and other auditory sensations of environmental origin (e.g., tools, machinery, music, animal sounds, nature; see Table 25).

Depending on the prevailing topic of multithematic neutralization, auditory phenomena may evolve as a prominent feature for brief episodes (e.g., 30 sec.), or auditory elaborations may assume a thematically leading role for much longer periods (see Case 70).

*Case 70:* A 42-year-old housewife (anxiety reaction, multiple psychophysiologic reaction, duodenal ulcer). For a period of 24 minutes processes of neutralization emphasized reality-related auditory elaborations in combination with a cinerama-type pattern, which is transitory and leads to the formation of a triple image.

TABLE 24.  *Auditory Phenomena Reported by Psychosomatic and Neurotic Patients during the First and the Second Autogenic Abreaction*

| Auditory Phenomena | Autogenic Abreactions | |
|---|---|---|
| | AA 1 (%; N = 100) | AA 2 (%; N = 96) |
| 1. Specific tones | 10.0 | 10.4 |
| 2. Music | 1.0 | 2.0 |
| 3. Spoken words | 6.0 | 7.3 |
| 4. Buzzing | — | 1.0 |

". . . this child is completely motionless . . . her hands are hanging limply by her side . . . she is completely still . . . her hands are quite relaxed . . . I am watching this girl . . . she is about six or seven years old . . . this girl is waiting for something . . . I think her hands should be clenched . . . but the hands are hanging loosely down . . . *there is such a humming in my right ear . . . no, it's morse code . . . and this girl is still standing there . . . m . . . s . . . c . . . l . . . ah, it's murderous . . . it's in my ears . . . I have got a head phone on my head . . . dit-da, da-dit-da-dit, da-dit-da . . . terribly fast . . . I keep missing something . . . da-dit-da-dit-da-da-dit-da . . . come, and very high speed . . . somebody else answers in high speed da-dit-da, da-dit-da, da-dit-da, da-dit-da, go ahead . . .* ah, this is quite exhausting . . . the little girl is still there . . . *this morse code is surrounded by interference . . . very high pitch . . . so difficult to pickout this very faint . . . e-b-o-a-t-s-, e-b-o-a-t-s . . . e-b-o-a-t-s . . . this morse code is going on,* and there is the child . . . and an erected wooden platform is going through my cheekbone to my ear, and this child is there . . . I got so many things here . . . the girl in the passage, the platform and something underneath the platform and I am sitting at a wireless set with earphones, and I am crouched and trying to hear something . . . *da-dit-da, da-dit-da, da-dit-da, clearly: c-o-m-e-h-o-m-e, c-o-m-e-h-o-m-e, interference: five, strength: 1 . . . m-a-k-e-m-a-k-e-m-a-k-e . . . it's just a humming sound now . . . it started again . . . this is horrible . . .* this brings back the war with everything . . . I still have this 'me' crouched down over a pad . . . the girl is still there in the passage in the upper part of the field . . . the platform is different . . . the person at the set is taken over by a mist . . . I can't say what is happening . . . I have to wait . . . *the morse code is humming away . . . it's automatic at such a speed . . .* I am supposed to listen to something . . . I can't get the set tuned in properly. . . ."

Generally it can be observed that the various modalities of auditory elaborations are adapted to the nature of the prevailing pattern and topic of neutralization. When, for example, brain-directed dynamics engage in neutralization of experiential material (e.g., car collision), the auditory elaborations tend to correspond to the reality-related thematic elements (e.g., "a noise like breaking glass"). During neutraliza-

TABLE 25.  *Auditory Phenomena Described during 50 Autogenic Abreactions by 20 Psychosomatic and Neurotic Patients*

| Categories of Auditory Phenomena | Frequency (N =75; 66 phases) | No. of Patients Reporting |
|---|---|---|
| 1. Speech | 15 | 7 |
| 2. Singing | 3 | 3 |
| 3. Laughing | 8 | 5 |
| 4. Crying, moaning, groaning, etc. | 14 | 6 |
| 5. Other human sounds or noises | 1 | 1 |
| 6. Music (instrumental) | 11 | 8 |
| 7. Occupational noise (tools, machinery, etc.) | 12 | 11 |
| 8. Animal sounds, nature | 7 | 4 |
| 9. Simple tones (buzzing, humming) | 4 | 2 |

tion of non-experiential material (e.g., tortures in hell), thematically corresponding auditory sensations may be noted (e.g., "echoes of diabolic laughter"). Since the brain-directed dynamics aim at neutralization of brain-disturbing material, it is not surprising that negatively loaded (e.g., anxiety, depressive) auditory sensations (e.g., crying, shooting, father's severe voice) are significantly more frequently encountered than positively loaded, agreeable ones (see Table 26; Case 71; Case 73, p. 168; Case 74, p. 169; Case 11, p. 53). Agreeable, calming, encouraging and other positively oriented auditory elaborations may occur as interjected antithematic elements (see Case 71, p. 167) of positively oriented antithematic phases (i.e., after or before neutralization of particularly difficult and disturbing material) or, this is more frequently the case, appear as an integral part of terminal phases (see p. 78 ff.). Furthermore, it is evident that various forms of thematic modification (see p. 292 ff.), such as thematic dissociation, are also reflected by variable degrees of self-involvement (see Table 44, p. 296) in auditory elaborations (see Table 26).

*Case 71:* A 39-year-old priest (anxiety reaction, multiple phobic and psychophysiologic reactions, ecclesiogenic syndrome). The first passage (A) is characteristic for auditory elaborations during neutralization of reality-related anxiety. The second example (B) illustrates the brain-directed interjection of antithematic auditory ellaborations and the third one (C) is a positively oriented terminal phase.

(A) "The profile of a round saw . . . I hear its grating . . . I'm afraid to get my fingers caught in the round saw. . . ."

(B) "Here I am again on the beach . . . alone . . . now, what's budging over to the right? . . . a frog, a turtle? . . . no, it's a snake with its mouth wide open and all red . . . I see its tongue . . . *I hear the clear laugh of a little girl* . . . I just have enough time to put a stick in between the

TABLE 26.  *Psychodynamic Aspects of Auditory Phenomena Described during 50 Autogenic Abreactions by 20 Psychosomatic and Neurotic Patients*

| Thematic Context of Auditory Phenomena | Frequency (75 auditory phenomena; 66 phases) | No. of Patients per Category |
|---|---|---|
| **1. *Thematic connotation*** | | |
| (a) Postively oriented (calming, encouraging, relaxing) | 22 | 12 |
| (b) Relatively neutral | 11 | 5 |
| (c) Negatively oriented (anxiety, depression, aggression, sadistic, masochistic) | 42 | 16 |
| **2. *Self-involvement*** | | |
| (a) Self-produced (e.g., own voice) | 5 | 3 |
| (b) Directed toward self (produced by others) | 8 | 6 |
| (c) No direct self-involvement | 57 | 19 |
| (d) Others (buzzing, humming, etc.) | 5 | 5 |
| **3. *Reality-unreality context*** | | |
| (a) Experiential | 24 | 13 |
| (b) Non-experiential | 47 | 17 |
| (c) Others | 4 | 2 |

snake's jaws to prevent it from closing its mouth, and from biting me. . . ."

(C) "I think of this line from one of Baudelaire's poems, one that I had cherished so much at one time: '*Le soleil s'est noyé dans son sang qui se fige*' . . . and again I think of Saint Francis of Assisi's 'The Canticle of the Sun' *all while listening to Raoul Jobin's beautiful voice singing this operatic aria: 'Ah! lève-toi, Soleil!'* . . . it's now dusk. . . ."

*Case 72:* A 35-year-old housewife, who at the age of 14 was very proud that she had not cried when her father died. The patient started swallowing soon after the therapist pronounced the introductory heaviness formulas. After 90 seconds (RAH, LAH, BAH, RLH), during "My left leg is heavy" the patient interrupted the therapist.

"I can hear my father chuckling . . . I miss him [crying] . . . I could also see his face, the way his left eye would close more than the right as he laughed . . . *I have often heard this sound whenever I thought of him* . . . I have always felt his presence . . . I didn't now . . . I didn't feel that he was there . . . maybe I have just realized that he is gone . . . [crying] . . . there was a bit of a headache when I came to stretch here . . . now it is cleared from the neck up. . . ."

*Case 73:* A 37-year-old technician (anxiety reaction, obsessive-compulsive reaction, hypothyroidism, ecclesiogenic syndrome). During the neutralization of accumulated aggression related to ecclesiogenic material, the following passage led to thematic elaborations of auditory phenomena.

"I see thousands of churches that I set fire to . . . what a beautiful bonfire . . . they're still crumbling down . . . I notice beautiful tabernacles, works of art burning away . . . sacred vases rolling about on the ground, all of them damaged . . . and a crowd rushes forth to pick up the gold and the remaining precious pieces . . . I'm looking at all of this from up there in the air, *laughing diabolically* . . . but the more I look at myself, the more it isn't me I see, I'm mistaking myself for another . . . *and the laughing continues . . . there's a lot of echo. . . .*"

*Case 74:* A 34-year-old priest (anxiety reaction, ecclesiogenic syndrome).
"A huge hall as in a castle . . . it's very big and high up . . . it's the hall for the Last Judgment . . . everyone is there . . . the chap solemnly walks in . . . *a trumpet sounds . . . a judge reads my record* . . . everything is written down . . . each accusation scandalizes the people . . . *I hear them shouting and calling me a bandit. . . .*"

As in other modalities of brain-directed elaborations, auditory sensations appear to be adapted to the patient's level of tolerance. Even in the few instances when auditory phenomena were described as being "loud," the intensity of the material released did not have a particularly disturbing effect. Painful sounds were not described. Of further interest is the high incidence of high-pitch elaborations. These are usually associated with specific phases focussing on neutralization of anxiety material.

TABLE 27. *Psychophysiologic Aspects of Auditory Phenomena Described during 50 Autogenic Abreactions by 20 Psychosomatic and Neurotic Patients*

| Psychophysiologic Aspects | Frequency (75 auditory phenomena; 66 phases) | No. of Patients per Category |
|---|---|---|
| 1. *Pitch* | | |
| (a) High | 26 | 13 |
| (b) Low | 6 | 4 |
| (c) Others | 43 | 14 |
| 2. *Intensity* | | |
| (a) Loud | 4 | 2 |
| (b) Faint | 3 | 3 |
| (c) Others | 68 | 17 |
| 3. *Auralization* | | |
| (a) Monaural (i.e., one ear only) | 1 | 1 |
| (b) Not specified | 74 | 19 |

# 12. Gustatory Phenomena

Gustatory sensations are occasionally reported by about 20 per cent (N=150) of psychoneurotic and psychosomatic patients. This is a significant increase in occurrence when compared with gustatory sensations reported during auotgenic standard exercises (see Table 14, p. 42[887,888]). The nature of the gustatory sensations which are usually closely adapted to the specific topic of neutralization includes the major categories of taste (i.e., sour, salty, bitter, sweet) and many other mixed sensations of particular flavors (e.g., pepper, cocaine, blood, chocolate) and related elements which specify the texture or the temperature of the food (e.g., hot milk, cold milk, bitter and slimy, cool and slimy like sperm).

Gustatory sensations may be of very brief duration and play an apparently complementary role in multithematic processes of neutralization (see Case 75, Case 76). In other instances gustatory sensations seem to serve as a point of departure for a brain-desired thematic shift (see Case 75).

*Case 75:* A 50-year-old priest (obsessive-compulsive reactions, multiple psychophysiologic reactions, ecclesiogenic syndrome). In the following passages the gustatory sensations play a specific role in bringing about a brain-desired thematic shift.

"Once again I fall on an oily surface . . . I'm floating vertically . . . submarine dive into the oil . . . dirty as it was, the oil becomes clearer . . . finally it turns golden . . . very thin oil . . . further down, further down it becomes white like milk . . . it has become milk, nice clean milk . . . I go down, everything is white, white, white . . . the milk gets thicker and I'm now swimming in cream . . . I'm floating on an inner lake of sweet cream . . . I'm rolling in it . . . *it's sweet* . . . *it tastes like the little tarts of my* childhood . . . which brings me to the family table where I'm eating bread soaked in cream . . . and strawberries . . . I go up to my room . . . under lock and key . . . I feel like masturbating. I have nothing else to do. . . ."

During neutralization of particularly disturbing material (e.g., almost choking on a mouthful of sperm) the brain-directed elaboration of specific gustatory sensations may play a central role during prolonged phases of thematic repetition (see Case 16, p. 66 ff.). Multiple occurrence of different gustatory sensations (see Case 76), are not unusual.

*Case 76:* A 35-year-old housewife (anxiety reaction, multiple psychophysiologic reactions). In AA 25, three thematically interrelated phases of neutralization with gustatory sensations occur: (A) childhood, with father in

170

kitchen and taste of his toast; (B) homosexual dynamics with antithematic interjection of gustatory sensation of sperm; (C) father's death, inadequate identification, taste of dust). Of particular interest is the patient's commentary, with questions indicating that the gustatory sensations were of particular thematic importance to her.

TABLE 28. *Examples of Gustatory Phenomena*
(25 Psychosomatic and Neurotic Patients)

---

"I float on a lake of soft cream. . . . I am rolling in it . . . it's sweet . . . it tastes like the little tarts of my childhood. . . ."

"Now I have a funny taste . . . it's like freshly grounded pepper."

"It tastes like alcohol . . . and oranges."

"I keep sucking her breasts . . . it tastes like milk. . . ."

"It tastes like honey. . . ."

"It tastes like milk . . . sour milk. . . ."

"I have a very strong sensation in my mouth. . . ."

"It tastes like varnish . . . like the wooden doll I had when I was a small girl. . . ."

"Now I start sucking her left breast . . . it is like milk. . . ."

"And now I have this taste, this taste of cocaine. . . ."

"It's like milk . . . it tastes like milk. . . ."

"I see a lot of blood . . . I see red rivers . . . and I have this taste of blood in my mouth. . . ."

"I suck the breasts . . . and the milk is coming . . . and this time it tastes good . . . and then . . . and now I am having intercourse. . . ."

"I scoop some water with my hands and drink and . . . it tastes very good . . . it feels a lot cooler now. . . ."

"I suck her breasts . . . and I taste the milk . . . sour, bitter. . . ."

"I keep sucking . . . and it tastes like peppermint. . . ."

"I swallow this stuff from the eye . . . and I feel it on my lips and it tastes bitter-sour . . . it tastes exactly like sperm. . . ."

"I am sucking the penis . . . the taste is not bad. . . ."

"And I drink the blood . . . and the breasts become normal and I suck . . . and the milk is too hot . . . I indicate this to my mother . . . and the milk is getting cooler . . . and it tastes a bit like chocolate. . . ."

"Mustard . . . it's choking me . . . burning sensation in my throat . . . the after-taste. . . ."

"It tastes bitter, it . . . it tastes like soot, it tastes like . . . like ash. . . ."

"And I start sucking, and I taste it . . . it is really very good. . . ."

"I just fell head first into a pile of cow shit . . . [retching . . . agitated] . . . I really tasted something bad . . ." [wiping his mouth].

"I suck his penis . . . he ejaculates . . . now I really have this taste. . . ."

"I am sucking his penis . . . it tastes salty. . . ."

---

| Transcript of passages from AA 25 | The patient's commentary (homework) |
|---|---|
| A. "Now it is Dad in the kitchen, we are making 'tire sur la neige' . . . he has the snow, everything is sticky . . . we are having a wonderful time . . . he insists we take a clean spoon every time in case we have mixed them up . . . his toast . . . [beginning to cry] . . . *I never tasted toast like that since* . . . [crying] . . . it is Dad . . . helping me with the mathematics . . . playing cards, his voice . . . singing . . . again in the cemetery. . . . | "Why did I have that gustatory sensation? Later I had the taste of sperm. Any connection? |
| B. I had this sensation of pubic hair against pubic hair and I thought that is impossible . . . but it is, I have that feeling . . . still sort of going on I think . . . I don't know how to describe it . . . it is vulva against vulva . . . there is genital awareness on my part but . . . all right the lips are opened somehow or other . . . touching . . . parts are sort of touching and rubbing . . . again I don't know what happened, I had . . . position change, person change and *I had sperm taste in my mouth . . . still there . . . sort of, the after-taste, the way it . . . pulls and gags when it goes near the throat* . . . now I see her on her back. . . . | What about the sperm taste? Does this mean or have something to do with being confronted with a penis when I want a breast? |
| C. It was the right arm that pushed it [a coffin] open . . . simultaneously, whoever was in, sat up . . . when I look, there is nothing . . . there is a body, there is somebody there . . . is it an outline . . . is it just a skeleton? I have the feeling there was no head . . . *I get the taste of dust* in my mouth . . . there is . . . as I said there is nothing. . . ." | Because of that dust taste in my mouth, I would say part of me wanted me in that coffin." |

Of particular interest are variations of gustatory sensations during chronologic regression to infancy through breast sucking. It has been repeatedly observed that aggressive dynamics are closely associated with breast sucking as such, and with gustatory sensations in particular. For example, it occurs that when a male patient finally engages in sucking the breast of a girlfriend, spontaneous regression to infancy follows, and his mother's milk "tastes bad" (sour, bitter). Such a combination of thematic elements easily triggers violent aggressive activity against the mother. However, after brain-desired levels of neutralization of these aggressive dynamics have been reached, and breast sucking is resumed, the milk tastes "good." Similarly it has been observed that resistance to engaging in intercourse appears to be reduced after sufficient breast sucking. The recuperative and "action-facilitating" role of breast sucking with or without gustatory sensations appears to have a biologically and developmentally understandable key position during certain dynamics of autogenic neutralization (see Case 77).

*Case 77:* A 24-year-old male graduate student (obsessive-compulsive and multiple psychophysiologic reactions, ecclesiogenic syndrome). The following patterns of antithematic alternation (i.e., aggression, breast sucking, aggression, breast sucking, aggression) includes variations in milk temperature in combination with the rather unusual flavor of chocolate. After an "action-facilitating" period of breast sucking, the patient continues the interrupted engagement in aggressive dynamics (i.e., father, therapist).

"I become a man again . . . and I kill myself . . . and I go to heaven . . . and I see myself as a little baby sucking my mother's breasts . . . and I bite the tip of her breasts . . . and I tear off the nipples with my teeth . . . and I drink blood . . . and the breast becomes normal, and I'm sucking . . . and *the milk is too warm* . . . and I signal this to mother . . . and *the milk becomes much colder* . . . *and it tastes a bit like chocolate* . . . and I kill my father with an ax . . . and I kill the doctor. . . ."

# 13. Olfactory Phenomena

During multithematic patterns of autogenic neutralization a variety of olfactory phenomena are occasionally described by about 30 per cent (N=150) of psychosomatic and neurotic patients. Only a few of these patients had experienced olfactory sensations before, during the practice of autogenic standard exercises (see Table 14[887,888]). The olfactory phenomena reported (during AA) may be of merely illustrative nature and actually void of olfactory sensations (not included in Tables) or they may consist of smells with variable intensities of olfactory sensation. Such brain-directed elaborations are of variable duration. Very brief olfactory episodes of thematically secondary nature and also longer phases (up to 10 min.) of thematic neutralization, during which olfactory sensations appeared to be of central importance (see Case 34, p. 201/I), have been observed. Although brain-directed elaborations of olfactory phenomena may occur without thematically corresponding elaborations in the visual field, they are most frequently encountered during cinerama-type patterns (see Table 33, p. 188). When the thematic content is of experiential nature (see Case 34, p. 201/I), the olfactory sensations tend to be at a corresponding level of realism, adapted however, to the re-experience. During thematic neutralization of brain-disturbing material of non-experiential origin (e.g., hell), the olfactory sensations appear to be composed of elements which are of experiential origin and other components which may be regarded as brain-desired products of thematic modification (see p. 292 ff.). Such brain-produced combinations often make it difficult for a patient to arrive at a clear distinction between olfactory impression and olfactory sensation.

*Case 78:* A 30-year-old priest (sexual deviation, obessive-compulsive manifestations, multiple psychophysiologic reactions, ecclesiogenic syndrome). During neutralization of anxiety material of ecclesiogenic nature (i.e., punishment in hell), the cinerama-type dynamics transitorily emphasize thematically synchronized (non-experiential) elaborations of an olfactory nature.

"And they are legions according to Saint Matthew . . . and I am at the end of the fork . . . they put the fork right in my pants . . . and I am hanging at the end of a devil's fork . . . he swishes his tail across my chin . . . *it stinks* . . . it is said that it stinks in hell, *it smells awful, ah, it's terrible* . . . *pfouah, ah, it stinks* . . . and I with my sensitive nose . . . well, you wanted to put your nose into the sex of lovely girls, all right you little pig, okay, now smell this . . . *ah, it's really awful* . . . *it's a suffocating stench,* it's . . . there isn't a word to describe this . . . it's a *diabolic stench* . . . eh, eh, ah . . . you can't even

174

vomit . . . *it smells awful*, really . . . ahhh, *these fumes* . . . fumes of shit are nothing in comparison with this . . . that's a kind of perfume . . . this . . . ahh, ehh . . . *it's awful*, and I am still hanging at the end of a devil's fork. . . ."

In attempting to put some order into the wide spectrum of olfactory phenomena encountered during autogenic neutralization, three large groups have been distinguished: (a) clearly pleasant and agreeable modalities (see Table 29), (b) clearly unpleasant and disturbing modalities (see Table 30) and (c) a variety of other olfactory phenomena which may be considered as less unpleasant or relatively neutral (see Table 31, p. 177).

TABLE 29.   *Examples of Olfactory Phenomena with Pleasant Connotations*
(20 Psychosomatic and Neurotic Patients)

---

"And now I see nicely packed soap . . . in gold and pink . . . and it smells, it smells like soap . . . all kinds of smell . . . like lilac . . . like violets . . . now like eau de cologne . . . and some lemon lime. . . ."

"The wind, the beach, the ocean . . . oh, it really smells good. . . ."

"It smells like perfume. . . ."

"It smells good . . . it smells like linseed oil in a barn. . . ."

"A very nice landscape . . . and it smells good. . . ."

"I see my grandmother, and she is making bread . . . it smells good. . . ."

"I am in a barn . . . and there is hay . . . and it smells good. . . ."

"I lie there and I am happy . . . I can even smell the forest . . . it smells very fresh . . . I can hear the birds. . . ."

"It smells good . . . it smells like perfume. . . ."

"I open the door . . . and there is this . . . smell of her perfume. . . ."

"His hair smells good . . . it smells like a strong hair lotion. . . ."

"It smells like a flower shop. . . ."

"It smells good . . . it smells like flowers. . . ."

"I am entering the kitchen . . . hmm . . . it smells good . . . they are preparing. . . ."

"And I put my nose into his hair, and it smells good. . . ."

"These flowers, I really do smell them. . . ."

"It smells like coffee, very agreeable . . . as if I am in a mountain of coffee . . . the same smell. . . ." [for about 4 min.]

"And I am biting her ear a bit, and smell the odor of her hair. . . ."

"We embrace each other . . . and I smell her perfume. . . ."

"I am in the dunes . . . and it smells good. . . ."

---

TABLE 30. *Examples of Olfactory Phenomena with Clearly Unpleasant Connotations*
(20 Psychosomatic and Neurotic Patients)

"It smells awful, it smells people, it smells what I detest. . . ."

"It's a suffocating stench, it's . . . there isn't a word for it . . . it's a diabolic stench. . . .''

"It stinks . . . nauseating acid odors . . . acids that burn, corrosive acids. . . ."

"It smells of rotten eggs . . . it stinks . . . it stinks. . . ."

"It's awfully smelly . . . I think it's garlic . . . garlic and beer. . . ."

"Now it is dark . . . and it smells bad . . . it smells like. . . ."

"It smells like paint, alcohol, oil . . . it's suffocating. . . ."

"It smells like roasted pig. . . ."

"It smells like shit. . . ."

"It's stinking . . . it stinks like shit. . . ."

"It smells like urine. . . ."

"It emanates a nauseating odor . . . *I like that . . . I think it smells good*. . . ."

"It smells bad. . . ."

"It smells like mud . . . like rotten mud . . . like rotten vegetables. . . ."

"It smells . . . it smells . . . it smells bad . . . it smells like decay. . . ."

"And I don't like to get closer . . . it stinks. . . ."

"This guy with the cancer and this thing in his throat . . . oh, the unbelievable awful smell. . . ."

"This yellow mustard . . . the smell just burns my nostril. . . ."

"I bash in the stomach of a dead cat . . . nausea . . . stink of decaying carcasses. . . ."

"And there is this sort of smell . . . of something rotten. . . ."

Particularly pleasant and generally agreeable modalities of olfactory sensations are elaborated in combination with other equally positively oriented thematic elements (e.g., visual, feelings) characteristic for interjected antithematic phases or brain-directed terminal patterns.

Negatively loaded, disagreeable olfactory phenomena appear to occur more often in connection with neutralization of anxiety material involving non-experiential elaborations (e.g., Case 78, p. 174). In such cases the participating experiential olfactory component appears to undergo certain thematic modifications which may result in undue amplification or exaggeration of the thematically related olfactory phenomenon.

The many variations of olfactory phenomena which are neither "very pleasant" nor "very bad" are not without disturbing or pleasing thematic connotations (see Table 31). In most instances these specific olfactory elaborations (e.g., chloroform, garlic and beer, sperm) appear as components of more complex thematic material which is of particularly disturbing potency (e.g., abortion, nostalgia, sexual trauma), which presented a particular problem (e.g., self-control, suppression of thematic reaction) or which provide a brain-desired antithematic effect.

TABLE 31. *Examples of Olfactory Phenomena with Less Unpleasant or Relatively Neutral Connotations*
(20 Psychosomatic and Neurotic Patients)

"And we are walking on paper . . . on sawdust . . . and it smells funny. . . ."

"And it's quite warm in the convent . . . it smells like the odor of wax, and it smells like nuns (*ça sent la bonne soeur*). . . ."

"It smells humid . . . and there are birds making some noise. . . ."

"And it is getting smoky . . . I smell smoke . . . like cigarette smoke. . . ."

"It is spring . . . and it is sunny . . . and there is this odor of old dry wood. . . ."

"And I am inside . . . and it smells musty and dusty. . . ."

"The room is filled with smoke . . . ah, ah . . . I don't smoke myself at the moment . . . [yawning] . . . tobacco smoke. . . ."

"I smell the odor of your hair . . . of your body. . . ."

"The [pubic] hair, there was this odor . . . I guess it is the lubricating liquid odor, substance . . . Okay . . . so I know. . . ."

"And it smells like chloroform or disinfectant or something. . . ."

"This odor . . . I think it smells like sulfur. . . ."

"The pigs in the mud . . . on each side of the fence . . . and they rub each other's snout . . . it smells like pig. . . ."

"It smells like sperm. . . ."

"It smells like sulfur . . . like gun powder. . . ."

"It smells like cattle. . . ."

"It smells like vinegar. . . ."

"The house is very old and has a musty type of odor. . . ."

"There is a strong smell in the room as if the room had been locked up for a long time . . . and I have the window open beside me. . . ."

"I smell . . . it smells like chrysanthemum, it smells like . . . flowers in a funeral home . . . it is just the smell and. . . ."

"We breathe the fresh air . . . and it smells fresh, like the ocean. . . ."

# 14. Vestibular Phenomena

During autogenic training, vestibular modalities of autogenic discharges are encountered frequently (SE I: 64%, N=100 pts.; see Table 12, p. 40[878,888]). They also play an important role as thematic elements during autogenic abreaction. Sensations such as sinking, floating, turning, lopsidedness and falling may appear for very brief periods as secondary elements of processes of multithematic neutralization, or they may be given thematic priority and dominate prolonged periods of the central abreactive phase (see Case 79, p. 181; Case 81, p. 182). Differentiated visual elaborations may or may not be associated with vestibular phenomena (see Case 16, p. 66; Case 79, p. 181). As in other instances, when certain physiologically oriented thematic elements (e.g., motor discharges, pain, crying) assume thematic priority, previously highly differentiated visual elaborations tend to undergo a functional regression to elementary levels (e.g., stages I, II; see p. 187 ff.) for transitory periods when certain types of vestibular modalities (e.g., falling, turning) related to brain-disturbing material of experiential nature (e.g., accidents) undergo phasic neutralization. Since it rarely occurs that particularly disturbing material (e.g., accidents, traumatic medical procedures, inadequate anesthesia, suffocation) appears in the beginning of brain-programmed processes of thematic neutralization, the occurrence of vestibular modalities remains at a relatively low level during the first few autogenic abreactions (see Table 32).

Later, as treatment with autogenic abreaction advances and participating brain mechanisms gain in functional flexibility, vestibular modalities tend to play an increasing role in the neutralization of thematically related material. Although many questions concerning the elaboration and release of vestibular modalities cannot be answered at this point, preliminary studies have provided some information which may be of interest for further investigations in this area. Generally, the release of vestibular modalities (e.g., sinking, falling, turning, spinning very fast) appears to be closely linked to thematically specific and particularly potent dynamics of anxiety. The anxiety dynamics may be related to specific material of experiential nature (e.g., fall from a ladder) or may be of non-experiential origin in association with inadequate brain-disturbing identifications (e.g., with somebody who fell from a ladder; with somebody going down to hell—*tomber en enfer*). The patient may or may not have been aware of the thematically related anxiety. During autogenic abreactions, brain-directed mechanisms of

178

TABLE 32.  *Vestibular Phenomena Reported by Psychosomatic and Psychoneurotic Patients during the First and the Second Autogenic Abreaction*

| Vestibular Phenomena | Autogenic Abreactions | |
|---|---|---|
| | AA 1 (%; N = 100) | AA 2 (%; N = 96) |
| (a) Dizziness | 2.0 | 7.3 |
| (b) Turning | 1.0 | — |
| (c) Floating | 1.0 | 2.1 |
| (d) Lopsidedness | 1.0 | 1.0 |
| (e) Sinking | 3.0 | 2.1 |
| (f) Falling | — | 1.0 |
| (g) Flying | — | 4.2 |

thematic modification (e.g., thematic disintegration, thematic dissociation; see p. 292 ff.) tend to keep the re-experience of the anxiety component at a very low level (e.g., some apprehension), and usually patients remain calm and relaxed while vestibular modalities undergo neutralization.

The release of vestibular modalities may follow a pattern of monothematic repetition (see p. 273 ff.), but alternating phases of antithematic vestibular modalities (e.g., ascending-descending, turning left–turning right) tend to occur more frequently. During neutralization of very complex material such as that related to severe traffic accidents, one or two vestibular modalities (e.g., turning, falling) tend to assume a dominating role while others (e.g., floating, lopsidedness, rocking back and forth) remain of secondary nature. So far no cases have been observed where the release of vestibular elaborations was restricted to one modality (e.g., falling). Studies of vestibular modalities released over longer series of autogenic abreactions have always been of multimodality nature. However, such pattern analyses showed that vestibular modalities are released in brain-programmed phases. Phases of relatively short duration may be scattered throughout the abreactive period of a given autogenic abreaction. Similarly, pattern analyses of longer series of autogenic abreactions which, for example, focussed on neutralization of a severe traffic accident showed that the brain-designed program of neutralization evolves in phases, each of which emphasizes the release of specific thematic components (e.g., crying, pain, vestibular; see Fig. 7). The phasic release of thematic modalities (i.e., vestibular and others) may follow a sequential or a rotational pattern of thematic programming (see p. 251 ff.).

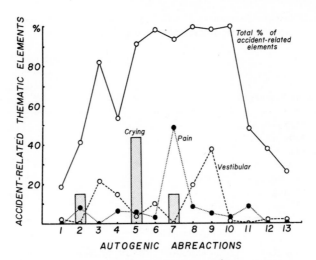

Fig. 7. Phasic release of thematically specific modalities (i.e., crying, pain, vestibular) during neutralization of a severe traffic accident (see Case 79, p. 181).

An increased occurrence of vestibular modalities has been observed in persons who have suffered accidents involving an unexpected and rapid displacement (see Case 79, p. 181). When such accidents involve the cranial area, and particularly when such episodes are associated with transitory loss of consciousness, more intensive elaborations of vestibular nature tend to ensue. Schizophrenic patients who received ECT had a significantly higher level ($P<$ .01) of vestibular discharges (e.g., floating, sinking) than other schizophrenic patients who had not received ECT (see Fig. 8c, p. 49/III). A high incidence of vestibular discharges was also observed in association with certain anxiety-promoting activities in sports (e.g., diving from high boards, waterskiing, judo) and so-called amusement machines which are known for "thrilling experiences" (e.g., rapid up and down .displacements, rapid rotation in horizontal and vertical directions; see Case 35, p. 202/I). Another area of brain-disturbing material which was observed as being associated with vestibular modalities were anxiety mobilizing episodes in combination with the use of inhalation anesthesia (e.g., ether, chloroform) and physiologically related variations of levels of conscious control and awareness (see Case 82, p. 183, Case 37, p. 203ff/I). When general anesthesia is brought about by intravenous injection of an anesthetic, the brain-disturbing effects appear to be of a different nature. In these cases there is no particular evidence indicating that the onset of anesthesia is associated with disturbances involving vestibular modalities in the same manner as in the case with inhalation anesthesia. However, it has repeatedly been observed that the transition from the state of general anesthesia to the normal state during the recovery period, with its peculiar stages of semiconsciousness, is of particular brain-disturbing significance. Similar brain-disturbing effects seem to result from events which occur during inadequate levels of general anesthesia. Closely related to this area of concern are brain-disturbing effects which occur in connection with fainting (or almost fainting), epileptiform seizures and insulin reactions. When brain-disturbing material of this nature undergoes neutralization, vestibular modalities (e.g., falling, sinking, turning, dizziness) tend to be more closely related with various intensities of motor discharges (e.g., twitching, spasms, jerks).

*Case 79:* A 29-year-old housewife was hit by a speeding car. On impact she was thrown up into the air, then fell back onto the hood and a little later down on the pavement in front of the car when it stopped (no loss of consciousness, no major injuries). The following passages are examples of phases of neutralization emphasizing vestibular modalities (see Fig. 7, p. 000). During these phases the cinerama-type elaborations underwent a compensatory functional regression to stage I (see p. 187 ff.).

*From AA 3:* "It's like a shadow and sort of blurred . . . and now it is turning . . . oh, it's going so fast . . . it's like hollow . . . like a sort of cavity . . . and something is turning in it . . . it's like a deep cavity and inside of it something is turning fast . . . or, I am turning . . . now it's getting bright . . . it's like flying sparks . . . now it's all gone . . . it's just an empty hollow space . . . but that is still turning . . . [This slower and faster turning in combination with "an empty space" which changes its illumination from dark to bright continued for 5 min.] . . . I cannot get any other image, I don't see anything . . . this is much worse as if I would see something. . . ."

*From AA 4:* "And it starts blurring again . . . it is all gray . . . all gray. . . . Now I have a feeling similar to when one sits in a swing . . . but I am not on a swing . . . I don't know where I am . . . I am standing while this is going on, forth and back, I have the feeling as if I am going to fall down . . . but there is nothing around me . . . it's the funny feeling . . . I am not standing on something . . . it's this feeling of swinging forth and back, of falling . . . I know I am holding back something . . . now I stopped this feeling and I feel very tense . . . I am so afraid of this swinging and falling feeling . . . it's such a peculiar feeling . . . I am holding it back . . . now I have a stomach ache . . . I don't see anything, just this feeling . . . this swinging . . . like a pendulum, swinging forth and back . . . very disagreeable . . . I am tense all over . . . I am afraid of this swinging . . . I am afraid to let go . . . [This feeling of swinging forth and back and falling continued for about 10 min. The visual elaboration remained at stage I].

*From AA 8:* "It's somehow like a top, turning . . . I don't know whether that thing is spinning or if I am turning . . . as I look longer at this I start feeling like passing out . . . it's slowing down now . . . it's like a turntable . . . I have a headache from this spinning . . . it's still turning . . . now a car comes right toward me . . . a big car . . . low and flat with a lot of chrome . . . again the accident spot . . . it now looks like a funnel . . . very deep . . . I have the feeling as if I fall into it, head first . . . and as soon as I am in the funnel, there forms a new funnel and I drop in again, head first, and again the same thing . . . there is a pressure in my stomach . . . now the car is coming again toward me . . . but it stops right before the funnel-shaped hole . . . again this funnel . . . now I am at the spot where I got up and I compare the distance between the two spots. . . ."

*From AA 9:* "My head is down again, I am very tired, it starts turning and then pulls me down to the left and then I don't see anything anymore . . . when I come up again, I am again sitting on the car . . . and this repeats itself over and over again, always the same thing [for 6 min.] . . . it's still going on, this being pulled down, this falling, that's terrible . . . and then when I look up I am somehow collapsing and it pulls me deep, deep, deep down to the left. . . ."

*Case 80:* A 24-year-old male student (anxiety reaction, moderate depression, ecclesiogenic syndrome). On various occasions during different autogenic abreactions brief phases of vestibular dynamics (e.g., turning) occurred in association with reference to alcohol intoxications.

"It starts turning . . . it is turning . . . it's as if one is drunk . . . exactly the same thing . . . it's still turning . . . toward the right . . . it's like the big circus wheel which turns from right to left, counterclockwise . . . I am still turning . . . still the same thing. . . ."

*Case 81:* A 32-year-old housewife (anxiety reaction). During AA 16 a phase occurs characteristic for neutralization of brain-disturbing effects related to alcohol intoxication. Vestibular modalities dominate and the visual elaborations remain at an elementary level of differentiation.

"It is uniform in color, homogeneous . . . it has not changed at all . . . physically I feel strange, again in motion . . . I think it is that horizontal spinning starting . . . vibration . . . there is pressure on the outside of the head, the left side . . . that has gone by now . . . but that movement, dizzying, with oscillation, is going on . . . I don't know if I am going to the right or to the left . . . and I think the jerking or oscillation is now on the longitudinal axis as the spinning goes on . . . I am still in motion . . . don't know which way I am going . . . I think I feel as if the left side is lower than the right . . . visually there has been nothing at all . . . I don't know how to describe the feeling . . . now it is as if I am just floating . . . now the legs feel very heavy . . . and they are higher than before . . . now I am perfectly horizontal . . . now it [the visual field] has a slant going up away from me . . . that there is what? a skylight on top of it? . . . it is not black . . . this might be . . . I was

figuring out the amount of alcohol I have been taking . . . one night I know I
took too much . . . I think that black I had seen before with what I thought
was the skylight, could be the . . . *goulot*, symbolic of that . . . now I think
there is a clearing up. . . ."

*Case 82:* A 33-year-old housewife (anxiety reaction, mild depressive reaction). The patient had not suffered any accidents, but at age 11 an anxiety-
producing tonsillectomy (*inhalation anesthesia*) was performed. Later inhalation
anesthesia was used again on three different occasions: (a) during delivery of
her first child, (b) before and during a Cesarean section (emergency) and (c)
in connection with a spontaneous abortion. During the patient's first autogenic
abreaction, brain-directed processes of neutralization emphasize (a) sensory
elaborations in combination with distortion of the body image (see p. 245) and
(b) various vestibular modalities (e.g., sinking, turning, sliding). The visual
elaborations remain characteristically restricted to stage I (see p. 187 ff., Table
33, p. 188) but show a progressive change in brightness (i.e., very dark in the
beginning, light toward the end). From thematic material elaborated during
subsequent autogenic abreactions, it is assumed that the traumatic tonsillectomy
at age 11 and the repeated use of *inhalation anesthesia* participated to a large
extent in the formation of this type of brain-disturbing material (see also
vestibular modalities occurring during neutralization of a paracentesis during
inhalation anesthesia of Case 37, p. 203/I).

"I feel absolutely calm. I feel very heavy, particularly my arms and legs.
I feel some tingling in my left hand, no in my right hand, and I have a feeling
as if my legs want to go up . . . my visual field is dark . . . I don't see anything
. . . I don't have any ideas . . . I feel completely relaxed . . . I don't feel anything else, I feel completely relaxed . . . there are no colors, I see nothing, I
feel nothing, I have no distractions, I have nothing else to describe . . . I feel
completely relaxed, heavy and everything is really black . . . now it is very
dark in the center and on the outside, it is a little bit lighter . . . but it does
not change . . . everything is calm . . . no change . . . I feel relaxed. . . . I
find it very difficult to talk when there is nothing to describe . . . the visual
field does not change . . . my impressions do not change . . . I feel heavy
particularly in my legs . . . no change . . . the visual field is a little bit brighter
. . . it does not change much . . . now there is some tingling in my left leg,
particularly in my foot . . . I still feel heavy, there is no change, but the visual
field is somewhat lighter . . . I feel perfectly relaxed, I have no ideas, I have no
distractions . . . well, I would like to terminate because I have nothing to say
. . . [*It is going very well, please continue to describe*] . . . There really is no
change . . . I can't invent something, I feel perfectly relaxed, calm . . . nothing
is going on, the visual field does not change . . . I feel heavy, particularly the
legs, the arms too, and my back . . . I feel some tingling in my back and in my
right hand . . . I feel completely relaxed, I have no distractions . . . I think
of what I am saying . . . that's all . . . I feel some muscular vibrations in my
left leg, I feel more and more heavy, particularly in my arms and legs . . . my
visual field has changed a little . . . everything is lighter . . . and I have the

impression which I have . . . which comes over me when I sleep . . . I have
the impression that I have *enormous arms, enormous legs, and enormous tongue*
. . . and dimensions of . . . I don't . . . of *terrible thickness* . . . I feel completely relaxed, completely calm . . . I would like to terminate . . . [*It is going
very well. Please continue to describe*] . . . I don't like this feeling when I feel
so heavy and so enormous and so thick . . . and I have the impression as if *my
tongue is about ten feet thick, and the same with my arms and legs* . . . I have
the impression that *I am enormous* . . . this happens to me quite often when I am
about to fall asleep, when I am in a sort of half sleep . . . at the moment I don't
feel like falling asleep, not at all, I only have *this funny feeling* . . . my visual field
did not change, it is uniform, it is lighter than in the beginning, I don't have
any distractions, I feel nicely relaxed . . . but this feeling of thickness and
heaviness . . . I feel as if *I am about to go down* into a hole, I am very very heavy
. . . I have the impression that *I am weighing tons,* particularly my hands, *they
pull* as if . . . *downward* . . . as if they were *enormous,* weights attached to
them, and the same for the back of my head, and that's not very agreeable,
and my back but particularly my hands . . . now I have this sensation also on
my lips and on my tongue . . . nothing else has changed . . . [*It is going very
well*] . . . now I feel tingling in both my hands . . . but I am feeling more and
more heavy and thick . . . when I had this feeling before, and now I have the
same thing, I have the impression of as if I am *going down* into something, I
*sink* into something . . . [*Well, that's all right, please continue*] . . . I have no
distractions, I have no ideas at the moment . . . everything is *turning* . . . I
feel like *turning* on a table . . . the turntable is *turning faster and faster* . . . I
am *quite dizzy* . . . like in a circus . . . the heaviness sensation doesn't go
away, but I feel it more in my hands, and particularly in my legs and my back,
on my tongue, everywhere . . . I *feel like an enormous block* which is *turning
faster and faster,* and that makes me *feel* dizzy . . . may I terminate now? . . .
[*No, it's going very well, your brain is discharging very nicely, please continue*]
. . . I feel some tingling in the back of my head, and I am *turning faster and
faster* . . . I . . . I am *spinning so fast* . . . I am *very dizzy* . . . I feel heavy as
before . . . the visual field did not change, but I am *turning fast* . . . I have
some tingling in my back and in the back of my head, I feel very heavy . . .
It doesn't change . . . my body is very heavy and I am *turning very fast* . . .
I have no distractions . . . I keep *turning* and I am a bit afraid . . . my head is
*spinning* . . . I don't feel this feeling of heaviness on my tongue anymore, only
in my body, in the back of my head . . . my back, my arms, my legs, my hands,
now I have the impression it diminishes, and the impression as if something is
*pulling in the opposite direction,* as if I am coming to a halt . . . there is strange
tingling in my hands . . . there is much less heaviness . . . I don't turn anymore, only *my head is turning* and the feeling of heaviness is only in my arms
and in my hands . . . the visual field didn't change . . . it's always light . . .
some tingling in the back of my head, going down the neck and my back, and
in my hands . . . now I am *turning in the other direction* . . . I feel much less
heavy, I feel relaxed and rested . . . Can I stop now? [*No, that would be a
technical error, your brain is discharging very well, please continue*]. The feel-

ing of heaviness went away, now it is only in my arms and hands . . . lots of tingling in my hands . . . I would like to stretch a bit . . . I am *turning in the opposite direction, but very slowly* . . . somewhat more around something, not around a fixed point as before . . . now I feel like *sliding* a bit, there is no feeling of heaviness except in the arms . . . I feel warmth in my legs . . . my visual field did not change . . . there are no distractions . . . I feel nicely relaxed . . . *I do not turn any more,* but now there is a spreading feeling of numbness . . . on all parts which are in contact with the bed . . . I feel very calm and relaxed . . . some tingling in my hands . . . I feel completely awake, I don't sleep at all . . . there is a feeling of freshness in my arms, my hands, in my legs too . . . I feel calm . . . my heart is calm, my respiration too . . . I feel very well . . ." (23 min.; termination).

While the close association between brain-disturbing events of experiential nature (e.g., accidents, certain types of sports and amusement, inadequate anesthesia) and processes of neutralization which emphasize thematically related modalities of vestibular nature are readily understandable from a physiologic point of view, there are other categories of brain-disturbing material where the physiologic relationship is less clear or obscure. In this connection note the psychophysiologic implications of certain anxiety-promoting effects resulting from negatively oriented forms of religious education. The unusually high incidence of vestibular modalities which occur during thematic neutralization of anxiety dynamics related to the fear of damnation and "going down to hell" *(tomber dans le péché, descenche en enfer)* indicates the brain-disturbing potency of thematically related non-experiential material (see Case 83).

*Case 83:* A 50-year-old priest (anxiety reaction, obsessive-compulsive reactions, multiple psychophysiologic reactions, ecclesiogenic syndrome). The following passages (first half of abreactive period) are an example of monothematic repetitions of vestibular modalities related to the non-experiential anxiety material of "going down to hell." Note interjected samatosensory and auditory phenomena.

"So I take the ladder again, I go back down again, 1 step, 2 steps, 3 steps, 4 steps, 5, 6, 7, 8 , 9, 10, 11, 12, 13, 14, 15, it's still . . . because the sounds are re-echoing in there . . . I go down, I'm still going down, Im still going down . . . another step, another step, another step, another step . . . I'm going down, I'm going down, I'm going down . . . now there's only a little opening up there, I've gone down so deep . . . there are still steps, still steps . . . I go down some more, I go down some more, I go down some more . . . now it seems that the hole is getting narrower . . . I feel the walls against my elbows, I feel them brushing against my back . . . now it's very narrow . . . there are no more steps on the ladder . . . I'm wedged inside the hole in which I can hardly manage to slide . . . now it's sliding . . . it's sliding inside, it's sliding

. . . with a little effort I manage to slide . . . and now the hole is getting wider now I'm falling . . . the fall has begun . . . another fall is beginning . . . I have a headache . . . so I fall, I'm falling feet first . . . feet first . . . I stretch my arms up above my head and now it's going down, going down, going down, going down very fast, going down very fast . . . and I'm down extremely straight because even if the hole isn't very big, I'm not getting caught on the sides . . . it's going down, still going down . . . it's rather smooth . . . it's not unpleasant . . . it's going down, going down, going down, going down, going down very fast . . . a bit like the sensation of going down an elevator rapidly . . . it's as if the blood, the blood was rising to the head . . . you lose your breath a little because it's going down too rapidly . . . still going down . . . and now the hole is quickly getting wider . . . and now I'm in an empty space . . . a big empty space, a big black empty space that apparently doesn't have . . . walls . . . if there are walls, they're very far . . . and now there are no more walls . . . it's as if I had sunk . . . as if I had sunk right through the earth and now as if I was falling in space, in absolute absence of all other things . . . I'm falling in space . . . I'm falling straight, feet first . . . it's going down, going down, going down for a long time . . . it's going down at a certain speed at such a point that it's as if I am hearing the noise of . . . of the air brushing against my clothes . . . all this going down fast . . . my trousers are floating on my legs . . . my shirt as well . . . at a very great speed, and it's still going down . . . I sink inside there, I plunge inside of there . . . feet first, arms up in the air . . . still going down, going down all the time, and I don't see any horizon . . . it's black, it's the blackness in which I'm going down . . . now I can go down horizontally with my body . . . and now face first . . . I'm falling like a bird, a bird, like a bird that was killed and which falls like a stone . . . and I can see the void in which I'm sinking, toward which I'm going . . . I'm still falling in this empty space all the time . . . I'm falling indefinitely . . . there's no reason to stop . . . because . . . there's nothing at the bottom . . . I'm going down, I'm going down, I'm going down . . . still going down, going down all the time . . . we continue . . . still going down, still down, still going down . . . it's surprising that I don't meet with meteorites . . . maybe there's a glow of stars down at the bottom, maybe the glow of stars . . . maybe I'll be passing through a sort of Milky Way . . . no, they're not stars, they're only sparks from lights . . . Im passing through a sort of cloud of these sparks from lights . . . I'm still going down . . . there are still sparks from lights . . . I'm passing through a sort of Milky Way, through this cloud of sparks from the lights . . . I went through one there . . . it lights up the way for me, in such a way that I see myself now, my suit, my shirt . . . I can see myself because it creates a certain, a certain flash of sparks from these lights in which I'm plunging . . . as if I was diving through bubbles in water . . . the descent continues . . . and now horizontally I can stretch out my arms, and I start soaring like a big bird with huge wings . . . I'm soaring, I'm soaring . . . ah, down there at the bottom is hell . . . down there at the bottom is hell. . . ."

# 15. Visual Phenomena

The variety of spontaneous visual phenomena which occur during the practice of autogenic standard exercises (see Table 6, p. 143/1), and studies of visual elaborations associated with the series of meditative exercises indicate that such visual phenomena may vary from very simple (e.g., monochromatic, cloud-like formations) to highly differentiated cinerama-type productions. In an attempt to put some order into these visual phenomena a distinction of seven general stages has been made (see Table 33).

Many of the visual phenomena considered in Table 33 correspond to those observed by J. H. Schultz (*Über Schichtenbildung im hypnotischen Selbstbeobachten,* 1920)[1245,2379] and earlier descriptions by, for example J. Müller (1826),[G*] J. H. Jackson (1870, 1873),[G] L. F. A. Maury (1878),[G] W. Robert (1886),[G] G. T. Ladd (1892),[G] O. Vogt (1897),[†] S. Freud (1900),[G] Dr. Bezzola (1902, 1906),[G] V. Urbantschitsch (1907)[G] and L. Frank (1913).[G] Later N. Krastnikov (1923, 1920),[2422,G] E. Caslant (1927),[G] R. Assagioli (1927),[G] K. Tuczek (1928),[G] C. Happich (1932),[G] R. Desoille (1938)[278,G] and many others[25,29,32,57,58,59,60,104,106,118,119,278,294,347,352,377,415,418,427,472,473,609,625,628,658,667,686,716,717,719,725,726,727,730,789,793,832-839,875,881,886,887,888,891,894,897,1051,1108,1110,1149,1204,1245,1259,1274,1484,1528,1551,1552,1629,1723,1724,1725,1726,1728,1733,1754,1761,1771,1790,1829,1900,1907,2059,2136,2147,2148,2170,2200a,2209,2284‡,2302,2318,2326,2341,2342,2379,2383,2399,2421,2422,2432] have elaborated in some detail on the nature and dynamics of visual phenomena in connection with a variety of *therapist-directed (non-autogenic)* approaches.

The seven general stages (see Table 33) can be grouped into three major categories: (a) elementary phenomena (stages I-III), (b) intermediary elaborations (stages IV and V) and (c) advanced degrees of differentiation (stages VI and VII). While such general distinctions are of some practical help for clinical purposes, they are inadequate for quantitatively oriented studies. Since it has become evident that the different components of visual elaborations (e.g., structural, chromatic, dynamic, brightness) may undergo desynchronized changes concerning the nature of the background and structure of images, more refined distinctions appear to be necessary.

---

* See Glossary, Vol. VI.
† Vogt, O.: Spontane Somnambulie in der Hypnose. Z. *Hypnotismus*, 1897, VI, 77–93 (80 ff.).
   Marcinowski, Dr.: Selbstbeobachtungen in der Hypnose. Z. *Hypnotismus*, 1899/1900, IX, 5–46 (14,29 ff.).
‡ Ishida, Y.: Psychosomatic Medicine, *Jap. J. Nurs. Educ.*, 1968, IX, 10, 15–36.

TABLE 33.  *Stages of Brain-Directed Visual Elaborations during Autogenic Training and Autogenic Abreaction*

Stage    I:  *Static Uniform Colors*
Elementary stage characterized by one-tone color filling the entire visual field (mostly dark shades). Frequently described as "just nothing," "a blank" or "as if my eyes are closed." Less frequent are lighter shades (e.g.; silvery gray, yellow, pink, light blue).

Stage   II:  *Dynamic Polymorph Colors**
Elementary stage with more differentiated elaborations of chromatic, structural (e.g., cloud-like, shadows, vague forms) and dynamic features (e.g., various simple movements).

Stage  III:  *Polychromatic Patterns and Simple Forms†*
Elementary stage with more differentiated and specific elaborations of forms (e. g., disks, ovals, rings, dots, lines, textile patterns), colors (e.g., purple, brown, blue, green) and dynamic features (e.g., turning, coming closer, getting bigger, undulating, "flying," "falling").

Stage   IV:  *Objects*
Further structural and chromatic differentiation of mostly static objects (e.g., utilitarian, ornamental, symbolic, faces, masks, monsters) which appear on a background of mostly dark shades of colors. Realistic or unrealistic dynamic features (e.g., "a turning coffee pot." "a moving candle") may occur.

Stage    V:  *Transformation of Objects and Progressive Differentiation of Images*
Development of differentiated images (e.g., interiors, outdoor) of progressively increasing complexity with gradual transformations, displacements and polychromatic features. Realistic and unrealistic components may be distinguished. "Self-participation": rare.

Stage   VI:  *Filmstrips*
Highly differentiated and complex elaborations of structural, dynamic and chromatic elements. During advanced phases of this stage the trainee may occasionally change from the role of a passive observer into an active participant (e.g., "Now I am looking out of a window"). Realistic and unrealistic features are distinguished.

Stage  VII:  *Cinerama*
Highest level of elaboration with prolonged periods of self-participation (e.g., "I am choking my father," "I am being eaten up by a huge monster," "I am driving along a road"). Realistic and unrealistic developments may alternate.

---

* Stimulation of the occipital lobes (areas 18, 19) of conscious patients produced visual phenomena which are in general agreement with visual elaborations of stages II and III (Penfield, W. and Rasmussen, T.: *The Cerebral Cortex of Man.* The Macmillan Co., New York, 1950).

† See also Penfield, W. and Jasper, H.: *Epilepsy and the Functional Anatomy of the Human Brain.* Little, Brown & Company, Boston, 1954, 116 ff.

A quantitative evaluation of the *structural aspects* of visual phenomena requires consideration of (a) the background and (b) the structures which appear on a given background. Furthermore, it appeared necessary to make a quantitative distinction between (c) the variable degrees of structural differentiation, (d) the vagueness or precision of the structures elaborated by the brain, and (e) the amount of surface (of the visual field) covered by relevant structures. In general agreement with the seven stages of visual differentiation as given in Table 33, a corresponding number of levels of structural differentiations ranging from O to VII has been used (see Table 34). Furthermore, to facilitate scoring procedures, each level (i.e., I-VII) has been divided into five sublevels,* thus permitting a maximum score of 35 points for each of the structural aspects under consideration. Following the same pattern of differentiation, corresponding distinctions were made for the evaluation of the *dynamic aspects* of visual phenomena (see Table 34). In this connection a distinction between two categories appears to be indicated: (a) the slowness or speed of movements, displacements and transformations and (b) the quantitative variable of the visual phenomena involved (e.g., a small bright point moving from left to right; a stormy ocean filling almost the entire visual field).

Variations in *chromatic (achromatic) differentiation* and *brightness* are evaluated in a corresponding manner. In this area, however, it is necessary to make a distinction between (a) the brightness of the background, (b) the spatial quantity of the background, (c) the spatial quantity of the structure (e.g., a small black dot, a huge monster), (d) the chromatic differentiation of the structure (e.g., bichromatic object, multichromatic natural landscape), and (e) the brightness of the structure (see Table 35).

The evidence obtained from detailed analyses of autogenic abreactions mainly involving elementary and intermediary stages of visual elaborations indicated that each of the different categories may undergo significant changes without affecting the features of other categories of visual elaborations (*desynchronized changes*). For example, a change in speed from static to slow and then to very fast may occur without a change in color, brightness, nature of the background or structure (see Case 88, p. 208 ff.; Fig. 8a, b, c). Such observations led to the tentative conclusion that functionally, relatively independent brain mechanisms participate in the elaboration of, for example, structure, color or dynamics.

---

* Details are available on request.

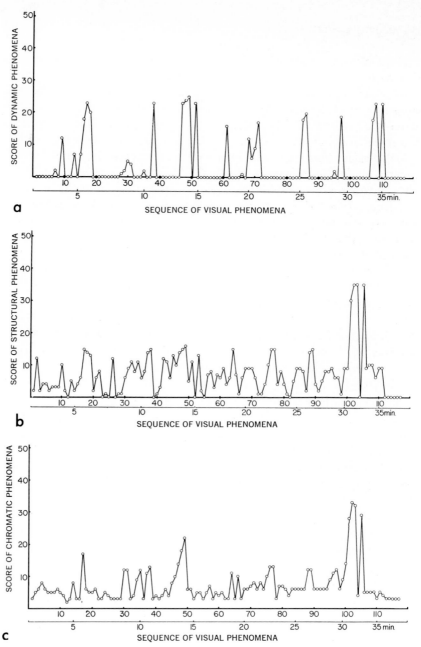

Fig. 8. Profiles of dynamic, structural and chromatic variations (AA 5, Case 88, p. 208 ff.) of largely elementary and intermediate stages of differentiation. A comparison of the three profiles conveys the relative functional independence of those brain mechanisms which participate in (a) dynamic, (b) structural, and (c) chromatic components of visual elaborations.

TABLE 34.  *Levels of Structural and Dynamic Differentiation of Visual Phenomena during Autogenic Abreaction*

| | Visual Phenomena | | | | |
| | Structural Differentiation | | | Dynamic Differentiation | |
| Levels | Surface of visual field involved | Structural differentiation | Precision of presentation | Quantitative aspects of involvement | Qualitative aspects (speed) |
|---|---|---|---|---|---|
| 0 | None (uniform) | None (uniform) | None (uniform) | None | None (static) |
| I | Up to 1% of visual field | Extremely simple | Very vague | Up to 1% of visual field | Extremely slow |
| II | 1–5% of visual field | Very simple | Vague | 1–5% of visual field | Very slow |
| III | 6–10% of visual field | Simple | Some lack of precision | 6–10% of visual field | Slow |
| IV | 11–25% of visual field | Medium | Medium (almost adequate) | 11–25% of visual field | Medium |
| V | 26–50% of visual field | Complex | Adequate precision | 26–50% of visual field | Fast |
| VI | 51–90% of visual field | Very complex | Very precise | 51–90% of visual field | Very fast |
| VII | 91–100% of visual field | Extremely complex | Microscopic precision | 91–100% of visual field | Extremely fast |

Since desynchronized changes of certain features tend to occur more frequently in the beginning of elementary and intermediary stages of differentiation, and since there frequently is a progressive development toward *synchronized changes* (i.e., different features undergo simultaneous changes in a functionally and thematically corresponding direction), it was assumed that there exist functional interrelations between each of the specific mechanisms (e.g., structure, color, dynamic) which are coordinated by another mechanism at a higher level of integration. In this respect it was noted that a decrease of desynchronized changes and a proportionate increase of synchronized changes appeared to be closely associated with a decrease of unreal features and a corresponding increase in the reality of features. This was viewed as an improvement of functional integration in a therapeutically desirable direction. It was therefore assumed that the brain-directed processes of autogenic

neutralization, while aiming at self-normalization, received their functional orientation and were guided by a participating *Reality Mechanism*. To facilitate quantitative evaluations, a tentative distinction of
unreality-reality levels (O-V) for each of the major categories of visual
components (i.e., structural, chromatic, dynamic) was made (see Table
36).

Information of a more general nature evolving from studies carried
out so far might interest the therapist who is confronted with a variety

TABLE 35. *Levels of Chromatic Differentiation and Brightness of Visual Phenomena during Autogenic Abreaction*

| | Visual Phenomena | | | |
|---|---|---|---|---|
| Levels | Brightness of Background | Surface of Visual Field Involved (background/object) | Chromatic Differentiation (object, structure) | Brightness of Object, Structure |
| 0 | Black | (Uniform/none) | None | Black |
| I | Almost black (e.g., purple-black, blue-black) | Up to 1% of visual field | Monochromatic | Almost black |
| II | Very dark (e.g., very dark purple, very dark blue, very dark brown or red, very dark gray) | 1–5% of visual field | Bichromatic | Very dark |
| III | Dark (e.g., dark blue, dark red, dark green, dark gray) | 6–10% of visual field | Trichromatic | Dark |
| IV | Medium (e.g., blue-green, red-orange, green, neutral gray) | 11–25% of visual field | Polychromatic with two predominant colors | Medium light |
| V | Light (e.g., yellow-orange, yellow, green-yellow, light blue, light gray) | 26–50% of visual field | Polychromatic with two predominant colors | Light |
| VI | Very light (e.g., yellow-white, white) | 51–90% of visual field | Polychromatic (very much diffentiated) | Very light |
| VII | Very bright (e.g., bright yellow, bright white) | 91–100% of visual field | Very high degree of chromatic differentiation | Very bright |

TABLE 36.  *Levels of Unreality and Reality of Visual Phenomena during Autogenic Abreaction*

| | Visual Phenomena | | |
|---|---|---|---|
| Levels | Structural Features | Dynamic features | Chromatic Features |
| 0 | No reality features | No reality features | No reality features |
| I | Very symbolic and deformed (e.g., shadows, spots, forms void of any particular meaning) | Very symbolic, highly artificial movements, very much deformed dynamics | Monochromatic |
| II | Very symbolic without deformation (e.g., nail, broomstick, ring) | Very symbolic but without deformation of reality dynamics | Achromatic or unreal |
| III | Symbolic but taken from reality (isolated from reality context; e.g., penis, breast) | Symbolic but taken from reality (isolated from reality context; e.g., umbrella, opening and closing) | Achromatic with some aspects of reality |
| IV | Some aspects of reality, but with certain modifications (e.g., deformed penis on normal body) | Some aspects of reality, but with certain modifications (e.g., empty sailboat on a lake) | Some aspects of reality, but with certain modifications |
| V | High degree of reality | High degree of reality | High degree of reality |

of problems of clinical management and for colleagues who are engaged in closely related fields of research.

The majority of psychoneurotic and neurotic patients who were selected for treatment with autogenic abreaction (see Table 37) report from the beginning of their first autogenic abreaction phenomena of advanced stages of visual elaboration (i.e., VI, VII). Another group (see Table 37) begins at elementary or intermediary stages and advances rather rapidly toward advanced stages with filmstrip or cinerama-type elaborations. Only about 20 per cent remain at elementary or intermediary stages (see Table 37, d, e). Although the patients who remained at elementary or intermediary levels were somewhat older and had practiced autogenic exercises for longer periods than the groups which began with advanced stages of visual elaborations, no criteria have been found so far which would permit a prediction of the nature of visual phenomena liable to occur during the first autogenic abreaction.

Once a patient's visual elaborations have reached stage VI or VII, functional regressions to lower levels of differentiation are infrequent (see Table 38, b; p. 195). In these instances brain-antagonizing forms of resistance (see Part I, Vol. VI) tend to interfere, and often the preceding autogenic abreaction (e.g., AA 1) had been particularly disagreeable or subject to premature termination. Others who remained at lower levels of differentiation during AA 1 tended to progress toward higher levels (see Table 38, a; p. 195). Of particular interest is the small group of patients who remain at, or regress to, elementary stages (i.e., I-III; see Table 38, b; p. 195; see p. 196 ff.).

TABLE 37. *Stages of Differentiation of Visual Phenomena during the First Autogenic Abreaction*
**(105 Psychosomatic and Neurotic Patients)**

| Stages of Differentiation of Visual Phenomena During AA 1 (Patients) | Visual Differentiation | | | | | | |
| --- | --- | --- | --- | --- | --- | --- | --- |
| | Elementary Stages | | | Intermediary Stages | | Advanced Stages | |
| | I | II | III | IV | V | VI | VII |
| (a) Begin immediately with cinerama-type elaborations (N=50) | — | — | — | — | — | — | **50** |
| (b) Begin immediately with filmstrip-type elaborations (N=13) | — | — | — | — | — | **13** | — |
| (c) Begin with elementary or intermediary stages of differentiation but who reach advanced stages (N=14) | 2 | 1 | 1 | — | 1 | ——→ **5** | |
| | 2 | 2 | 3 | — | 2 | ——→ **9** | |
| (d) Begin with elementary elaborations and reach intermediary stages (N=10) | 1 | — | 3 | 1 ——→ **5** | | | |
| | 1 | — | 4 ——→ **5** | | | | |
| (e) Remain at elementary levels of elaborations (N=10) | 3 | 3 ——→ **8** | | | | | |
| | 1 —→ **1** | | | | | | |
| | 1 | | | | | | |
| (f) Considerable variations of levels of differentiation (N=8) | ←——————— **8** ———————→ | | | | | | |

TABLE 38.   *Stages of Differentiation of Visual Phenomena during the Second Autogenic Abreaction*
**(104 Psychosomatic and Neurotic Patients)**

| Stages of Differentiation of Visual Phenomena During AA 2 (Patients) | Visual Differentiation | | | | | | |
|---|---|---|---|---|---|---|---|
| | Elementary Stages | | | Intermediary Stages | | Advanced Stages | |
| | I | II | III | IV | V | VI | VII |
| (a) Reach higher levels of differentiation in AA 2 than in AA 1 (N = 28) | | | | 1 | 1 | 1 | 9 → **12** |
| | | | | | 5 | | 5 → **10** |
| | 1 | | | 1 | 1 | → **3** | |
| | | | | 2 — → **2** | | | |
| | 1 ——— → | | 1 | | | | |
| (b) Regress to lower levels of differentiation in AA 2 (N = 11) | | | | | 2 | 5 ← **7** | |
| | | | | | 2 ← **2** | | |
| | | 1 ← ——— | | 1 | | | |
| | | 1 ← —— | 1 | | | | |
| (c) Remain at the same level of differentiation as in AA 1 (N = 57) | 1 | 3 | | | | 7 | 46 |
| (d) Considerable variations of levels of differentiation during AA 1 and AA 2 (N = 8) | | ← ————————— **8** ————————— → | | | | | |

Another relatively independent component is the "feeling tone" (i.e., pleasant, unpleasant) which is associated with autogenic abreaction involving visual elaborations. The effective component may be as unpleasant or pleasant during elementary stages as it may be at advanced stages. However, autogenic abreactions at the cinerama stage tend to have a better possibility of engaging in processes of thematic neutralization which appear to facilitate the experience of more positively oriented or agreeable feeling tones.

A rather close relationship exists between the frequency and forms of self-participation (see Table 44, p. 296) and the general level of differentiation of visual phenomena. The highest frequency with more direct forms of self-participation occur at the cinerama stage, significantly less frequently at the intermediary stages IV and V; and higher degrees of dissociation prevail during elementary stages (i.e., I-III).

## ELEMENTARY STAGES

Stages I, II and III are characterized by comparatively low levels of reality-related structure, dynamic and chromatic differentiation. The brain-desired use and the brain-designed nature of these elementary visual phenomena appear to serve different purposes. In certain instances elementary forms of elaborations are clearly associated with positively oriented brain-directed dynamics (e.g., "Bright Light Phase"). Under other circumstances they are associated with or, a consequence of *brain-antagonizing* forms of resistance (see Part I, Vol. VI). Other variations of elementary forms of visual phenomena are found to be a component of specific brain-desired maneuvers or they may appear in combination with certain forms of *brain-facilitating* forms of resistance (see Part I, Vol. VI). They may appear as a significant or as a marginal thematic element of a more complex topic of neutralization. Certain categories of elementary elaborations seem to serve recuperative purposes; others precede certain functional readjustments (e.g., thematic shift), or seem to be an expression of compensatory silence during periods where the brain-desired program of thematic priorities emphasizes other "channels."

These preliminary observations indicate that the elementary stages of visual elaborations cover a wide area of psychophysiologically important functions which are of therapeutic significance.

In many patients, phases of elementary elaborations occur in the beginning of treatment with autogenic abreaction and seem to play a preparatory role for brain-desired functional readjustments which are required to engage in elaborations of thematically more specific material. However, as the number of autogenic abreactions increases, such preparatory phases of elementary elaborations become shorter and finally disappear.

### Stage I: Static Uniform Colors

The lowest level of differentiation of visual phenomena is a uniform very dark or black visual field, devoid of any structure and lacking in dynamic features (stage I). Such monochromatic (achromatic) visual fields are encountered in all kinds of achromatic or chromatic variations. Generally seven groups of uniform visual fields can be distinguished:

A. Uniform visual fields which are a functional component of patterns which are restricted to elementary levels.

B. Uniform visual fields which are a manifestation of occasionally interjected, brain-designed antithematic functional regressions, which are assumed to serve recuperative purposes or which appear to be designed to allow a brain-desired functional readjustment (e.g., thematic shift).

C. Uniform visual fields which result from brain-antagonizing forms of resistance (usually dark).

D. Uniform visual fields which tend to occur when brain-directed processes of neutralization give particular priority to other thematic elements (e.g., massive motor discharges, intensive and prolonged vestibular modalities, intellectual elaborations, crying, pain).

E. Uniform visual fields which are indications for brain-desired termination (e.g., "Now it is as if everything has stopped . . . it is just gray . . . light gray . . ."; "Now it is just empty . . . nothing seems to come anymore . . ."; "It is light blue . . . very light blue . . .").

F. Unusually bright uniform visual fields associated with positively oriented feeling tones (Bright Light Phase) which tend to occur after advanced levels of neutralization of specific brain-disturbing material has been achieved.

G. Uniform visual fields which form a thematically related part of the topic undergoing neutralization (e.g., "Now I am lying on the pavement and I see the blue sky . . .").

*Stage II: Dynamic Polymorph Colors*

This stage of visual differentiation clearly distinguishes itself from stage I in various respects. The visual field may largely maintain the same color, but certain dynamic, spatial, structural characteristics indicate that various brain-directed mechanisms participate more actively. The "surface" may appear granulated, uneven, "far away," or "very close." There may be small flickering spots, rays of light (see Color Plate 1, No. 3, 12), cloud-like formations moving slowly, concentric movements (see Color Plate 1, No. 10, 11) or shadows which have a vague resemblance to something (see Color Plate 1, Color Plate 2, Color Plate 4). The participating chromatic components are usually relatively restricted and may follow an antithematic pattern of alternation (see Color Plate 3, No. 2 and 3, No. 7 and 8). These elementary phenomena, which are frequently observed during inital phases of the abreactive period, tend to be of transitory nature, leading to the more differentiated phenomena of stage III. Elaborations characteristic for stage II have been observed under the following circumstances:

A. As a normal component of elementary patterns which either may remain restricted to stages I, II and III, or which may be part of a preparatory phase with subsequent development toward higher degrees of differentiation.

B. In association with brain-antagonizing forms of resistance which induce a functional regression (usually with emphasis on darker shades of colors).

C. When brain-directed processes of thematic neutralization give functional priority to other thematically related modalities (e.g., motor discharges, vestibular phenomena, intellectual elaborations).

D. During developments which precede or follow a Bright Light Phase, or phenomena which come close to reaching the characteristics of a Bright Light Phase but actually cannot be considered as such. In these instances light colors (e.g., light yellow, silvery, very light gray) associated with agreeable affective components are predominant.

E. During terminal phases as part of brain-directed elaborations indicating self-regulatory termination (see Case 88, p. 208 ff.; Color Plate 4).

F. As a thematic component of more complex processes of neutralization (e.g., "I am lying on the beach and look at the sky . . . there are a few clouds . . . they barely move. . .").

*Case 84:* A 38-year-old female teacher (sexual deviation, depressive reaction, affective deprivation). During her first autogenic abreaction the visual elaborations remain restricted to alternating elementary stages I-III with emphasis on darker colors (see Color Plate 1). A progressive change toward lighter colors and more differentiated elaborations (stage IV) is reflected by the sequences of visual phases in AA 3 (see Color Plate 1).

*AA 1:* "The sky is getting blue and there is a bright spot in the center, this spot is golden (Color Plate 1, No. 1) . . . the color is becoming more yellowish and the blue is receding (No. 2) . . . now there are irregular circles and their lines are crossing each other (No. 3) . . . it's getting purplish-blue . . . this week I was more sensitive, and lying on my back arouses a readiness for a certain pleasure . . . everything continues to move around and changes from blue (No. 5) to red (No 6), then to yellow (No. 2) . . . there are always these circles (No. 3, 4, 12) . . . the lines are crossing each other (No. 3, 12) . . . when the colors are bluish there are no particular forms (No. 8) . . . when they are yellow (No. 2), the overlapping circles start again (No. 3, 12) . . . the blue is now darker and in the center it's purplish (No. 5) . . . the center is bright blue like a beautiful gem (No. 7) . . . now it's lighter . . . the circles are crossing each other . . . I really feel a deep desire to enjoy myself . . . now it's all blue and in the center it's green (No. 8) . . . now it's a mixture of colors . . . they always move around a bit (No. 9) . . . I would like to be on a meadow now, somewhere . . . with somebody whom I could love . . . caress . . . now the circles are getting bigger and seem to go further away (No. 10) . . . and they are sort of shrinking (No. 11) . . . and the colors get darker (No. 12) . . . now it stabilizes for a moment . . . the movements start again and the colors are getting brighter . . . on and off there is this golden spot in the center of a blue background (No. 1) . . . and then it changes to orange (No. 2) . . . now it's darker . . . blue, but not clear blue . . . the forms are crossing each other (No. 12) . . . they form sort of decorative patterns (No. 4, 12) . . . the colors are getting lighter and lighter . . ." (15 min.; termination).

*Case 85:* A 36-year-old female teacher (postoperative hypothyroidism, anxiety reaction, reactive depression, ecclesiogenic syndrome). In this case visual elaborations progressed very slowly toward more advanced levels of differentiation. AA 8 is still largely restricted to elementary levels II and III. Of particular interest are the characteristic chromatic differences between rather dark initial sequences (see Color Plate 2A) and the lighter shades of the terminal phase (see Color Plate 2B).

A. *Initial sequences:*

"The visual field is dark . . . almost nothing . . . two big circles, half dark in the upper part of the visual field (Color Plate 2, No. 1) . . . a darker circle in the center with a clear line under it which goes on each side (No. 2) . . . and now there is a lighter circle on the left (No. 3) . . . the rest is dark . . . and now there is a big half-circle on the bottom, from one corner to the other (No. 4) . . . half dark, and small bright spot on the left side . . . the background is half dark (No. 4) . . . all kinds of circles (No. 5) . . . a few big ones pass and are replaced by a small one in the center (No. 6) . . . which disappears very fast . . . more big circles which are moving from the center toward the top (No. 7) . . . a light ball on the right which moves down, below the center . . . all the rest is dark (No. 8) . . . a little lighter in the center . . . a brighter line which crosses obliquely from left to right . . . the visual field is dark with a lighter circle in the upper part, on the left . . . and there is a black dot in the center of the circle (No. 9) . . . a darker shade from the top comes down on each side to form a kind of a triangle (No. 10) . . . the triangle disappears slowly and is replaced by a lighter circle, which is on top at the right (No. 11) . . . now a lighter line which crosses diagonally from the left to the right . . . the rest is dark (No. 12). . . ."

B. *Terminal sequences:*

"A small black dot which gets bigger and forms an oval (No. 46) and then joins another long and very narrow oval on the other side . . . half dark with a light spot on the right part of the center . . . and a triangle from left to right

. . . pointing to the center, only two sides are visible . . . on the left there is a circle at the height of the point of the triangle (No. 47) . . . now the visual field is half dark (No. 48) . . . with a triangular shade on the right which comes down, passes the middle in the center and which diminishes at the bottom, on the right (No. 48) . . . a vague circle in the center (No. 49) . . . a dot which goes up to the left in a less darker area (No. 49) . . . the visual field becomes lighter on the right . . . three small dots above the center . . . a shadow appears on the left . . . below the center (No. 50) . . . it is less dark . . . the visual field is not clear . . . there are lights at the bottom on the right side going up to the top on the right . . . it's dark in the middle (No. 51) . . . it is lighter with a dark spot in the center (No. 52) which disappears . . . clear lines from left to right . . . which cross the visual field a little bit above the center . . . sort of curves . . . the left side is lighter than the right one (No. 59) . . . lighter at the bottom . . . there is a shape in the center which has two diagonal lines which meet . . . the small dot comes back very small and very dark (No. 54) . . . the left side is lighter . . . the lighter colors go up on the right with a slanted line (No. 54) . . . now the visual field is lighter . . . there is a curve going down toward the left . . . and the black triangle in the center comes back (No. 55) . . . the upper part becomes lighter . . . bright circles . . . bright lines going down to the center and to the left (No. 56) . . . it is lighter on the top part of the left side and below the center . . . the light part spreads to the right (No. 57) . . . now the visual field is brighter . . ." (54 min.; termination).

*The patient's commentary:*

"I think it is again the whole sexual area which expresses itself with less precision or, with more fear and anxiety. Generally the images are darker and rather vague, but the sex organs always come back in more or less recognizable shapes. The small black dot keeps coming back, like an obsession. What does that mean? A preoccupation? Anxiety? Fear? Does it mean that an entire dimension is still not free enough to come up or to show itself? Toward the end the light comes again, but it is slow and sort of timid in coming and penetrating the darkness or the half tones which seem to indicate fear and uncertainty."

*Stage III: Polychromatic Patterns, Simple Forms and Dynamics*

This stage is characterized by more concise structural elaborations of simple forms (e.g., ring, vertical bar, disks, ovals, geometric forms, organized series of dots, lines, textile patterns; see Color Plate 1, No. 4, 6, 7, 9; Color Plate 2, No. 2, 3, 9, 10, 46, 47, 50, 54; Color Plate 3, No. 6, 7, 9), more specific dynamics (e.g., rotating, coming closer, undulating, getting bigger) and an increase of chromatic elements. Patterns of monothematic repetitions and antithematic alternations may involve structural, dynamic and chromatic features. During initial phases of autogenic abreactions which emphasize elaborations at this level of differentiation, desynchronized antithematic changes (e.g., dark to light, yellow to purple-blue) can be observed (e.g., chromatic: Color Plate 3, No. 2 and 3, No. 7 and 9). When the dynamic component engages in antithematic dynamics, the following patterns are frequently described: centripetal–centrifugal (see Color Plate 1, No. 10 and 11), going further away–coming closer, getting bigger–getting smaller, turning clockwise–turning counterclockwise, and moving up–coming down. Similarly, antithematic elaborations of structural phenomena are encountered (e.g., disk–triangle; ring–bar). About five per cent of psychosomatic and neurotic patients (see Table 37, p. 194) tend to remain for a series of autogenic abreactions at this level. Although certain forms of brain-antagonizing resistance were present in each of these cases, other variables appear to be involved, the nature of which requires further investigation. In some cases, for example, it became evident that the patients did not give *carte blanche* to their brain, but used the description of the visual field as a convenient maneuver to help them avoid engagement in other less convenient topics (e.g., Case 85, p. 199 ff.). It is in this connection that it must be emphasized again that visual elaborations are only one sector among many others. It is therapeutically important that the patient understands clearly that passive acceptance means giving *carte blanche* to whatever the brain wishes to elaborate.

A unilateral preference or restriction to a description of visual phenomena implies therapeutically unfavorable restrictions, reduces the self-curative potentialities of the brain's self-regulatory mechanisms and may easily induce a variety of undesirable after-effects which are normally associated with program-related resistance and thematic avoidance (see Part I, Vol. VI).

In the majority of cases who begin with phases of elementary elaborations, stage III is preparatory for a progressive development toward more differentiated levels (see Case 86, p. 203; Case 87, p. 207, Case 86, p. 208; Color Plate 3; Color Plate 4). In other instances stage III elaborations may occur when brain-directed indications for termination are not respected (i.e., delayed termination, p. 84 ff.) or brain-antagonizing forms of resistance do not permit the brain to follow its own courses of thematic neutralization.

Patterns of autogenic neutralization which are largely restricted to elementary levels I-III (see Fig. 18, p. 304) are of therapeutic value. The opinion that only advanced stages of visual elaborations are therapeutically effective has not been supported by clinical observations. In this connection it is of psychophysiologic and therapeutic interest to remember that a variety of positively oriented progressive changes occur during autogenic abreactions restricted to elementary stages.

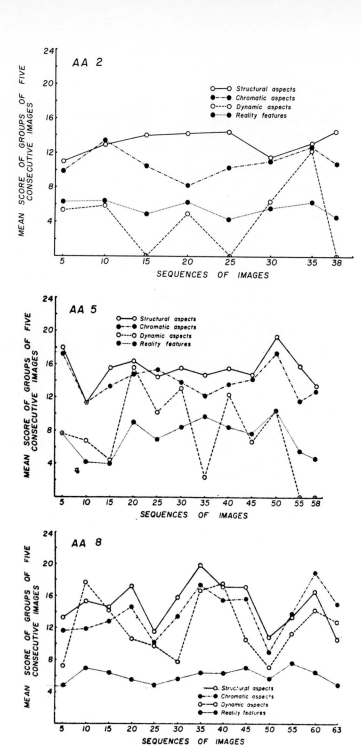

One of these changes is the significant difference in brightness of initial and terminal sequences of visual phenomena (see Case 85, p. 199; Color Plate 2A and B; Fig. 10). The progressive trend toward an increase of chromatic, structural and dynamic differentiation in each autogenic abreaction is also evident in longer series of autogenic abreactions. The brightness score is considered as one of the indications which reflect the progress of the therapeutic process (see Fig. 10).

As the brain-directed dynamics are permitted to continue their activities at elementary levels as long as they wish, there invariably comes a point of transition toward stage IV. This important transition, which usually is followed by a more rapid development toward advanced stages VI and VII, announces itself in a very gradual manner (see Case 86, elaborations indicating a transition to intermediary levels are in italics).

*Case 86:* A 31-year-old social worker (anxiety reaction, situational stress reaction, mild depression). In the following autogenic abreaction (AA 3) there occurs a characteristic development from an initial emphasis on stages I and II to a progressively increasing appearance of more differentiated visual elaborations of stages III and IV (see *italics*).

"Nothing special yet . . . [coughing] . . . it's rather blue . . . little light to the right [big sigh] . . . it's still rather blue-green, *like a blue-green circle toward the left* . . . [sigh] . . . *like lines of . . . like a sun with rays all around* . . . *a pale blue glow, a . . . a circle in the center, very pale blue, another one* . . . *another sun* . . . [sigh] . . . mmm . . . toes . . . it's black but it's like little, little white dots, very small . . . little white dots continuously moving on the black . . . *a pale blue opening* . . . [sigh] . . . it's much clearer much clearer glows . . . [cough] . . . oh, it's that again, it moves, I can't explain it, it's, it's rather black, *like white glows moving about* . . . [sigh] . . . as if something was, it's very black . . . [sigh] . . . it's still black . . . [sigh] . . . it's darker in the center . . . [sigh] . . . *it's darker in the center and lighter all around* . . . [sigh] . . . *somewhat green, turquoise . . . very green, black* . . . [sigh] . . . *it's still green . . . mmm . . . rather black* . . . [cough] . . . mmm *it turns green again, black* . . . [sigh] . . . *it's lighter toward the center, like in the distance, like a, a white circle in the distance that gets smaller and bigger,*

---

Fig. 9. Variations and progressively oriented changes of structural, dynamic, chromatic and reality components in AA 2, AA 5, and AA 8 (Case 85, p. 199 ff.). The closer correspondence of the profiles of structural, chromatic and dynamic components in AA 8 is considered as an indication of improvement of functional integration. The reality component does not yet participate in this progressive development and remains relatively stationary at a symbolic level of elementary unreality–reality features (see Color Plate 2).

it's still there . . . it gets smaller as it nears me, then no, it gets smaller as it goes farther away . . . [sigh] . . . it gets bigger . . . like a mauve glow around it . . . that moves back, the mauve glow comes nearer, still a dot in the distance, a mauve glow that's closer up, like a sort of horn more to the left . . . there's still a white dot in the distance, a mauve glow coming nearer, getting bigger . . . a white dot in the distance . . . the mauve glow is very close . . . [sigh] . . . disappears . . . nothing . . . like two eyes, turquoise-blue, mauve . . . a circle with rays . . . [sigh] . . . [sigh] . . . I feel more relaxed . . . it's rather blue . . . still blue, green with a few rays . . . blue-green and clouds . . . *fingers* . . . pale green, lighter, nearly white . . . it's still nearly white . . . [sigh] . . . eh . . . [big sigh] . . . gray-white . . . [cough] . . . a white circle in the distance, pink, black and white, between the two, a trefoil . . . darker . . . *steering-wheel, steering-wheel of a car* . . . [sigh] a paler circle that gets smaller, that gets bigger, that that gets smaller, gets bigger, gets smaller, gets bigger gets smaller, gets bigger, gets smaller . . . gets bigger, gets smaller . . . gets bigger, gets smaller . . . there's some pale blue in the middle that stays put, but it's all around that that gets bigger, that gets smaller, like the black that gets bigger then that gets smaller, and the blue circle stays put . . . gets bigger then gets smaller . . . the black gets smaller, gets bigger . . . [sigh] . . . the blue gets a bigger nothing more, it gets smaller . . . it's green, it's gray . . . gray, white clouds, blue . . . blue clouds then down below it's black . . . green . . . rays from the sun . . . [sneezing] . . . gray, gray, nothing, blue-gray, it's as if it was the sky, clear sky, nothing it's still the sky, blue sky . . . darker, still the sky . . . eh . . . blue-gray . . . *a white horn*

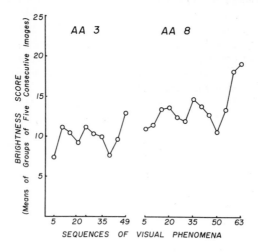

Fig. 10. Progressive increase of brightness during autogenic abreactions emphasizing visual elaborations at elementary stages (AA 3, AA 8, Case 85, p. 199; Color Plate 2A and B). Of particular interest is the low score of brightness during initial sequences, and the characteristic increase in brightness during terminal sequences.

in the center . . . like a gray sky with white clouds . . . [sigh] . . . it's still the gray sky with a black cloud in the distance . . . [big sigh] . . . still the gray sky, blue-gray, a black shape, I don't know what, the shape gets smaller . . . it's moving, gets smaller, gets still smaller . . . it starts off big then gets small like a circle, it's pale blue in the middle and black all around, it gets smaller, it gets smaller . . . lightning to the right . . . [sigh] . . . a pale blue sky . . . still a pale blue sky . . . a sprinkler toward the left . . . a nose . . . [sigh] . . . gray . . . a black circle that gets smaller . . . a white circle in the middle that also gets smaller . . . still the same thing, it's getting smaller all the time . . . [sigh] . . . it starts off big, it gets small like the opening of a horn that is getting smaller, that is getting smaller . . . [sigh] . . . it's gray . . . sad tones . . . mauve, black clouds, black dots moving about . . . blue sky with rays of the sun in the middle . . . [very big sigh] . . . rather dark but not black . . . again the dark sun with its rays in the middle, the rest is lighter . . . a much happier tone . . . still the same thing, the dark circle with dark rays on a light background . . . [sigh] . . . the rays are turning . . . still turning . . . fixed . . . aurora borealis . . . a bottle . . . a nose . . . [sigh] . . . clouds . . . a clear dot that showed up at the right, but that disappeared as soon . . . dark up above lighter down below . . . a few mountains down below . . . a blue-gray sky . . . a darker sky . . . a sadder tone . . . another circle that's getting smaller, that's diminishing . . . [sigh] . . . still the same thing . . . it gets smaller still the same thing, still the same thing, still the same thing . . . the background it blue-black . . . still the same thing, still the same thing, the background is blue-black, and it's a white circle that becomes, that diminishes, that diminishes like a horn . . . [big sigh] . . . [anxious voice] . . . it's rather blue . . . a nose . . . gray . . . *a rolling pin* . . . rather blue, like a road that gets smaller in the distance, that is wider up this way, it was white on a black background . . . a *telescope* . . . *a nose* . . . *a face, like the silhouette of a woman,* but eh . . . horizontal . . . forms that are moving about, but I don't know what . . . forms that are moving, that are getting smaller . . . again the sky which is blue, blue, blue . . . *a happy tone* . . . again a blue sky . . . [sigh] . . . darker . . . [tired tone] . . . *piano notes, fingers, corn on the cob, molded Jello,* forms that are moving toward the left . . . *a hand* . . . *a road that gets wider up this way, a white road on a black background* . . . [dull voice, sigh] . . . vague . . . [big sigh] . . . *nose* toward the left . . . circle that gets smaller, that gets bigger . . . pale circle on a black background, gets bigger . . . the background is pale, black forms disappearing . . . pale blue background . . . *a nose* . . . *boats or steeples on edge of a bank* . . . [sigh] . . . darker . . . sad . . . darker and a white square like a window up above . . . gray, but less dark . . ." (38 min.; termination).

## INTERMEDIARY STAGES

The intermediary stages IV and V cover the area of those visual elaborations which have not yet developed characteristics of a film-like nature (e.g., continuity, dynamics, higher degrees of self-involvement)

and which are no longer dominated by low reality level components
encountered during the elementary stages. During the first autogenic
abreaction, about 14 per cent of patients (see Table 37, p. 194) pass
rather rapidly through the intermediary stages and reach higher levels
of differentiation (i.e., stages VI or VII). Another ten per cent gets
temporarily arrested at stages IV or V, but most of these patients progress relatively fast to stages VI and VII during subsequent autogenic
abreactions. More detailed pattern analyses have suggested that stages
IV and V are levels of a preparatory nature which facilitate the transition from stage III to the highly differentiated stages VI and VII. When
a functional regression of the overall pattern from further advanced
stages (i.e., VI and VII) occurs, then these patterns of functional regression tend to remain at stage V and only rarely for brief periods
continue to stage IV. Furthermore, a number of observations have indicated that functional regressions from stage IV to elementary elaborations (i.e., I-III) occur more easily than functional regressions from
stage V to, for example, stage III.

*Stage IV: Transformation of Objects, Multichromatic and Dynamic
Differentiation*

As the patient's brain is given the opportunity to continue its self-
regulatory work of neutralization, the initial emphasis on elementary
elaborations diminishes. Increasingly more objects and reality features
(e.g., chromatic, dynamic) tend to appear. The time devoted to elementary elaborations decreases and the first objects tend to appear
during earlier phases of each abreactive period. Following a characteristic pattern of functional progression and regression (see p. 318), a
shift from isolated elaborations of objects to small series of objects can
be noted. Antithematic patterns become evident (see Case 87, Color
Plate 3, No. 15-18; 28, 30; p. 207 ff.), the series of objects becomes longer
and finally a continuity of objects with increasing complexity appears
and disappears as in an automatic presentation of slides. Initially all
kinds of objects (e.g., utilitarian, ornamental, symbolic, faces, masks,
monsters, animals, products of nature) are elaborated on a usually dark
background. As the process of neutralization advances, the background
colors become lighter or more realistic. The dynamic components (e.g.,
a rotating chandelier, an undulating bicycle) become less frequent, and
a progressively more realistic agreement between structural, chromatic
and dynamic elaborations indicates a development toward more adequate levels of integration (see Case 87; Fig. 9, p. 202 ff.; Case 88, p.
208 ff., Color Plate 4).

*Case 87:* A 38-year-old female teacher (see Case 84, p. 198). The visual elaborations during the patient's third autogenic abreaction begin with sequences (see Color Plate 3, No. 1-14) which in certain respects are very similar to the structural, chromatic and dynamic features observed during AA 1 (see Color Plate 1). However, the background colors are lighter. Later the initial emphasis on elementary elaborations (stages I-III) subsides, and a characteristic progressive development toward more differentiated structural and chromatic features with symbolic connotations (e.g., No. 15-17) becomes evident (compare also with Case 88, p. 208; Color Plate 4).

"I see absolutely nothing . . . there is a sort of intensive itchiness in both my hands and around the left wrist . . . I still don't see anything . . . it's a neutral color . . . as if one has the eyes closed . . . it's not gray and it's not white . . . this is not at all like the other times . . . I wonder if this is because of my psychological state . . . now there appears a blue center on a pale background (Color Plate 3, No. 1) . . . it turns but without changing its color . . . it is always the same thing . . . it's always a dark blue circle which is turning a little bit . . . that's all what I am seeing . . . the blue disappears all of a sudden . . . and I don't see anything anymore . . . it's hard to describe nothing . . . there isn't even any form . . . now there is a lighter spot in the center (No. 2) . . . it becomes lighter, like a sun going up . . . it becomes yellow, quite strong (No. 3) . . . always with a darker center . . . the yellow color is gone . . . the dot stays but it remains dark (No. 4) . . . now it's a neutral color, a faded color . . . gray, purple, very pale (No. 5) . . . certain parts of the purple become lighter (No. 6) . . . then the colors meet and form a purplish circle, the surrounding colors are lighter, yellowish (No. 7) . . . the colors inverse, the center is yellow and all around it's purplish (No. 8) . . . this varies between purple and yellow . . . purple in the center, yellow around . . . yellow in the center, purple around . . . without particular shape . . . the circle is not clear . . . a darker yellow with a few red lines across (No. 10) . . . all is gray without precise shape (No. 11) . . . the center becomes yellow again . . . with a darker spot in the center and there are rays all around (No. 12) . . . and all disappears . . . light gray in the center (No. 13) . . . a little bit of red mixed with the gray (No. 14) . . . the center becomes yellow again. . . . I see a wooden disk (No. 15) . . . now I see as a stick, something like a broomstick but without a broom (No. 16) . . . in natural wood . . . the colors become lighter and everything disappears. . . . I see the page of a catalogue with physics tools on it . . . very small pieces which make contact in electricity (No. 17) . . . I looked often at this page this week. . . . Now I see the corner of a gray stone house (No. 18). . . . A pink center which become luminous . . . (No. 19) . . . I have the impression of smelling something like vinegar . . . everything is gray again (No. 20) . . . the colors are transparent . . . they have an octagonal form with the opposed sides equal, two to two . . . it is similar to a table mirror (No. 21) . . . [*Can you look in this mirror?*] . . . it is already gone . . . now it is red (No. 22) . . . yellow, it looks like nice natural wood (No. 23), pale yellow and there are lines in the red . . . everything is neutral, almost white . . . lighter, then dark . . . nothing . . . it is as if the dot in the center is becoming an eye . . .

(No. 24) . . . not very clear . . . and it disappears . . . the tones are darker . . . a few rays of purple across (No. 25) . . . the center is purple and everything disappears again . . . now I see a timetable in front of me (No. 27) . . . like the one in our classes at the college . . . and it disappears . . . again it's yellow with an eye in the center . . . last time it was in the horizontal position, and now it is slanted (No. 28) . . . now it's purplish again (No. 29) . . . and it disappears . . . a newspaper folded in half (No. 30) . . . a sheet with problems to correct or to solve, I don't know (No. 31) . . . these things disappear very fast . . . on a gray background, I can see a cross with wide and short arms (No. 32) . . . the cross becomes yellow (No. 33) . . . and disappears . . . blue-gray in the background . . ." (termination).

As the progressively oriented development continues, the elaboration of isolated objects (e.g., a book on a dark brown background) tends to shift toward an increase of object-related environmental elements (e.g., a book on a table). Such increases in structural differentiation is usually associated with correspondingly higher levels of chromatic, dynamic and reality features which are approaching the characteristics of stage V (see Case 89).

### Stage V: Progressive Differentiation of Images

During this stage the images are no longer elaborated on an "artificial" out-of-context background but impress by their complexity (e.g., landscape, interiors, underwater scenes). The images may be a mixture of thematically distorted or symbolic elements and reality features. Generally, in comparison with stages IV and III, a further increase of reality elements (e.g., structural, chromatic, dynamic) ensues. The images tend to stay longer, and certain transformations of structural or chromatic features may occur. These dynamic features are regarded as preparatory manifestations of brain-directed functions which later participate in filmstrip and cinerama productions. Dissociative functions are decreased and certain forms of self-participation (see Table 44, p. 296) may occur on rare occasions for very brief periods. Such advanced degrees of self-involvement and very short interjected phases with filmstrip qualities indicate that the brain-directed pattern of functional progression and regression approaches stage VI (see Case 88; Color Plate 4; Case 89, p. 220).

*Case 88:* A 31-year-old student of theology who had recently discontinued his studies at a foreign university because he felt unable to work and practically unable to adapt himself to the new environment. Other complaints: fatigue, tension, difficulty in concentrating, reduced capacity to memorize, fear of not being able to study successfully, doubt about his future, indecision about his specialization, apprehension and fear when confronted with groups, difficulties in social contact, difficulty in praying, compulsive manifestations, feeling of inferiority and great need of approval, avoidance of responsibilities (anxiety reaction, mild depression, ecclesiogenic syndrome, hypotension, brady-cardia). Physical examination: B. P. 98/64, P. 56 reg., otherwise normal.

Details of the patient's history are reserved for research purposes except for the following: he grew up in a bourgeois, conservatively minded religious family setting with an authoritarian father. No auto-, homo- or heterosexual activities reported. During his college period he had superficial contact with a few girls, one of them "Jacqueline." After two minutes of passive concentra-tion on the standard formulas of the First Standard Exercise, he started de-scribing (see left column). The interpretation and comments (see right column) and the drawings (see Color Plate 4) are part of the therapeutic program which the patient carried out himself at home.

The pattern of visual elaborations (AA 5, Color Plate 4) shows a characteristic trend from initially static, structurally and chromatically rather undifferentiated phenomena of symbolic nature (stages I-III; e.g., Color Plate 4, No. 1-12) to more colorful, more dynamic (e.g., No. 37, 52-54), more reality-related struc-tural elements (stages IV and V). Toward the end (e.g., No. 82-85) more com-plex images with transitory self-involvement (i.e., No. 82: "And now I am looking out of a window") indicate that the development of visual elaborations approaches stage VI. This is followed by a self-regulatory terminal phase with functional regression to stages II and I with emphasis on light shades of colors (see No. 88-93).

The generally progressive trend is composed of alternating phases of func-tional progression and regression (see p. 318 ff.). The frequent occurrence of desynchronized changes of chromatic dynamic and structural features are viewed as indications that functionally interrelated although relatively inde-pendent brain mechanisms participate in the elaboration of such visual phe-nomena (see also Fig. 8, p. 190; Fig. 9, p. 202; Fig. 10, 204; Color Plate 3).

| The patient's verbal description during autogenic abreaction | Watercolor drawings of the various phenomena observed* | The patient's comments and interpretations of the phenomena observed during autogenic abreaction |
|---|---|---|
| "I see something like a dark ball in the center. . . . | —1— | "It is something static, something blocking, it is related to tension, rather non-specific. |

*See Color Plate 4.

| The patient's verbal description during autogenic abreaction | Watercolor drawings of the various phenomena observed* | The patient's comments and interpretations of the phenomena observed during autogenic abreaction |
| --- | --- | --- |
| Now this changes into something like a rather narrowed frowning eye . . . the background color is rather pale grayish brown . . . the eye is somewhat unrealistic. . . . | —2— | The eye is always there, it is disagreeable, perhaps my father's eye, the eye of authority, the eye of God; to the feeling of being observed, perhaps by myself, by my own conscience. I am rather inclined to think of my father. It is the type of narrowed, sort of frowning eye he had when he questioned us on certain delicate things. The oval shape makes me think of the vagina. |
| Now there is just a purple ball . . . it is in the center. . . . | —3— | The persisting reappearance of the circular shape strikes me. |
| And a vertically oriented oval form appears . . . changing into a horizontal oval while the purple ball in the center is getting darker. . . . | —4— | The oval forms have a female sexual connotation. A vagina with a tendency to close up, an entrance ready to close. It could be a mouth, a mouth ready to close, impossibility of talking, difficulty of communication. It could be a disguised eye. There is tension related to it. I think the vertically arranged ovals are more disturbing, more revealing—vagina—anxiety. The images with sexual connotation create some anxiety. It is as if I was waiting for them and fighting them at the same time. The fact that I feel unbalanced or retarded in that respect humiliates me undoubtedly. There certainly is anxiety in me. A lack of easiness in that direction. I believe that I have the impression that a woman who is a little smart would turn my head. This makes me afraid. I would like not to be impressed by all that. I wish I would not be so vulnerable as I think I am. |
| This is followed by forms . . . rather mixed up . . . the background has a tendency to change to purple. . . . | —5— | Purple is a funeral color. It seems to indicate the end of something. It is a background color, dark, not very appealing, a color which I respect but |

*See Color Plate 4.

| The patient's verbal description during autogenic abreaction | Watercolor drawings of the various phenomena observed* | The patient's comments and interpretations of the phenomena observed during autogenic abreaction |
| --- | --- | --- |
| A dark outline of a disk appears in the right section of the visual field . . . and there is a sort of purple current. . . . | | which I do not like. The Easter colors. A rest of attention seems to go with it. A sort of intermission. Resistance? A circle is the outline of a hole—Am I in the hole? |
| And now there another oval form like an eye. . . . | —6— | The eye is the most hostile image, that gives me the impression of being observed or, that one is aware of the fact that one is under observation. It is related to shyness and anxiety. |
| A light green oval is coming down from the upper part . . . it is rather mobile. . . . | —7— | Pale green is more peaceful, calmer, less anxiety. The mobility of the oval seems to indicate more vitality which at the same time is unstable. Green is a natural color. I like green, I like nature very much. 'Green' may also mean: not yet mature, lack of knowledge and experience—myself? |
| Now a dark form like a bird's neck . . . or, it could be a horse. . . . | —8— | It is a dark aggressive form, something mysterious, rather big. Penis? |
| A dark disk in the center . . . on a purple background changing into gray. . . . | —9— | The dark disk in the center is something blocking, one cannot look through it, it is dark and threatening, anxiety, inhibition, regression, resistance? |
| And now a wedge-like form is moving in . . . from the left side . . . it is rather pointed and becoming black. . . . | —10— | A breast? A penis? something agressive. |
| Now there is a purple round in the center and the whole upper part is purple . . . the upper part is still purple. . . . | —11— | (see 3, 4) |
| Now a sort of point came in from the right . . . it splits open. . . . | —12— | Something aggressive and persistent. |
| Like a mouth of a crocodile. . . . | —13— | A ferocious animal, threatening. |
| Now it looks more like the mouth of a viper with a small red tongue and many small teeth in a whitish jaw. . . . | —14— | An aggressive snake, a wide open mouth, an opening full of danger, anxiety. Something of electric quality, something like a trap which could |

*See Color Plate 4.

| The patient's verbal description during autogenic abreaction | Watercolor drawings of the various phenomena observed | The patient's comments and interpretations of the phenomena observed during autogenic abreaction |
| --- | --- | --- |
| | | cause death or hurt—forbidden fruit. The pasty white: sensuality, foam, sperm. |
| This changed suddenly and now I see something like an arm and three fingers like a claw with long nails. . . . | —15— | Something which becomes more aggressive, a claw-like hand—female? or anonymous or non-identified power. The devil? |
| Again there is a purple round in the center . . . it is still purple. . . . | —16— | (see 3, 5) |
| Something black . . . it looks like hair . . . like fur. . . . | —17— | Something sexual, hair, fur, the vagina. |
| Now something . . . I have the impression it looks like a heel seen from below. . . . | —18— | A strong heel, masculine, but not precise, male genital organ? |
| Again purple . . . it is still purple . . . the purple disappears . . . some gray . . . in the lower part. . . . | —19— | (see 5) |
| And flesh-color follows. . . . | —20— | The color of flesh, of a human body, not differentiated, disguised, sexual desire, something not yet differentiated, not acceptable. |
| And now there is the narrowed eye again . . . nothing special. . . . | —21— | The frowning eye appears again. One could say it is already enough to think of it, for it to appear readily as an image. |
| It is all purple . . . still purple . . . as if there are clouds . . . like currents of purple shades. . . . | —22— | (see 5) |
| Something like a nose . . . a whitish nose . . . and something red and green . . . and the nose is getting smaller and smaller. . . . | —23— | Something aggressive. Penis? Breast? I am often scratching my nose and put my fingers up into it. I do this in my room and I avoid doing it in public as much as I can. A hole in which someone likes to fumble around, a substitute for a vagina which one likes to visit, an unconscious desire, a pleasure. The red and green are not identified and may be related to the red lancet of the viper (see 14). The whitish color of the nose may be re- |

| The patient's verbal description during autogenic abreaction | Watercolor drawings of the various phenomena observed | The patient's comments and interpretations of the phenomena observed during autogenic abreaction |
|---|---|---|
| | | lated to the breast like shape—milk. There is something infantile and sensual about it. |
| I see something like a copper coin . . . with bright rays radiating from it in all directions. . . . | —24— | Something brilliant, radiating, round, a hole, attractive . . . a female symbol? |
| Many oval forms . . . with an eye in the center of the arrangement. . . . | —25— | (see 2 and 4) |
| Now it is a sort of black trumpet . . . as if seen from above . . . as if facing me. . . . | —26— | An attracting hole, something round and bent, leading nowhere, black and dark—why? An opening and a funnel shaped hole: vagina? Something which produces sound—the voice of the conscience which is crying something? |
| Now a bluish greenish round mass . . . with many small whitish dots in it . . . this changes into a diffuse bright something . . . like a source of light . . . rather diffuse illumination. . . . | —27— | Something green with small round structures, like ovules or seeds in an ovary, or perhaps drops—ejaculation? A fruit? A female symbol, forbidden fruit? (see 7) Something getting lighter, more vital, sort of vitality. |
| Something like legs . . . a funny sort of legs . . . like legs of a chair . . . they are wooden legs and rather strong. . . . | —28— | Legs of a chair, legs: sexual symbol. Also a symbol of force and prestige. Legs of a woman with the upper part missing. Dark like rubber gloves— boots. |
| Now there is an oval form with a big coated tongue . . . the tongue is changing from a flat into a hollow shape. . . . | —29— | Vagina and a coated tongue. Penis? This has a sensual attraction similar to the whitish nose-like structure of 23. Symbol of a penis which penetrated whatever that may be or rather something coming out of an opening, 'French kiss'? |
| The image disappeared and now it is purple . . . the purple is more intensive in the upper and in the central part of the visual field. . . . | —30— | Again purple: interruption, rest period, intermission. |
| Now there is a black vertical bar on a grayish background. . . . | —31— | Clearly a phallus. Obstacle, resistance? |
| Again there is the strongly frowning eye. . . . | —32— | Again the hostile, always observing eye (see 2 and 4). |

| The patient's verbal description during autogenic abreaction | Watercolor drawings of the various phenomena observed | The patient's comments and interpretations of the phenomena observed during autogenic abreaction |
| --- | --- | --- |
| A starfish in bright orange . . . the starfish disappeared . . . and. . . . | —33— | A living water creature, its somewhat rough texture is clearly defined. A human person? A woman with arms and legs? The color is attractive like the color of the copper coin (see 24). |
| Now I see something like a huge dark rock. . . . | —34— | Something mysterious, impressive, powerful, obstacle, blocking the view, resistance? |
| This has changed . . . and now there is an eye on the left side . . . looking upwards into the air . . . the colors are beige and purple. . . . | —35— | A side-view of an upward looking eye, rather delicate, a triangular structure as seen before but not in this particular way—as if looking from below at the rock, trying to see beyond the things. Myself? Hope, desire, looking far away. |
| Now it looks like skin . . . as if a blanket has been partly removed from a person lying somewhere. . . . | —36*- | Sexual connotation. |
| I see something like falling water . . . one can see the water running . . . it is running quite well . . . it is running quite well . . . it is still running down . . . it is a sort of a fountain-like spring . . . it is still running . . . and one can see rays in the falling water . . . the foam is rising into the air. . . . | —37— | A running source, very clearly reflecting water: ejaculation. It is running from top to bottom. The blue color is a problem. It is running in the vagina for a rather long time. A flowing river, healthy water. I always liked water. I do not remember any disagreeable experience with water. Waterfall: something natural and powerful. |
| Now I see a form like a nose changing into something like an arm . . . the arm is moving . . . and there is something which looks like a shape of a waist. . . . | —38*- | Female quality, sexual connotation. Something which is not dangerous. |
| The picture disappeared and it is all purple . . . and now I see a side-view of an eye . . . the eye is on the left side . . . the eyebrows seem to be rather close. . . . | —39— | Again purple and the hostile eye—the censoring eye follows. |
| Now just broken lines . . . the color is now pale . . . sort of brown beige . . . it could be flesh. . . . | —40*- | Undifferentiated. Background more neutral. Sexual connotation. |

*The patient did not draw this image.

| The patient's verbal description during autogenic abreaction | Watercolor drawings of the various phenomena observed | The patient's comments and interpretations of the phenomena observed during autogenic abreaction |
|---|---|---|
| And now I see a spoon resting on something. . . . | —41— | Male and female qualities—'*Manger à la même écuelle*' (to live on intimate terms together). |
| A bigger spoon . . . like a soup ladle. . . . | —42— | Something bigger and brighter with a lightning-like effect: attractive, '*chatoyant.*' |
| Now a triangle pointing down. | —43*— | Related to a female genital area, a breast of a lying person, something aggressive. Perhaps a disguised penis. |
| Another triangle pointing down . . . something like a ribbon. . . . | —44*— | |
| And now it looks like the legs of a red spider arranged in a triangular form. . . . | —45*— | I was always afraid that spiders would sting me. It is a disagreeable symbol. |
| Now I see a sort of chandelier in red . . . it is turning horizontally around a sort of axis. . . . | —46— | It is something which is producing tension. The inconsistent red seems to be related in some way to the red lancet of the viper (see 14) |
| This disappeared and in the center there is a sort of stick or something like a statue. . . . | —47— | A phallic symbol. Something without life, artificial, unreal. |
| Now there is a head of a seal with two big teeth . . . it is looking upward . . . and one can see its mouth. . . . | —48*— | A menacing animal, related to 14. |
| Now two wooden legs. . . . | —49*— | Related to 28. |
| A mixture of red and orange like a sort of garland . . . with spots of pale purple. . . . | —50— | A colorplay: impression of animation and more vitality. |
| A small wheel. . . . | —51— | Something round, female quality, with a hole in the center for an axis: sexual connotation. |
| And now I see a small bicycle moving up and down in front of a horizon which is moving in a wave-like fashion . . . the bicycle disappeared. . . . | —52— | Two wheels and two triangles seem to be related to the elementary forms I have seen before. There are no pedals, they are not necessary. The horizon is dynamic. |
| And now I see something like a balloon . . . the yellowish balloon is | —53— | The yellow images seem to start here. Yellow: lighter, brighter, less hidden, |

*The patient did not draw this image.

| The patient's verbal description during autogenic abreaction | Watercolor drawings of the various phenomena observed | The patient's comments and interpretations of the phenomena observed during autogenic abreaction |
|---|---|---|
| ascending . . . it is going up and down . . . one can see the yellowish cables very clearly . . . the yellow is getting brighter . . . | | more objective? Purple and yellow are in a way complementary colors The yellow is more peaceful and neutral and also more stable. The balloon is a combination of a round and triangular structure. Why are the cables (holding a sphere-like structure) of particular interest? There seems to be a relation with the legs seen before (see 28, 49). The whole thing is going up, up into the air—away from reality? |
| And now I see a star . . . turning very fast toward the left. . . . | —54— | The form seems to have a female quality (see 33 and 24). It is very dynamic and full of tension. Why is it turning toward the left? |
| Something dark in a bright yellow field, which has a tendency to become pale . . . it is still yellow. . . . | —55— | Something dark in a yellow field, something mysterious, not clear in my mind. |
| And in the center there are two forms arranged like the outline of an hour-glass . . . it is still yellow. . . . | —56— | A very schematic form, barely visible, on a yellow background. Sexual connotation. |
| One can see the abdomen of somebody . . . it is rather vague . . . yes . . . that's it . . . the abdomen with a sort of dress covering the genital region. . . . | —57— | A sort of red dress but with fittings like the dress of the Middle Ages. The attention is focussed on the lower triangle, the lower abdomen. |
| It has changed a bit. . . . | —58— | The transformation reveals very clearly a male lower abdomen with enlarged genital organs, at times covered with something dark; ambiguous situation, attraction, inhibition, rejection, resistance? |
| Round forms in a vertical superposition. . . . | —59— | I am not sure of the meaning 'two.' |
| Now I see a sort of stone . . . a sort of crystal . . . mica . . . it is lemon-yellow. . . . | —60*– | Related to 54 and 24? |
| An inclined oval with another oval form superimposed on it . . . it is yellow. . . . | —61— | Related to 4, 5, 6 etc.? |

*The patient did not draw this image.

| The patient's verbal description during autogenic abreaction | Watercolor drawings of the various phenomena observed | The patient's comments and interpretations of the phenomena observed during autogenic abreaction |
|---|---|---|
| It is quite yellow . . . like the sun. . . . | —62— | Related to 24, 33, 54? |
| In the center it is now rather dark. . . . | —63— | Related to 1, 4, 9, 17, 47? |
| A sort of purplish shade changing into yellow. . . . | —64— | |
| The entire field is yellow. . . . | —65— | |
| There are round forms . . . which now look like yellow mountains. . . . | —66— | Female connotation. Obstruction on a road to the horizon. I always wished to climb a mountain, to go up to the top, to dominate the landscape and to embrace the horizon. Yet, I still have to climb the mountain. All mountain adventures seem to have a sexual component. |
| There is a huge mountain . . . it looks like a pyramid with a sort of castle on the top . . . the mountain changes its shape and rises. . . . | —67— | Something blocking the view, something hard, something unaccessible, barren and forbidden, the mountain of Sinai 'où Dieu parle d'une façon terrible.' A pyramid could be a firm breast. I also think of the mountain of Sinai where the Ten Commandments were proclaimed. A sort of symbolic superego, a call to order. There is something important on the top, nipples? Something rising up into the air: erection? |
| There is a sort of pole rising on top of the mountain. . . . | —68— | Clearly a phallic symbol. |
| Now it is all yellow. . . . | —69*- | |
| And now there is a dark spot in the center. . . . | —70*- | Something blocking, it is dark and threatening, anxiety? Inhibition? Resistance? |
| Now it looks like ears and the neck . . . the hairline of somebody seen from behind. . . . | —71— | I think it is a man seen from behind, afraid to face something, or an enormous genital organ? |
| The picture is changing . . . and now one can see the ears and the chin particularly well . . . it is a sort of caricature. . . . | —72— | Sexual connotation, afraid to face somebody. The ear may be a symbol for somebody who listens, who is submissive, who does not talk, who receives orders, who is tired and disgusted with this. Unnatural attitude. |

*The patient did not draw this image.

| The patient's verbal description during autogenic abreaction | Watercolor drawings of the various phenomena observed* | The patient's comments and interpretations of the phenomena observed during autogenic abreaction |
|---|---|---|
| Now there is a sort of big point . . . pointing downward . . . the field is still yellow. . . . | —73*– | Something aggressive, phallic symbol, sexual aggression? Related to 8, 12, 31, 43? |
| The field is yellow with a round form in the center. . . . | —74*– | Related to 63? |
| Now it looks like small hills . . . like the mountains I saw before. . . . | —75*– | Related to 66? |
| A sort of pyramid reappears. . . . | —76— | Related to 67 and 68? |
| Now it looks as one may see it from a flying airplane . . . and on top of the mountain there are sorts of trumpets . . . and one can see the shafts of the trumpets particularly well. . . . | —77— | Now I am flying over the mountains, this is a sort of domination of something I have overcome? The trumpets are sort of mysterious outgrowths, sexual connotation, attractive vagina, penis? Related to 14, 26, 28? |
| The field is yellow and now there are very thin legs . . . they become sort of deformed . . . the legs are still there and very long . . . the color is whitish. | —78— | Legs leading nowhere or, leading toward something which is veiled. The whitish color has sexual quality. Related to 28? |
| Now there is a rather vague spot in the center. . . . | —79— | Something dark, mysterious, not clear. |
| Now there is a rear part of a car . . . of a modern car. . . . | —80— | We never had a car at home. To me it seems symbolic, something strange, something which could make me afraid, the modern way of living, the life I do not know. The pointed fins seem to be of particular interest. A stopped car, it could be a disguised rear of a person. Why the fins? It is somewhat impressive. A car means success in life and is related to virility, self-assertion. |
| Now there are roofs of houses . . . covered with snow. . . . | —81— | The houses are not clear. The white snow on the roofs is very thick. The cool snow covers something. |
| And now I am looking out of a window and see a landscape with trees. . . . | —82— | A peaceful country house landscape seen from inside through a window, trees and leaves, something attractive, green is dominating (related to 7, 27?). However, it is still a view through a window. |

*The patient did not draw this image
*See Color Plate 4.

| The patient's verbal description during autogenic abreaction | Watercolor drawings of the various phenomena observed* | The patient's comments and interpretations of the phenomena observed during autogenic abreaction |
|---|---|---|
| Now a woman near a tree . . . the person is sitting and wears a large and very surrealistic dress . . . the arms and breasts are also very surrealistic. . . . | —83— | There is a lot of green, a tree, and lying on the meadow a very surrealistic or cubistic woman in a long wide and colorful dress which covers her feet. Anxiety, no doubt she is waiting for me. I do not remember the face, it was unexpressive. |
| Now it looks somewhat like Christ in agony . . . drooped forward. . . . | —84— | It is much closer now. The dress has still many colors but the head is sort of hidden, as if not to frighten somebody. Related to 71? |
| The field is yellowish, pale . . . and now I see a smiling face of a Mrs. Kennedy-type girl. . . . | —85— | Now only the face appears from behind the tree: a Mrs. Kennedy-type, dark hair, smiling, an inviting face, not frightening, creating a feeling of easiness, with a somewhat protective expression. The tree as a phallic symbol is also there. I once met a girl, her name was Jacqueline and I was quite impressed by her natural ease. |
| The picture disappeared and on a yellowish-green background I see a shape like a small 's' . . . like a curl of hair and this is getting bigger and bigger . . . and the lower part of the 'S' is twisting. . . . | —86— | The 'S' seems to convey vigorous power. It is aggressive and appears exactly in the genital area of the preceding image. Snake? Tapeworm? |
| Now a sort of a triangular structure forms and starts rising like a mountain . . . or like a rocket . . . and inside of it there is a form like a stick . . . and one can distinguish two sorts of legs. | —87— | Penis? Erection? Discharge? |
| Now it is all purple. . . . | —88— | A phenomenon of illumination accompanied the image. |
| And it changes into a beautiful blue. . . . | —89— | The blue was like a summer sky, quite striking, considerable luminosity, almost blinding the eyes. |
| It is still blue . . . the blue is getting less beautiful and pale. . . . | —90— | |

*See Color Plate 4.

| The patient's verbal description during autogenic abreaction | Watercolor drawings of the various phenomena observed | The patient's comments and interpretations of the phenomena observed during autogenic abreaction |
|---|---|---|
| It is more yellowish . . . a dirty yellow. . . . | —91— | 90–93: Variations of background, less pleasant, instability. |
| And it turns more to yellow. . . . | —92— | |
| Now it is yellowish-greenish. . . ." | —93— | |
| (Termination, total time: 38 min.) | | |

*Case 89:* An 11-year-old student who had learned the standard exercises and who occasionally experienced some anxiety in school. In AA 5 the visual elaborations show an alternating pattern of functional progression and regression involving stages I to VI with emphasis on stages IV and V. After about 15 minutes a few short filmstrips (*italics*) appear. In contrast to the preceding case (Case 88, p. 208 ff.) a significantly higher level of reality elements is noted.

"I see a chess board . . . it is all orange . . . I still see orange . . . I see my teacher's face in orange . . . I still see orange . . . I feel warm all over . . . except my feet are a bit cooler . . . I see green [yawning] . . . I still see green . . . I see green with purple in the middle . . . I still see green . . . I see black hair on the back of a head . . . I see a black hat . . . purple . . . yellow . . . I see purple with yellow in the middle . . . I see a crocodile's mouth, opened . . . a person sitting on a chair . . . it is all blue . . . purple . . . a pair of black pliers . . . an old building . . . [yawning] . . . a young boy in a fireman's suite . . . I see the back of a car stopped at a stop sign . . . I see purple with yellow in the middle . . . [yawning] . . . yellow with purple in the middle and now it is all yellow . . . [eyelids twitching] . . . I see orange . . . a face of a man in a sort of stagecoach window . . . the face of a rough looking man with a beard . . . a car . . . a middle-aged lady sitting on a sofa . . . two gingerbread men . . . [yawning] . . . [twitches in various parts of the body] . . . purple . . . purple with yellow in the middle . . . a purple mask . . . a shovel in a blue pail . . . and old man . . . trees . . . and bushes like a hedge and a road . . . *a person riding on a bike on the same road* . . . a telephone pole . . . a big wheel of a stagecoach . . . a modern train . . . a train station . . . *another train moving across the country* . . . telephone pole . . . a truck . . . buildings . . . a ladder on whitish-grayish background . . . a wagon . . . the rigging of a ship . . . the white hull of a ship seen from above . . . a motorboat . . . a bench . . . a wheelbarrow full of earth . . . my little sister lying on a field . . . and there is a big box beside her . . . a girl's face . . . *two people wrestling seen from above* . . . purple with yellow in the middle . . . [yawning] . . . a red mailbox . . . three or four toy poodles; they are gray . . . *a man walking across the street* . . . a bus stop . . . two shovels leaning against the wall . . . building

. . . a car . . . a screwdriver . . . a chair . . . two boys . . . a picture . . . wrapped up soap on shelves . . . a shoe . . . a glass . . . a paper clip on gray-whitish background . . . [yawning] . . . I feel tired . . . a gray carpet . . . my mother . . . a basket . . . an egg . . . my mother again . . . a ringbook full of paper . . . a girl's face . . . a pair of scissors . . . a big coil of rope hanging on a hook . . . [yawning] . . . a book . . . a car . . . [right shoulder twitching] . . . a small calendar . . . a dog . . . *a man shoveling* . . . [both legs twitching] . . . I see numbers . . . I am feeling very tired . . ." (31 min.; termination).

When during advanced developments of stage V, active self-participation occurs for the first time, other progressively oriented changes tend to follow (see Case 90). For example, the images tend to become more complex and stay longer. Frequently one is left with the impression that the brain elaborates such relatively neutral and comparatively long-lasting "exposures" to facilitate and encourage further episodes of "self-participation" (see Case 90).

*Case 90:* A 23-year-old student (anxiety reaction). The following passages are characteristic for changes toward more complex and more differentiated visual elaborations after "self-participation" (sequence 70) has occurred.

| A. Before "self-participation" | B. After "self-participation" had occurred for the first time |
|---|---|
| *(sequences 50-69)* | *(sequences 71-90)* |

"A mountaingoat . . . I see part of a box . . . it could be a table . . . wood construction . . . a barrel . . . headlight of a car coming toward me . . . a swordfish . . . an octopus . . . the eye . . . it's closed now . . . green on black, changing continually . . . a building, a square building . . . a hand . . . a white piece of paper . . . checkers . . . many, many little things . . . like modern art . . . windows dark outside . . . some legs . . . cuckoo clock . . . trees . . . flashes of blue on black . . . I see a window with a bright sky outside and red mountains . . . I see a horse grazing in the grass. . . ."

*"I see a banquet, it's a very large room with tables, people sitting and a very high ceiling. The tables are very long with lots of food and candles . . . I see a house, a brown house with windows with white rim and the roof with white rim . . . a geometric figure . . . I see a church, the door is open but it is black inside, inside it is a black-red color . . . up at the altar there are candles burning . . . I see a wooden wheel . . . a white card . . . a knife . . . a knife with a black handle . . . sticking in the wall . . . I see a cart, a luggage cart at the airport . . . a trailer with a tractor pulling it . . . I see a labyrinth . . . I see figures, mathematical figures . . . just abstract drawings . . . I see a room with a picture on the wall, a modern picture, it looks very comfortable, beige color, and furniture and there is a black sort of padded bench . . . newspaper . . . I see a notebook, a pile of notebooks . . . a thermometer . . . newspaper again . . . a triangle . . . a hand with long nails."*

## ADVANCED STAGES

The most obvious features distinguishing the visual phenomena of stages VI and VII from the intermediary stages IV and V are the film-like dynamics and the continuity of such visual elaborations. Indications of increasing self-involvement are closely related and, during cinerama patterns, tend to develop toward prolonged phases of "active self-participation" (see Table 44, p. 296). Associated with such manifestations of higher levels of functional integration is a further increase of reality features with thematic reproduction of experiential material.

About 75 per cent of patients (see Table 37, p. 194) reached advanced levels of visual elaborations during the first autogenic abreaction, and only 4 patients of this group regressed to stage V during AA 2. Over 80 per cent of psychosomatic and psychoneurotic patients tend to remain at advanced levels during their second autogenic abreaction (see Table 38, p. 195). This percentage increases with the number of subsequent autogenic abreactions. These figures indicate that visual phenomena at advanced stages of differentiation are an essential component of brain-directed processes of neutralization. However, it must be remembered that the processes of brain-directed neutralization are multithematic in the psychophysiologic sense, and it is unusual that processes of neutralization are confined to visual elaborations. In many instances and sometimes for prolonged periods, depending on the brain-designed program of thematic priorities (see p. 251 ff.), thematically related visual elaboration are of secondary or marginal importance. It is therefore a technical error to give a patient the impression that visual phenomena are therapeutically more important than other brain-directed elaborations (e.g., motor discharges, crying, intellectual elaborations, vestibular modalities). Undue emphasis on visual phenomena interferes negatively with brain-desired self-regulatory readjustment of other modalities of brain-disturbing material which may be of greater pathofunctional potency than those thematic components which are participating in determining the nature of visual elaborations.

### Stage VI: Filmstrips

Brief phases of film-like elaborations, such as "a train moving across the country," "a waterfall with lots of water coming down," "cars driving along the highway," animals or persons in action are initially interjected in functionally progressive and regressive patterns which emphasize visual phenomena of the intermediary stages (see Case 89, p. 220). These short filmstrips tend to occur more frequently and are of longer duration as the brain-directed processes of neutralization are given adequate opportunity to continue their self-regulatory work. Finally, a filmstrip may last several minutes or even fill a large portion of the central abreactive period. The chromatic features are usually highly differentiated and generally realistic. Achromatic (black and white) filmstrips are rare. When phases of such exceptional elaborations are reported, the relative lack of color is usually associated with vagueness of structure and blurring, or they are described as "a washed-out film." As the visual elaborations gain in complexity and differentiation (i.e., dynamic, structural, chromatic, realistic) there appears to be an increased tendency toward more active forms of self-involvement (see Table 44, p. 296). Mostly during relatively neutral phases patients describe the functionally important change from the role of a "passive observer" into an "active participant." This transition toward self-participation comes about in a matter-of-fact way. The patient simply describes, for example: "Now I am driving along the road," "I am getting into the car," "I am looking out the window," "I try to open that door," or "I am going up to the house." These simple and relatively neutral modalities of self-participation are initially limited to phases of brief duration. However, as the brain-directed developments aim at larger functional flexibility at lower levels of dissociation, a shift to a predominance of cinerama-type elaborations comes about (see Fig. 11).

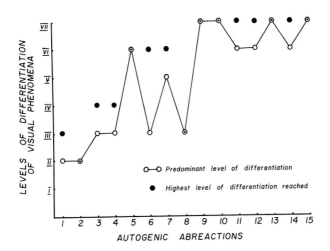

Fig. 11. Evolution of progressively increasing levels of differentiation of visual phenomena during 15 autogenic abreactions (24-year-old student; sexual deviation, anxiety reaction, multiple psychophysiologic and phobic reactions, ecclesiogenic syndrome).

## Stage VII: Cinerama

This highest level of differentiation of visual elaborations is usually associated with correspondingly high degrees of functional flexibility, providing optimal conditions for differentiated and multithematic processes of brain-directed neutralization. Spontaneous age regressions and spontaneous age progressions, transsexual transformations, engagement in violent dynamics of aggression or all imaginable activities of a sexual nature occur at this level of differentiation. Material of experiential nature (e.g., fight with a teacher) and disturbing material of non-experiential origin (e.g., suffering in hell, dying) may participate in highly complex and variable cinerama productions. Initially, cinerama patterns are of shorter duration, and functional regressions to stage VI tend to occur easily. Later these cinerama elaborations may continue for one or two hours or even longer.

Brain-antagonizing and brain-facilitating forms of resistance may participate in bringing about temporary functional regressions to stage VI, to intermediary or even elementary stages (see Part I, Vol. VI).

# 16. Motor Phenomena

From a series of polygraphic studies and other observations it is known that variable intensities of motor impulses are released during the practice of autogenic standard exercises (see Table 3, p. 28[887,888]; Table 2, p. 31/I; Table 4, p. 37/II; Fig. 3, p. 20/III, Fig. 5, p. 25/III; Fig. 6, p. 26/III; Fig. 8a, p. 48/III.[1022,2019,2021,2073,2093,2094] The brain-directed phasic activity of striate muscles may be limited to a certain muscle, to a specific group of muscles or may be of a more generalized nature involving larger portions of the *somatomotor system.* The intensity and duration of such motor discharges is variable. Since electromyographic studies have verified that during the autogenic state motor discharges occur which the trainee does not notice, it appears appropriate to make a general distinction between *subliminal* motor phenomena and other motor discharges of which trainees are aware. A similar distinction is applicable to a variety of spontaneously occurring *visceromotor* phenomena (see Table 5, p. 31[887,888]; Table 2, p. 31/I; Table 7, p. 9/II; Table 5, p. 38/II, Fig. 2, p. 6 ff./II; Fig. 4, p. 20/II; Fig. 7, p. 42/II; Fig. 8, p. 46 ff./II; Fig. 17, p. 97/II; Fig. 18, p. 99/II; Fig. 10, p. 40/IV; Fig. 11, p. 42/IV; Fig. 12, p. 46/IV, Fig. 13, p. 48/IV; Fig. 23, p. 64/IV.

Furthermore, episodes of more complex *reflexmotor* activities, such as spells of coughing, sneezing, laughing, yawning, swallowing, vomiting, sucking or crying (see Table 4, p. 30[887,888]), may be a part of brain-directed processes of unloading occurring during autogenic exercises.

All these different modalities of motor discharge are also encountered during autogenic abreaction. However, as distinct from the comparatively brief and thematically dissociated occurrence of motor discharges during autogenic training, the release of motor impulses during autogenic abreaction is usually of a more systematic manner which follows a recognizable pattern closely connected to specific topics in the process of multithematic neutralization. The thematically related release of motor impulses tends to occur in phases, or sometimes in connection with brain-antagonizing forms of resistance (see Part I, Vol. VI). Since thematic engagement in particularly disturbing material tends to occur more often during advanced phases of treatment with autogenic neutralization, the incidence of motor phenomena remains relatively low during the initial series of autogenic abreactions (see Table 39).

TABLE 39.   *Somatomotor and Reflexmotor Phenomena Described or Observed during*
*the First and the Second Autogenic Abreaction*
(Psychosomatic and Neurotic Patients)

| Phenomena Described by Patients or Observed by the Therapist | Autogenic Abreactions | |
|---|---|---|
| | AA 1 (N = 100; %) | AA 2 (N = 96; %) |
| 1. Trembling | | |
| (a) Body | — | — |
| (b) Upper extremities | 3.0 | 1.0 |
| (c) Lower extremities | — | — |
| (d) Cranial region | — | — |
| 2. Twitching | | |
| (a) Body | 1.0 | 6.2 |
| (b) Upper extremities | 4.0 | 6.2 |
| (c) Lower extremities | 3.0 | 4.2 |
| (d) Cranial region | 10.0 | 9.4 |
| 3. Movements | | |
| (a) Body | 1.0 | 1.0 |
| (b) Upper extremities | 3.0 | 3.1 |
| (c) Lower extremities | 2.0 | 2.1 |
| (d) Cranial region | 9.0 | 10.4 |
| (e) Opening of eyes | 7.0 | 8.3 |
| 4. Muscular tension | | |
| (a) Body | 12.0 | 4.2 |
| (b) Upper extremities | 2.0 | 2.1 |
| (c) Lower extremities | 1.0 | — |
| (d) Cranial region | 7.0 | 5.2 |
| 5. Sitting up | 1.0 | 1.0 |
| 6. Swallowing | — | 1.0 |
| 7. Vomiting | — | 1.0 |
| 8. Biting lips | — | 1.0 |
| 9. Sneezing | 1.0 | 2.1 |
| 10. Yawning | 1.0 | — |
| 11. Crying | | |
| (a) Crying spell | — | 2.1 |
| (b) Lacrimation | 5.0 | 8.3 |
| 12. Grimacing | — | 1.0 |
| 13. Smiling, laughing | 8.0 | 4.2 |
| 14. Coughing | — | 1.0 |
| 15. Sighing | 3.0 | 5.2 |
| 16. Deep respiration | 5.0 | 4.3 |
| 17. Pulling hair | — | 1.0 |
| 18. Borborygmus | 3.0 | — |

## SOMATOMOTOR PHENOMENA

Perceptible motor discharges in topographically discernible areas of the skeletomuscular system may be described as a *feeling of tension.* Such feelings of tension in topographically specific areas (e.g., right shoulder, left thigh) tend to follow an "on" and "off" pattern of repetition. Occasionally, feelings of tension in specific topographic areas develop into brief phases of muscular fibrillation or twitching of the same group of striated muscles. The thematic relationship of such topographically specific motor discharges requires further investigation. Only in certain instances, such as during the neutralization of accidents, traumatic deliveries, certain categories of brain-disturbing material of non-experiential nature and in connection with certain forms of brain-antagonizing resistance, there appears to be a close functional relationship. In many other instances the thematic context of such feelings of tension in specific muscle groups remains obscure.

Topographically nonspecific *diffuse and generalized muscular tension* does occur during phases of apprehension related to specific themes of neutralization, but rarely as a consequence of brain-antagonizing forms of resistance.

More intensive and *well-localized motor discharges,* for example, *twitching, trembling,* or *jerking,* involving a particular group of skeletal muscles tend to follow a phasic crescendo and decrescendo pattern. Such motor disharges are often a thematic component of more complex material accumulated in connection with specific traumatic episodes (see Case 91).

*Case 91:* A 43-year-old physician reported topographically specific motor discharges which were associated with a childhood trauma.

"The visual field was dark blue, with clouds of darker shades moving about. Then I started having the impression that I was lying on my left side and my right foot started twitching occasionally. The twitching of the foot increased and became at times very rapid and completely automatic. There was also a funny feeling around the ankle of my right foot. This twitching and wiggling was accompanied by occasional violent jerk-like movements of my right leg. After about ten minutes all calmed down and the right leg and foot were relaxed. I somehow tried to start the motor discharges again, but it did not work. While the violent twitching and wiggling was going on, and perhaps because of this peculiar feeling around my right ankle, I remembered my mother telling me the following story: When I was about two years old, my parents went out for the evening and had left me with our maid. When my parents came home, the maid was asleep in her room and I was lying buried, face down in my pillows, and looked bluish. My right foot was caught between two wooden bars of the bed-railing in such a manner that my parents were unable to withdraw my foot. My father had to get a saw in order to remove one of the vertical bars. I do not remember any other incidents which would explain the motor discharges in my right leg and foot. Later during the week, two similar, however very brief, episodes occurred. But whenever I tried to get the motor discharges going again, only a few 'artificial' movements resulted and I was unable to trigger a typical discharge pattern."

*Massive generalized motor discharges* involving the trunk, the extremities, head and face have been observed occasionally. The repetitive pattern of such discharges usually starts unexpectedly and may be quite surprising for both the patient and the therapist. In such situations immediate verbal support by the therapist is indicated to avoid brain-antagonizing surprise reactions (e.g., opening of eyes, sitting up, premature termination). Passive acceptance must be maintained so that the stormy motor discharges can drain off without resistance.

Such generalized motor discharges tend to come in waves with intermittent periods of relaxation and a feeling of calmness. There is some indication that the number of wave-like motor discharges varies with the nature of the triggering theme and the anxiety associated with it (see Case 93, p. 230, Case 92).

As the brain is given *carte blanche* to discharge whatever it needs, the intensity and duration of these generalized motor discharges decrease. Depending on the nature of the accumulated material and the thematically related need for motor discharges, brain-desired levels of neutralization may be reached in the course of one or two autogenic abreactions. In other instances many repetitions spreading over a considerably larger number of autogenic abreactions have been observed (see Fig. 12).

*Case 92:* A 49-year-old priest (anxiety reaction, obsessive-compulsive and phobic reactions, ecclesiogenic syndrome). The following excerpt of one of the patient's autogenic abreactions shows that certain thematic components (e.g., lice, sucking spiders, centipedes, octopus, lion, dogs, crabs, lizard, devil) seem to have a triggering effect on series of major and minor motor discharges (see also Fig. 12). Particularly strong motor reactions simultaneously involved muscle groups in the neck and shoulder area and both legs.

"I sprinkle you with boiling water . . . I burn your cunt with a torch . . . I slash your chest open with one stab of the knife and I tear your heart out . . . I have you burned with bundles of wood . . . I commit suicide . . . a bullet through the heart . . . off to the devil . . . the hell of fire . . . I'm in the fire . . . it burns me through and through . . . I'm broiling . . . I'm roasting . . . it comes in through my eyes . . . a fork stabs me in the buttocks, cunt and eyes . . . there are spiders and lice all over my body . . . *[jerk in the shoulders, 3 times]* a real hysterical fit . . . *[9 twitches, shoulders, thighs, legs]* . . . there are spiders on my chest biting and sucking me *[10 twitches]* . . . centipedes

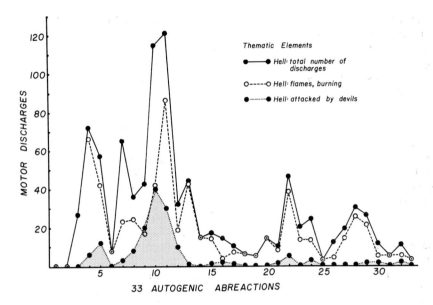

FIG. 12. Thematically related motor discharges (jerk-like movements and twitching of arms, shoulders, head, upper trunk) during a series of 33 autogenic abreactions which focussed on neutralization of brain-disturbing material of ecclesiogenic nature (e.g., damnation, being tortured by devils and thrown into the eternal fire of hell). These motor discharges occurred (a) when the patient was confronted with or attacked by devils, (b) when brain-designed developments brought him closer to the flames of hell, (c) when he was thrown into the fire and burning, and (d) during occasionally interjected confrontations with giant spiders and slimy snakes (49-year-old priest; see also Case 92).

[4 twitches] . . . the octopus wraps its tentacles around me and clings to my chest [twitch] . . . wraps them around my arms and paralyzes me, fixes itself to my thighs . . . my two legs . . . the snakes . . . a boa wraps itself around my body and bites my sex . . . [twitch] . . . centipedes run about all over my body . . . every so often there are twitches in my shoulders and throughout my body . . . we have the fireplace there . . . [3 twitches] . . . a lion throws itself on me . . . [3 twitches] . . . I'm telling you it's jumping around here . . . enraged dogs [4 twitches] . . . bite me, it's no fun . . . a ferocious fox throws itself at my throat to strangle me [twitch] . . . the fire is as of a very somber greenish black . . . the . . . the crabs are advancing [3 twitches] . . . it's jumping . . . crawfish are cutting off my toes [6 twitches] . . . it's jumping . . . [moderate nervous discharge, 15 twitches] . . . the snakes in my paintings . . . the fantastic lizard in my painting . . . oh . . . [3 twitches] . . . the damned . . . [5 twitches] a devil charges down on me . . . my shoulders are jerking . . . I think there are flaming jets . . . there are streaks at the top left . . . it's pinkish . . . it's fire . . . not perfectly distinguishable yet, but it's coming . . . it seems to me that it smells of sulfur . . . a pool of sulfur and fire . . . I think of the fire in hell and my shoulders jerk . . . these are violent imageries, this is dynamite . . . the lizard is walking all over my body [8 *twitches*] . . . a devil throws himself on me with his pitchfork [5 *twitches*] . . . it's jumping . . . now there's nothing going on. . . ."

*Case 93:* A 37-year-old male patient (anxiety reaction). Shortly after the therapist started reciting "My right arm is very heavy," massive motor discharges occurred. These motor discharges (about 1/sec.) involved jerk-like contractions of the trunk, lifting the patient's shoulders and his head off the couch. Associated with these major motor discharges, there were minor twitches of both arms, both legs, tenseness around the mouth and twitching of the eyelids. The motor discharges which lasted about 90 seconds were described as being accompanied by a wave-like display of red-yellow, mustard-like colors in the visual field. It is assumed that a preceding discussion about the patient's declining interest in flying his own aircraft, his mentioning of a recent fatal crash of a person who had criticized the patient's aircraft as unsafe, and the patient's anxiety as related to the theme of sudden death and hell participated in mobilizing relevant brain-disturbing material and helped to trigger these motor discharges.

### Reflexmotor Phenomena

During treatment with autogenic abreaction a number of physiologically rather complex reflexmotor activities such as crying, sucking, coughing, laughing, vomiting and yawning are frequently encountered and are of particular therapeutic interest.

From many observations of brain-directed dynamics of neutralization involving thematically related modalities of reflexmotor reactions, it was assumed that these biologically important activities play a significant role in two functional directions. They appear to participate in bringing about or in reinforcing certain brain-disturbing functional disorders in cases where repeated voluntary efforts at suppression of one or several of these reflexmotor activities have resulted in a functional block which prevents the biologically normal function of relevant brain-mechanisms. On the other hand, there is impressive evidence indicating that the brain-directed unloading of suppressed and accumulated reflexmotor modalities contributes effectively to advances in brain-desired functional readjustments. This positively oriented functional role is generally accepted concerning the beneficial effects of crying spells. However, the clinical and therapeutic significance of other reflexmotor modalities appear to be underestimated.

Depending on the case-specific nature of the accumulated brain-disturbing material, a brain-desired amount of crying may be as important as, for example, a brain-desired number of episodes of vomiting, or sucking, or laughing. When brain-antagonizing forms of resistance (see Part I, Vol. VI) interfere with the brain-desired activities of these reflexmotor modalities, a variety of modality-related functional disturbances tends to ensue. For example, suppressed or inadequate crying is in many instances followed by frontal headache. The headache promptly disappears after a brain-desired amount of crying has occurred. Similarly, gastric and other abdominal complaints (e.g.,cramps, nausea, anorexia) tend to increase as brain-desired vomiting (e.g., accident-related) is not permitted, and surprisingly quick improvements have been noted after the brain-desired release of vomiting impulses has taken place. These two brief examples may suffice to show the necessity of giving the patient ample opportunity to understand the therapeutically beneficial nature of such brain-desired processes of thematic unloading and that, for example, intentional forms of brain-antagonizing resistance in this area are to the detriment of himself and the treatment process. This therapeutically important orientation is more readily understandable to those who have had the opportunity to observe the amazing persistance or perhaps insistence with which brain-directed forces aim at overcoming or dissolving functional barriers which inhibit the normal function of reflexmotor modalities. In many instances it has been observed that considerable slowdown of the brain-directed processes of neutralization occurs when, for example, brain-desired crying or vomiting is not yet possible. Inversely, rapid progress is noted after previously blocked reflexmotor functions have regained their normal level of biologically determined functional possibilities.

During autogenic abreactions, productive engagement in flexible multithematic processes of neutralization is frequently preceded by crying. Repeated observations of this nature have led to the impression that crying assumes a functional key position in certain types of thematic neutralization (see Fig. 7, p. 180). Brain-directed elaborations of visual nature are usually reduced to elementary stages I and II (see Table 33, p. 188), while monothematic priority is given to crying. After crying spells an increase in brightness of colors and other manifestations of positively oriented nature tend to follow (e.g., increase in dynamic and realistic features). An impending need for crying is sometimes expressed by thematically corresponding elaborations in the visual field. During elementary and intermediate stages, globular or drop-like structures may appear in association with relatively dark background colors. In filmstrip or cinerama-type elaborations, initial phases may emphasize, for example, a dark cloudy rainy sky or a stormy ocean on a rainy day. Other indications may involve confrontations with crying persons, with particularly saddening thematic elements or with an image of oneself crying. In other instances, when brain-desired crying is inhibited, it has been repeatedly observed that brain-directed dynamics keep elaborating pain, which is often localized in topographic areas which were affected during certain accidents (e.g., right shoulder: hockey accident; right arm: fracture; right thorax: ski accident). Such brain-directed elaborations of pain may continue for prolonged periods (e.g., 20 min.) and assume disturbing intensities which appear to aim at the facilitation of crying. In such cases it has been consistently observed that the pain subsides and disappears after brain-desired crying has occurred (see Pain-Crying Mechanism, p. 240).

Brain-desired engagement in breast sucking is frequently accompanied by cinerama-type elaborations and brain-directed age regression (see Case 96, p. 234; Case 99, p. 235). In other instances, however, breast sucking activities, including the oral motor components may, similar to other motor discharges, start and continue for prolonged periods (e.g., 20 min.) without differentiated visual phenomena (e.g., remaining at stage I or II). Interjected breast sucking phases appear to have a particular recuperative and activating effect which, depending on the central theme of neutralization, may be reflected in many positively oriented ways (e.g., engagement in intercourse with mother becomes possible; killing of father follows).

Repeated episodes of coughing may be thematically related (see Case 97, p. 234) or may be a disguised form of crying which cannot yet assume its brain-desired functional role.

Of particular importance are brain-designed indications that the brain wishes to engage in a release of accumulated impulses designed to produce vomiting. Such indications may be conveyed by visual elaborations of, for example, seeing someone vomiting or by a series of images which are nausea-promoting. In other instances, abdominal discomfort and feelings of nausea are the only indications. Since the onset of vomiting is not always predictable, it is advisable to foresee such eventualities in relevant cases (e.g., pail, towels, deodorizer ready to use). Of practical importance is that the patient feels absolutely free to engage in vomiting whenever his brain wishes to release such forms of reflexmotor discharges. Episodes of vomiting tend to occur in phases and must be permitted to undergo the brain-desired number of repetitions. In most instances episodes of nausea and vomiting are thematically related to material of experiential nature such as states of shock (e.g., after fractures), accidents in connection with transitory loss of consciousness, concussions, and other non-accidental situations where the urge to vomit was energetically suppressed. After a brain-desired amount of vomiting impulses have been released through adequate function, patients tend to enjoy a very agreeable feeling of well-being.

Another reflexmotor modality of practical concern is laughing. Since this modality is more easily expressed during actual situations, spells of laughing due to a voluntarily suppressed need to laugh occur less often (see Case 94, p. 233). Therapeutically it is of importance that patients feel free to laugh whenever the brain wishes to engage in this modality. In other instances laughing may be preparatory for engagement in crying. In these cases the thematic relationship permits a clear distinction from those others where laughter arises because of accumulated situation-related voluntary suppression of laughing impulses.

Repeated yawning may be a manifestation of actual fatigue, but it may also be related to an undue accumulation of yawning impulses which resulted from voluntary suppression of yawning during certain situations (see Case 98, p. 235). Similarly, repeated episodes of "unexplained" sneezing have been observed. However, it must be remembered that both repeated yawning and sneezing may be preparatory brain-designed maneuvers aiming at a progressive facilitation of an inhibited crying mechanism.

Fluttering of the eyelids which may be related to the palpebral reflex tends to occur particularly at the beginning of autogenic abreactions. Apart from the assumption that this type of motor discharge reflects an increased level of tension, no other more specific thematic relationships have been noted.

Sequences of swallowing have been also observed. This reflexmotor activity tends to occur before the onset of crying, when a need for crying is being suppressed, and occasionally during thematically related phases of neutralization (e.g., sucking, drinking, eating).

*Case 94:* A 26-year-old female teacher (anxiety reaction, moderate depression). After thematic neutralization had focussed on a variety of anxiety-promoting childhood episodes (e.g., being left alone at home and feeling scared, ghost stories, nightmare) an antithematic shift toward more agreeable material occurs (see below). During this antithematic phase the brain aims at the release of laughing impulses which had been voluntarily suppressed during the actual event.

"I remember a nightmare I once had . . . my legs seem to be moving up and white phantom-like shapes such as knives were going through the door. I can't recall I ever screamed . . . [sigh . . . starts smiling] . . . I can see my aunt and my mother bringing in my Easter basket . . . I was not sleeping, but I pretended to be . . . I listened . . . I was furious to find out there was no bunny . . . I just listened to them drinking the milk and eating the cookies I had left for him . . . then I thought I would laugh . . . *I remember wanting to burst out laughing* when my aunt said that she thought I was not asleep and that I was hearing everything [smiling] . . . *I feel like laughing* . . . *[laughing spell]*. . . ."

*Case 95:* A 40-year-old priest (anxiety reaction, moderate depression, multiple psychophysiologic and phobic reactions, ecclesiogenic syndrome). The passage given below is one example of many similar episodes where dynamics of neutralization emphasize brain-desired engagement in breast sucking. As breast sucking is permitted to continue, a characteristic recuperative effect and feeling of well-being ensues. This is frequently accompanied by a feeling of warmth.

"I am again a baby clinging to my mother's breasts . . . now I am seeing the beautiful breasts of a woman . . . at first it was somewhat vague . . . now it becomes Marylin Monroe . . . [laughing] . . . and *I start sucking with avidity* . . . [sucking movements] . . . and I feel warmer . . . the feeling of warmth is increasing. . . ."

*Case 96:* A 38-year-old teacher (anxiety reaction, moderate depression, hypothyroidism). During thematic developments which focussed on the patient's mother relationship a prolonged period of breast sucking occurred.

"I feel blocked, I cannot take her clothes off, and I cannot get at her breasts . . . I caress her hips . . . and the breasts through her dress . . . I am kissing the upper part of her breasts . . . where the breasts start . . . to be able to caress a breast one has to suck . . . that's where my problem is . . . I have to suck . . . now I undress her . . . I pull the dress away . . . she is naked . . . I would like to suck her breasts . . . one has to become a baby to do that . . . *I suck* . . . it is difficult . . . *I am sucking* . . . *[noise of sucking]* . . . she becomes unreal when *I suck* . . . *[sucking continued with typical noise]* . . . I caress her a bit while *I suck* . . . *[sucking is louder than before, for about 4 min.]* . . . she covers her lower body . . . she is waiting . . . she is immobile . . . I would like her to pay attention to me . . . *[sucking continues]* . . . I would like her to do something . . . actually she does not think of me at all . . . she looks at me somewhat bemused . . . she remains passive . . . she does not appear to be interested in me . . . *[sucking continues]* . . . one hand on her forehead, on her breast . . . her shoulder . . . she isn't interested in me . . . I don't exist for her . . . I don't exist for her . . . for my mother I never existed . . . for her I was just another burden. . . ."

*Case 97:* A 50-year-old male patient (anxiety reaction). Thematically related spells of coughing occurred before and during engagement in neutralization of an abortive attempt to commit suicide at the age of six.

"Ah to be an accountant is my most profound desire, but in another context of time, at 20 years old . . . *[coughing spell]* . . . *it's funny, I'm coughing and I'm hoarse* . . . it's probably because I strangled my mother and Luthe . . . *[coughing]* . . . well now, that's odd . . . like being strangulated by a rope . . . it's my hanging . . . my neckties that I tightened around my Adam's apple. . . ."

*Case 98:* A 39-year-old businessman (anxiety reaction).

"Swirling about like a lot of ghosts . . . thinking of that joke about wrapping paper . . . I don't know why *I'm always yawning during all these* 'trips' . . . specially on a fairly good night's sleep . . . yes, I'm still seeing this chap who has a gift shop. . . ."

## VISCEROMOTOR PHENOMENA

The variety of visceromotor and related autonomic phenomena which occur for brief periods and in an apparently incoherent manner during autogenic training (see Table 5, p. 31[887,888]; Table 2, p. 31/I; Table 1, p. 9/II; Table 5, p. 38/II) are also encountered during autogenic abreaction. Changes of intestinal motor patterns as conveyed by borborygmus, precordial palpitation, changes of respiratory movements, increase or decrease of salivation, and manifestations of vasomotor changes may occur without evident thematic relationship. In other instances, specific visceromotor and autonomic reactions tend to coincide with more specific dynamics of thematic neutralization. It is hoped that further research in this area may yield some information which may be of particular interest in the area of psychosomatic medicine. Spontaneous urination is rare and defecation during autogenic abreaction has been observed in only one case. Cyanosis and "frothing at the mouth" did not occur.

Phasic activation of genital mechanisms is usually closely associated with thematic neutralization of, for example, brain-disturbing effects resulting from relative or absolute affective and sexual deprivation. In these cases variations of bloodflow into the corpora cavernosa and corresponding variations of erection are reported during thematically related phases of neutralization. Ejaculation of semen is relatively rare. A significantly greater facility in experiencing orgasm has been observed in female patients (see Case 99).

Of particular interest are occasionally occurring phases of uterine contractions. This specific type of motor activity has been observed in connection with thematically related material of experiential nature (e.g., traumatizing deliveries, abortions; see Case 100) and also in women who for various reasons had not been pregnant (see Case 99).

*Case 99:* A 29-year-old married nurse (personality disorder, anxiety reaction, moderate depression, functional sterility). During the following initial part of a prolonged autogenic abreaction which largely focussed on neutralization of brain-disturbing material accumulated over several years while working in operating rooms, the disagreeable dynamics are preceded by an agreeable antithematic "introduction." While engaging in homosexual activities, breast sucking and orgasms are thematically integrated. Later uterine contractions were experienced.

"And there is a girl with blond hair, and I take her and *I suck her breasts* . . . I am thirsty, and *I suck her breasts* and *I come off [orgasm]* . . . and I let my hands wander down her back, on her hips, her thighs . . . oh, her feet are tickling me . . . and we are rolling in the grass and I feel her skin against mine . . . and her skin feels warm . . . and it is sunny and warm, and the trees are moving a bit . . . and she puts her hands around my back and I take her into my arms and rub my breasts against her back . . . ah, I rub my breasts against her back and *this makes me go off [orgasm]* . . . and I put my hands into her vagina, and she puts hers into mine, and I have *more orgasms* . . . I have *more orgasms* . . . ah, I feel her hair in my face, and I go with my hair between her legs and I tickle her and she is writhing and so do I . . . ah, she is sucking my vagina . . . oh, *my uterus starts contracting* . . . oh, *my uterus is contracting* . . . ah . . . and we are going to rest a bit . . . we are walking to a nice beach . . . lying in the warm sand. . . . I see children, and while I say that I become pregnant and I hope to give birth to a baby . . . well I am pregnant and I have this funny feeling in my abdomen . . . oh, ah, and it pushes right and left on my coccyx . . . the baby is coming down and close to my vulva . . . ah, and I push, and this girl is going to help me with the delivery . . . and I push, I push hard . . . *[actually doing this in delivery position on the couch]* . . . the head just passed, the head just passed, then the shoulders, then the placenta . . . the placenta is as bad as the head, the placenta . . . that reminds me of the operation room in obstetrics . . . the terrible things I saw there . . . the placentas . . . and the blood, the surgeons and the sutures, and the women, they were writhing and felt hot and thought they were going to die . . . ah, now it's me who is going to die . . . I have a hemorrhage, and the blood is all over the place, and the blood is everywhere and I am under tension, and my blood pressure is going down and. . . ."

*Case 100:* A 24-year-old secretary (anxiety reaction). The following passage was taken from the central abreactive period of an autogenic abreaction which largely focussed on neutralization of anxiety accumulated in connection with a medical abortion (inadequate anesthesia). The topographically specific motor discharges are thematically associated with the medical intervention and the fear of impending death. Positively oriented antithematic elements (e.g., orgasm, agreeable feelings) are interjected.

"And I am afraid to have an orgasm and to die and he penetrates and I am afraid to have an orgasm and to die, and he penetrates, and he penetrates, and he penetrates . . . *I have all kinds of contractions in my lower abdomen* . . . and I die and I am afraid of dying and I die and I am afraid of dying and I die . . . *I still have these contractions,* and I am a bit afraid of having another abortion and to die . . . oh, it's good . . . he penetrates . . . it's funny that orgasms are like that . . . *I have quite violent contractions* and after, I don't know, one feels nothing at all, anyway *these contractions feel good* . . . I don't know it's funny . . . *very rapid series of contractions and some are stronger than others.* . . ."

# 17. Sensory Phenomena

During autogenic abreaction an almost endless variety of combinations of sensory phenomena involving topographically different portions of somatosensory and viscerosensory areas have been encountered. Sensory phenomena may dominate large portions of the abreactive period or may occur for brief phases as secondary components of thematically more complex processes of autogenic neutralization. In many instances differentiated visual elaborations undergo functional regression to elementary levels of differentiation when a brain-desired priority is given to sensory elaborations (see Case 101, p. 237; Case 102, p. 242). The incidence of sensory phenomena is relatively low in initial autogenic abreactions (see Table 40) and tends to become more intensive during more advanced treatment periods, when thematically more disturbing and more complex material is submitted for neutralization. All somatosensory and viscerosensory modalities encountered during the practice of autogenic standard exercises are also noted during autogenic abreaction (see Table 9, p. 36[887,888]; Table 2, p. 31/I; Table 3, p. 58/I; Table 4, p. 62/I; Table 1, p. 9/II; Table 4, p. 37/II; Table 5, p. 38/II; Table 8, p. 87/II; Table 9, p. 88/II; Table 14, p. 166/II, see Table 40).

As distinct from the sensory discharges occurring during autogenic standard exercises, the sensory phenomena observable during autogenic abreaction are of longer duration and tend to follow a pattern of sequential or rotational repetitions which usually appear as a thematic component of more complex processes of neutralization. The brain-directed release of sensory modalities may be monothematic (e.g., feeling of numbness) or may consist of multithematic combinations of a variety of sensory phenomena which may also include distortions of the body image and closely related somesthetic elements (see Case 101).

Case 101: A 40-year-old teacher (anxiety reaction) who at the age of 23, was kicked in the head during a soccer game (loss of consciousness for 3 days). The following passage is a good example of multisensory processes of neutralization.

"I am in a nice warm place, very nice . . . oh . . . inside a kind of room, or sort of container . . . and it's all pink . . . and my heart is beating and I am feeling every beat of my heart . . . and I have kind of muscular fibrillations, contractions . . . my left hand is cool suddenly . . . as if I was putting my hand in cool water . . . now I feel itchy all over . . . very itchy . . . very itchy all over . . . can I scratch? [yes] . . . [scratching face, chest, arms, lower trunk, laughing] . . . I feel more comfortable, but very funny . . . as if collapsing inside . . . as

TABLE 40.   *Sensory and Related Phenomena Described during the First*
*and the Second Autogenic Abreaction*
(Psychosomatic and Neurotic Patients)

| Phenomena Described by Patients | AA 1 (N = 100; %) | AA 2 (N = 96; %) |
|---|---|---|
| **1. Heaviness** | | |
| (a) Body | 2.0 | 3.1 |
| (b) Upper extremities | 7.0 | 4.2 |
| (c) Lower extremities | 3.0 | 6.2 |
| (d) Cranial region | 4.0 | 4.2 |
| **2. Warmth** | | |
| (a) Body | 6.0 | 6.2 |
| (b) Upper extremities | 5.0 | 1.0 |
| (c) Lower extremities | 3.0 | 2.1 |
| (d) Cranial region | 2.0 | 1.0 |
| **3. Burning (genitals)** | — | 1.0 |
| **4. Itching** | | |
| (a) Body | 1.0 | — |
| (b) Upper extremities | — | 2.1 |
| (c) Lower extremities | — | 2.1 |
| (d) Cranial region | 2.0 | 2.1 |
| **5. Tingling** | | |
| (a) Body | 1.0 | 1.0 |
| (b) Upper extremities | 4.0 | 2.1 |
| (c) Lower extremities | 2.0 | 2.1 |
| (d) Cranial region | 1.0 | 1.0 |
| **6. Swelling** | | |
| (a) Body | — | — |
| (b) Upper extremities | 1.0 | 1.0 |
| (c) Lower extremities | 1.0 | — |
| (d) Cranial region | — | — |
| **7. Numbness** | | |
| (a) Body | 2.0 | 3.1 |
| (b) Upper extremlties | 2.0 | 2.1 |
| (c) Lower extremities | 1.0 | 4.2 |
| (d) Cranial region | — | — |
| **8. Pulsation** | | |
| (a) Body | — | — |
| (b) Upper extremities | 2.0 | 2.1 |
| (c) Lower extremities | 1.0 | 4.0 |
| (d) Cranial region | — | — |
| **9. Electrical sensations** | | |
| (a) Body | — | — |
| (b) Upper extremities | 2.0 | — |
| (c) Lower extremities | 1.0 | 1.0 |
| (d) Cranial region | — | — |

TABLE 40. Continued

| Phenomena Described by Patients | AA 1 (N = 100; %) | AA 2 (N = 96; %) |
|---|---|---|
| 10. Coldness | | |
| (a) Body | — | — |
| (b) Upper extremities | 2.0 | — |
| (c) Lower extremities | — | 1.0 |
| (d) Cranial region | — | — |
| 11. Detachment (body) | 1.0 | — |
| 12. Feeling of displacement | | |
| (a) Body | — | 1.0 |
| (b) Upper extremities | — | 1.0 |
| (c) Lower extremities | — | 1.0 |
| (d) Cranial region | 3.0 | — |
| 13. Pressure | | |
| (a) Body | 2.0 | 2.0 |
| (b) Upper extremities | 1.0 | — |
| (c) Lower extremities | — | — |
| (d) Cranial region | 4.0 | 2.1 |
| 14. Pain | | |
| (a) Body | 3.0 | 4.2 |
| (b) Upper extremities | 2.0 | — |
| (c) Lower extremities | 2.0 | 1.0 |
| (d) Cranial region | 2.0 | 2.1 |
| 15. Distortion of body image | 2.0 | 4.2 |
| 16. Nausea | 2.0 | 1.0 |
| 17. Depression | 6.0 | 4.2 |
| 18. Drowsiness | 2.0 | 1.0 |
| 19. Tiredness | 5.0 | 6.2 |
| 20. Sleep | — | 1.0 |
| 21. Need to urinate | 3.0 | 2.1 |
| 22. Sexual arousal | 4.0 | 3.1 |
| 23. Cardiac sensations | 3.0 | 2.0 |
| 24. Respiration more difficult | — | 1.0 |
| 25. Weightlessness | — | 1.0 |
| 26. Feeling of restlessness | 1.0 | 3.1 |

if my body is shrinking, deflating . . . my skin was tight . . . and now I have an agreeable sensation, as if my flesh is getting firmer . . . I was under tremendous sort of pressure from inside, that eased up now . . . and I have pain in my right hand, like in the center of the bone . . . it's like a decompression . . . not disagreeable . . . the pressure goes away and the blood is coming back . . . but my fingers are numb . . . now I feel good. . . ."

Since research is not far enough advanced to provide data which would permit a better understanding of the clinical significance and psychophysiologic dynamics which participate in the accumulation and brain-programmed release of the many different sensory phenomena encountered during autogenic abreaction, a detailed discussion of these thematic components will be a major subject of a future publication.

## PAIN

The occasional experience of various modalities of pain (e.g., dull, sharp, pressure-like, sting-like) is a well-known phenomenon associated with the practice of autogenic training (see Table 2, p. 31/I; Table 1, p. 9/II; Table 4, p. 37/II; Table 5, p. 38/II). Such sensations of pain are usually of brief duration and rarely assume intensities which oblige the trainee to interrupt his autogenic exercises. In many instances such sensations of pain are well localized and may follow a phasic "on and off" pattern, unless elaborations characteristic for the *pain–crying mechanism* are given brain-designed priority (see Vol. VI). Studies of such discharge activity during autogenic exercises indicate that certain sensations of topographically localized pain are related to accidents during which the same bodily area was affected. In many instances no satisfactory explanations were found. Of particular interest were different modalities of pain and pain-like sensations involving the cranial region (see Table 8, p. 87/II; Table 9, p. 88/II).

The brain-directed elaboration and release of various modalities of pain during autogenic abreaction requires further investigation. For the time, a tentative distinction of five major categories of pain has been made:

A. Pain or pain-like sensations which are clearly related to experiential material and which occur as one of the psychophysiologic features of multithematic processes of neutralization. In these instances tolerable intensities of pain and related psychophysiologic reactions may be related to, for example, accidents, medical conditions (e.g., biliary colic) or clinical procedures (e.g., bone marrow aspiration).

B. Pain or pain-like sensations which are in some way related to the central topic undergoing neutralization, but which do not show a direct but perhaps a symbolically disguised relationship to specific material of experiential nature.

C. Pain or pain-like sensations which seem to be elaborated or released without recognizable thematic context.

D. Pain or pain-like sensations which tend to occur in association with certain forms of brain-antagonizing resistance (e.g., pain–crying mechanism, aggression–heart pain mechanism, frontal headache–suppressed crying or other thematic resistance).

E. Pain or pain-like sensations which appear to result from physiologic reactions related to specific brain functions participating in processes of neutralization. This category includes, for example, various modalities of pain or pain-like sensations which are described as being localized "right above my left ear on the surface of the brain," "here, directly under the skull" or "exactly here on the outside of the left frontal lobe." These topographically well-localized sensations are mostly noted over frontal, temporal, and parietal areas. They are of bothersome but transitory nature and may or may not follow a pattern of phasic repetition. The reactive nature of such localized pain or pain-like sensations appears to be different from other more diffuse types of headaches (e.g., occipital, frontal, "all over").

From more detailed studies of case material it is evident that there are considerable variations in the elaboration and release of pain or pain-like sensations during autogenic abreactions. In certain patients pain or pain-like sensations occur rarely or never in spite of a case history which reliably shows that disturbing modalities of pain had been experienced in a variety of pain-producing situations. In other patients the brain keeps emphasizing and repeating the same thematically related modalities of pain, while other experiential material with subjectively equally disturbing experiences of pain remains "silent." Although there is some evidence supporting the hypothesis that pain was not subjectively experienced at the time of the accident, and it is given thematic priority during autogenic neutralization, it is felt that the "subjective non-experience" is only one variable among others which seem to participate in guiding processes of neutralization involving sensations of pain. Other observations have led to the hypothesis that originally recorded sensations of pain undergo thematic modification (e.g., thematic disintegration, "splitting up for release," thematic dissociation; see p. 292 ff.) and reappear during autogenic abreaction, for example, as a sensation of pressure, as "mild burning sensation," or perhaps as numbness. The assumed participation of neutralization-facilitating processes of brain-desired thematic modification is viewed as one manifestation of a variety of self-regulatory adaptational functions which characterize the self-promoting nature of autogenic neutralization. In fact, intensities of pain which correspond to the pain experienced in the thematically related reality situation have not yet been observed.

During brain-directed neutralization of accumulated material involving sensations of pain, the same patterns of phasic repetition observed in other modalities (e.g., motor, vestibular) are noted. When the thematic emphasis is on pain, previously differentiated visual elaborations usually undergo compensatory functional regression to elementary levels (see Case 102). Pattern analyses of longer series of autogenic abreactions involving accident material indicate that the thematic emphasis on pain or pain-like sensations is more marked during certain autogenic abreactions than during others (see Fig. 7, p. 180), and that brain-designed thematic priorities may be given to other modalities (e.g., crying, vestibular) before processes of neutralization are permitted to focus on pain. Pain, pain-like sensations and psychophysiologically related reactions disappear progressively as the brain-directed processes of neutralization are given an adequate opportunity to pursue their self-normalizing activities.

*Case 102:* A 29-year-old housewife who was hit by a speeding car (see Case 79, p. 181; Fig. 7, p. 180). The following passages are examples of brain-directed thematic emphasis on various types of pains and aches which the patient did not feel during or after the accident.

*AA 6:* "I see the car only . . . the car is very fast, it turns me around . . . the car is six feet in front of me . . . I hold it away from me . . . it is very big . . . my back is hurting . . . I don't see anything anymore . . . I feel choked, strangled . . . now the car is driving over me again . . . but it is very light. . . ."

*AA 7:* "I see the street-corner again . . . the cars are still driving on this side [left] . . . I don't mind all this . . . I can't concentrate well today . . . in spite of the fact that I don't see anything particular, my backache and the pain in the upper abdomen and the soreness in my arms is getting worse . . . I am so preoccupied with my aches and pains that I come to nothing else . . . now my stomach really hurts, I feel sick . . . there is a tearing sensation in my left arm, down from the shoulder, my right hand is burning, I have cramp-like sensations in my stomach, feel kind of nauseated, a stabbing pain in my back, as if something is pressing very hard against it and is going to break my back, headache . . . and now the cars are driving over me again . . . but they don't touch me . . . they are all driving in one direction, sometimes slow, sometimes fast, sometimes over me, sometimes around me . . . and it has become dark, it's quite dark now and all the cars have no lights on . . . I have pains all over . . . mostly my back, the stomach and the abdomen and the arms . . . a feeling as if I am going to break into pieces . . . the street became still darker and all the cars are dirving on the wrong side . . . oh, my back is hurting . . . it hurts so much, it's almost indescribable

. . . as if my back is going to break [groans] . . . it hurts so much . . . as if my back is going to come out in front, and it hurts as if my spine is about to break . . . my right hand stopped burning and there is no tearing sensation anymore in the left arm [starts crying] . . . and my abdomen hurts . . . but the back is much worse . . . the cars still keep driving . . . the pain in the back comes in waves . . . I ony see the one side of the street . . . oh, my back . . . [moaning, sobbing] . . . my back, my back [crying louder] . . . the pain radiates to the front . . . this is much worse than a delivery . . . [sobbing] . . . now a stabbing pain in my left axilla and in my left shoulder . . . now my whole back hurts . . . it is slowly getting better . . . now it's getting worse again . . . the picture of the East/West Street blends in occasionally, on and off, on and off, but I am so busy with my aches and pains . . . this takes such a long time . . . the pain in the back keeps increasing and decreasing . . . I have to go to the bathroom. . . ." (technical termination).

*AA 8:* "And I have a feeling as if I dissolve into the car . . . now a feeling as if falling forward, deeper and deeper . . . I am still falling . . . I want to keep hold of something . . . a terrible feeling . . . I catch my breath . . . my stomach is cramped . . . it's deeper and deeper . . . terrible . . . it is as if I am squeezed together, my whole body . . . this is the feeling I had when it hit me, when I thought: "Now I am finished" I know I am holding it back . . . I see the hole . . . the car . . . I start falling again . . . as if I am torn apart . . . again the car . . . my back is getting worse and my head . . . and again the car . . . this is terrible, these pains and the feeling of sinking . . . there is the car again . . . when the car is very close then everything starts turning and I fall and that is very painful . . . and again the same thing over again . . . and again . . . it is hurting everywhere . . . the car again and it takes me up into the air, I start turning and then it's going deep down, the deeper it goes the more painful it is . . . and the same thing over again . . . and again, and again . . . and this time it took me high up into the air and I fell deep deep down . . . I am sore all over . . . I have so much pain [moving on couch as if in pain, holding her left elbow] . . . the pain in the back comes in waves . . . and there comes the car again . . . and again . . . the car continues to come . . . but I don't turn any more . . . I tense up all over . . . and this repeats itself a number of times . . . my back is hurting so much and my left arm and elbow . . . I don't see anything any more . . . I am so occupied with my pains . . . the car is still coming, but that does not bother me any more . . . *during the accident I felt nothing at all* . . . and now all this . . . my left foot is hurting . . . everything is hurting . . . when the car comes everything is even hurting more than before. . . ."

*Case 103:* A 33-year-old secretary (anxiety reaction, depressive reaction). The following two passages are examples of thematic modifications involving pain and probably other sensations related to a traumatizing procedure which was carried out without anesthesia.

"I am walking down the path and looking around at the trees and suddenly I hit a branch and it goes right through me . . . through my stomach and I

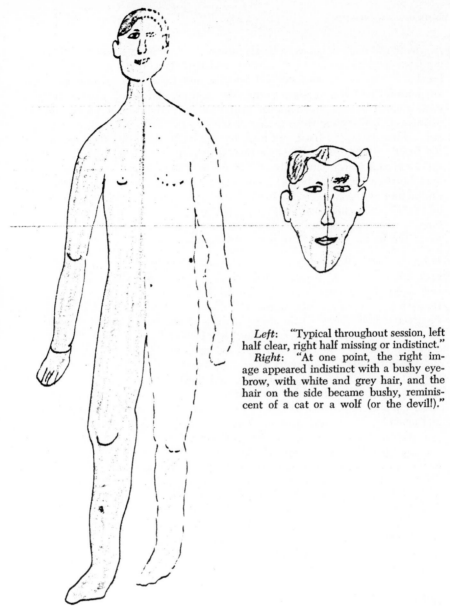

*Left:* "Typical throughout session, left half clear, right half missing or indistinct."

*Right:* "At one point, the right image appeared indistinct with a bushy eyebrow, with white and grey hair, and the hair on the side became bushy, reminiscent of a cat or a wolf (or the devil!)."

FIG. 13. Disturbance of self-image (37-year-old male patient, personality disorder). For prolonged phases of cinerama-type processes of neutralization which emphasized engagement in self-concept-disturbing material with ambisexual components, the brain-directed visual elaborations confronted the patient with disturbed images of himself. The right side of the body was always clear and realistic, while the left side remained indistinct or appeared to be missing.

feel a very sharp piercing pain in my stomach . . . I feel terribly weak and I lie there. . . ."

"I can't seem to get up and the horse runs over me and keeps running over me, back and forth, and I can feel his hoofs beating into me . . . and I can feel it on my stomach more than anywhere else . . . then the horse runs away and I lie there and feel sore all over. . . ."

## COENESTHETIC PHENOMENA AND BODY IMAGE

From clinical observations during autogenic standard therapy, it is known that the regular practice of autogenic standard exercises contributes to therapeutically desirable adjustments of certain functional disorders involving coenesthetic phenomena,[1404,1531] which are symptomatic for discrepancies between the body schema and the body image.[348,1047,2104,2140] Patients tend to express such improvements as a "more like-a-unit feeling" (see Case 15, p. 135/I; Case 37, p. 92, 95/III). Initially existing disturbances of the body image (e.g., detachment of the limbs, disproportions) are also known to decrease as autogenic exercises are practiced regularly over prolonged periods (see Fig. 1b, p. 9). Similar positively oriented developments occur during autogenic abreaction.

Depending on the nature of multithematic processes of neutralization, a variety of negatively or positively oriented coenesthetic phenomena (i.e., sensations derived from the body as a whole without precise localization) are frequently reported. When disturbing coenesthetic phenomena are prominent, brain-directed processes keep aiming at neutralization of such negatively oriented disturbing coenesthetic elements (e.g., thematic repetition) and bring about progressively more neutral and positively oriented sensory phenomena. Such positively oriented coenesthetic elaborations (e.g., "feeling more like myself," "particular feeling of well-being," "feeling completely relaxed and clean") may occur during the central abreactive period after brain-desired levels of neutralization in thematically specific areas have been achieved (e.g., during or after a Bright Light Phase), or they form a part of positively oriented terminal phases.

The brain-directed elaboration of negatively or positively oriented coenesthetic phenomena may or may not be associated with other synchronized elaborations involving the body image (see Table 41). When negatively oriented disturbing coenesthetic phenomena appear in combination with equally negatively oriented distortions of the body image, brain-directed processes of neutralization tend to go through thematic repetitions until brain-desired readjustment is achieved (see Case 101, p. 237). The brain's persistence in attempting to reduce and eliminate

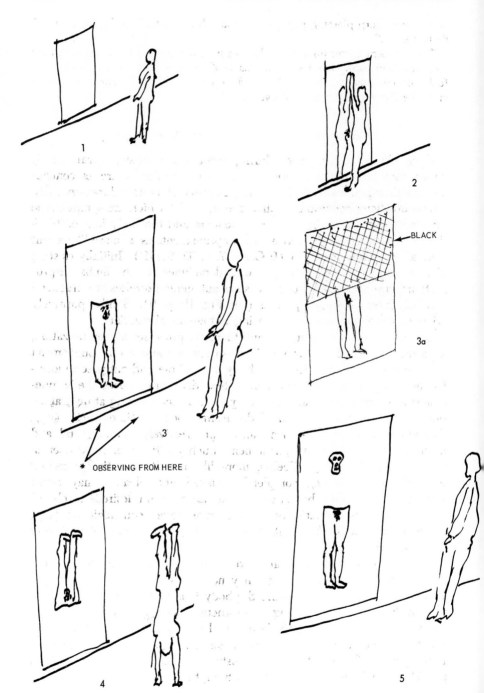

TABLE 41.  *Examples of Deviations of the Body Image during*
*Autogenic Abreaction*
(10 Psychosomatic and Neurotic Patients)

"I changed . . . I became a woman, black and big . . . I am sucking a penis and I imagine that my lips are big. . . ."

"I am at least as tall as the Place Ville–Marie building . . . I kick the C. I. L. building with my foot . . . I jump a bit, the buildings are shaking and they collapse. . . ."

"I feel as if my legs are separated from my body and as if I am floating at two different levels. . . ."

"I feel dead . . . I feel very narrow . . . it's as if I have no body anymore . . . Its as if my hands could touch each other across my body . . . I feel very long . . . it's always the same thing, I feel very long . . . like a corridor . . . with a small door at the end. . . ."

"I have funny hands, well, I think my hands . . . my hands are . . . my hands are right at my shoulder . . . I don't know . . . the arms are missing . . . that's a funny feeling . . . I feel only my hands. . . ."

"I feel very big and heavy . . . my hands seem particularly heavy and ready to . . . ready to . . . I don't know . . . they seem to be twisting and taking the shape of a stranglehold . . . I rather look like a demon, a monster going after somebody. . . ."

"I am stuck at the end of the pitchfork . . . I can't get off . . . I am very tiny . . . I am like a small pea on a fork. . . ."

"My arms feel very heavy, extremely heavy . . . and I feel very big, enormous. . . ."

"I am a little dog, sniffing around in the dead leaves in a park . . . I am sniffing the earth . . . and I fall on my side and I am dead. . . ."

"I am in a bed, in a hospital, and my belly is like a huge mountain . . . I am very big . . . oversize . . . enormous . . . the proportions are not normal . . . I am in a bed which is much too high and I am too big. . . ."

FIG. 14. Disturbance of self-image (37-year-old male patient, personality disorder). During a cinerama-type autogenic abreaction the patient observed himself looking into a mirror and (as observer on the scene) described intricate dynamics of brain elaborations involving anxiety-related disturbances of the body image. While looking into the mirror from a distance, he cannot see himself (No. 1). As he approaches the mirror the image becomes clearer and he can see himself (No. 2). The mirror image vanishes again as he moves a little away from the mirror. As he lowers his pants and underwear, the mirror image shows only his naked lower half (No. 3). On attempting to visualize the upper part of his body in the mirror, he experiences anxiety, and the upper part of the mirror becomes black (No. 3a). In a vain attempt to test the mirror image, he performs some acrobatics (No. 4). However, even in an upside-down position, the upper part of his body does not appear in the mirror (No. 4). After this (patient-directed) maneuver, he adopts a more passive attitude. After a while he recognizes a white skull (No. 5). As he keeps describing the skull and maintains a passively accepting attitude, the upper part of his trunk starts forming gradually, the skull fades away and is replaced by an image of himself.

disturbing interferences from material which generates unfavorable coenesthetic elements and distortions of the body image may be considered
as an indication for the biologic (or pathofunctional) importance of a
body image which is in favorable agreement with the body schema.

Observations in this area of autogenic neutralization support in many
respects the well-known studies by P. F. Schilder.[1204] Such phenomena
as macro- or microparesthesia, multiplicity of limbs, all kinds of distortions of the shape of the body, frequent involvement of erogenous zones
(e.g., eyes, mouth, nipples, genitals, urethra, anus), various manifestations of identification and phenomena of "appersonization"* are frequently
of central thematic importance during autogenic abreaction. However,
in certain other respects material obtained during autogenic neutralization raises the question whether P. F. Schilder's contemporary emphasis
on the libidinous aspects of the structure of the body image[1204, p. 170 ff.]
may need a reevaluation in a direction which coincides with the orientation of C. Vogt and O. Vogt† (see Case 101, p. 237), and which P. F.
Schilder pointed out himself: "It would be erroneous to suppose that
phenomenology and psychoanalysis should or could be separated from
brain pathology. It seems to be that the theory of organism could and
should be incorporated in a psychological doctrine which sees life and
personality as a unit."[1204, p. 7]

---

* Schilder's definition, p. 251, ref. 1204.

† Vogt, C. and Vogt, O.: Gestaltung der topistischen Hirnforschung und ihrer
Förderung durch den Hirnbau und seine Anomalien. *J. Hirnforschg.* 1953, 1, 1-46.

# PART IV.  BRAIN-DIRECTED MECHANISMS
## OF NEUTRALIZATION

## 18. Introduction

To facilitate an understanding of the seemingly endless possibilities of variations and combinations of brain-directed functions of autogenic neutralization, Part IV focusses on a discussion of the dynamics of the most important mechanisms which may participate to a variable extent in promoting a variety of brain-desired processes of neutralization. The physiologically oriented use of the term "mechanism" in connection with certain brain-directed functions of autogenic neutralization appears to be justified, since it has become evident that in different persons the same categories of biologically given brain functions systematically combine in such a manner that individually specifically adapted brain-desired functional changes aiming at progressive self-normalization are facilitated or brought about. Only a thorough knowledge of the psychophysiologic features of habitually occurring patterns of combinations of these self-regulatory brain mechanisms permits the clinically and therapeutically important distinction between positively oriented (i.e., self-curative) neutralization-facilitating dynamics and various negatively oriented (i.e., self-destructive) brain-antagonizing forms of resistance (see Vol. VI, Part I). Since positively oriented neutralization-facilitating dynamics may often appear to be very similar, or may suddenly shift to brain-antagonizing dynamics, extensive use of cross references to case material used in other parts of Vol. V and VI is designed to help the reader develop his ability to discriminate between neutralization-facilitating and neutralization-antagonizing dynamics of autogenic abreaction.

The various brain-directed mechanisms of neutralization may be considered as the basic therapeutic elements which the brain applies with sophisticated ingenuity while striving to re-establish functional harmony in its own system by attempting to reduce and eliminate disturbing effects resulting from accumulated neuronal material and relevant biologically unfavorable dynamics.

As one follows the brain in its attempts to reach its self-curative goal and observes the way in which biologic wisdom applies self-generated forces to very complex therapeutic tasks with computer-like precision, one cannot help wondering about the usefulness and the comparatively limited therapeutic efficiency of various therapist-designed forms of psychotherapy which have been in vogue for many years.

Brain-desired selection of disturbing material, timing and limitation of release of specific neuronal records, brain-directed management of multidimensional thematic combinations, gauging the dynamic force of material released and its correct adaptation to the system's level of tolerance, thematic repetitions and changes, self-confrontations and integrative dynamics, verification of its own progress and efficiency, programming and self-termination are only a few examples suggesting the complexity of interacting functions which are coordinated, guided and controlled by the patient's brain mechanisms. Being confronted with such naturally given potentialities of self-curative activity it appears to be an obvious conclusion that a therapist's brain cannot match the resourcefulness, sophistication and precision of biologic forces existing in the patient's brain. In consequence, during treatment with autogenic abreaction, a therapist's task is to give specifically adapted technical support which is designed to overcome brain-antagonizing forms of resistance and to help the patient's brain to carry out its own program of self-normalizing activities. To perform this therapeutic role correctly while respecting a positively oriented application of the *principle of non-interference*, the dynamics of the brain-directed mechanisms of neutralization presented in the following sections require careful consideration.

# 19. Thematic Programming

Systematic studies of autogenic discharges occurring during the practice of autogenic standard exercises over longer periods have revealed
that the profile of autogenic discharges undergoes progressive changes
which are reflected by quantitative and qualitative differences of the
modalities (e.g., motor, sensory, vestibular) released by the brain. The
phasic nature of the patterns of modalities discharged during certain
periods of autogenic standard training (see Fig. 7, p. 180; Case 15, p.
15/III; Fig. 3, p. 20/III) were taken as an indication that modalities of
autogenic discharges are released according to a brain-designed program
of functional priorities.

Pattern analyses of various categories of autogenic abreactions (see
p. 252 ff.) provided further evdience supporting the assumption that brain-
directed processes of self-regulatory discharge follow a brain-designed but
case-specific sequence of programmed thematic priorities. Similar to observations of phasic changes of autogenic discharges occurring over longer
periods of autogenic training which may involve different kinds of
physiologic and psychophysiologically oriented discharge modalities,
there appears to be no qualitative (e.g., motor, olfactory, sensory, vestibular, visual) restriction of brain-designed programming concerning the
possibilities of releasing a great variety of modalities during autogenic
abreaction.

These observations imply that the brain mechanisms which participate
in coordinating and controlling psychophysiologically multidimensional
processes of neutralization occupy a key position with commanding
access to various types of neuronal records accumulated in the central
nervous system. The evidence of a hierarchy of thematic programming
can be followed back from the organization of thematic sequences as
reflected by longer series of autogenic abreactions to the organization of
thematic neutralization within each autogenic abreaction and the structure of various thematic phases and their elements which constitute the
complex processes of autogenic neutralization.

While it is relatively easy to understand the sequence of brain-designed
programming in retrospect (e.g., after termination of a given AA; after
a series of AAs) it is generally difficult or in many instances impossible
to predict the precise course of self-curative action for the autogenic
abreactions to come. However, the patient's case history (e.g., traumatic
events, accidents), his actual clinical condition (e.g., depressive reaction,
obsessive-compulsive reaction, phobias), the thematic nature of the

preceding autogenic abreaction, and perhaps certain events which have occurred during the interim period (e.g., heart attack, death of father, car accident, ski accident, confrontation with stimuli which are known to be potent mobilizers of certain dynamics) may provide general clues for eventual processes of neutralization. It is in this connection that the nature of a patient's first (and perhaps second) autogenic abreaction requires particular consideration. Frequently, the content of initial auto-genic abreactions is composed of all kinds of more or less disguised elements which on first sight may impress by a lack of logic and coher-ence, but which in retrospect actually contained, as in a table of con-tents, many or all of the thematic elements which came to assume a central role during later phases of treatment with autogenic abreaction. A thorough study of the content of the first and second autogenic abreaction has been of particular value in determining the possibility of *thematic avoidance* (see Vol. VI, Part I) during later series of autogenic abreactions. Considering the forecasting value of the thematic elements composing the first and second autogenic abreaction, it was assumed that the brain already knew at this point what it intended to release for detailed neutralization during later phases of its self-curative program. Of similar forecasting significance are seemingly unrelated thoughts or images which tend to flash by during the inductive phase, before the patient begins to describe. Such telegram-style thematic announcements, which also may occur in the beginning of the initial abreaction phase (see Case 104), usually assume particular importance during the brain-programmed developments which characterize the dynamics of neutral-ization of the central abreactive phase.

*Case 104:* A 37-year-old technician (sexual deviation, obsessive-compulsive manifestations, ecclesiogenic syndrome, hypothyroidism). In the beginning of the initial abreactive phase, while the thematic dynamics are still rather un-differentiated, the patient describes himself alone on a golf course. The in-terjected image of a car refers to a girl friend who owns such a car. Later, during the central abreactive phase, thematic neutralization focuses for long periods on the patient's relationship with this girl friend.

"There's a landscape of trees in the background and through the branches the sky is blue . . . it's also very hot out . . . for a moment the picture is fixed . . . *the image of a car intervened and disappeared immediately* . . . once again I'm on the golf course. . . ."


## ROTATIONAL AND SEQUENTIAL PROGRAMMING

A series of alternating enagements in a brain-determined number of interrelated areas of disturbing material (i.e., rotational programming) in combination with periods of straight-forward consecutive changes of thematic neutralization (i.e., sequential programming) are the most frequently encountered forms of many varieties of brain-designed types of programmed neutralization.

The varieties of rotational programming can be reduced to the following simplified example of phasic multithematic neutralization: A-B-C-D –B-C-D-A–B-D-A-C–D-A-B-C. Such phases of rotational processes of thematic neutralization tend to go through a series of modified versions of thematic repetition until a brain-desired level of neutralization has been achieved and a thematic shift to the next multithematic phase (e.g., E-F-G-H-J) is brought about. While observing the dynamic changes which are habitually associated with rotational patterns of thematic neutralization, one is left with the impression that relevant brain mechanisms engage in systematic activities which aim at a lowering of disturbing potency in series of specific areas which for unknown reasons have priority over other areas of disturbing material. As the brain mechanisms continue their peculiar pattern of multithematic rotational neutralization from A to Z, they may start all over again with a somewhat modified combination of rotational sequences (e.g., A-B-F-B-C-H or AC-BE-F-GD). Such processses are repeated in a dynamically or thematically progressive manner (see Table 11, p. 57). In the course of such processes, certain thematic elements which were emphasized in the beginning may undergo modifications in a more normal direction (e.g., symbolic, less symbolic, reality) or disappear from the phases of rotational neutralization.

The sequential type of programming proceeds in a fairly straight-forward manner of progressively modified monothematic seqeuences of repetitions (e.g., A-A-Aa-A-Aa$_2$-Aa$_3$-AAaa). Only after brain-desired levels of thematic neutralization have been reached (e.g., versions of A) does a thematic shift to B follow. However, as the brain follows this pattern of sequential programming, interjected phases with greater thematic flexibility and similarity with features characteristic for the rotational type of programming tend to occur more frequently. As the brain-directed functions gain in dynamic flexibility, many other forms of program-related combinations are encountered.

## STRATIFUNCTIONAL PROGRAMMING

In patients who appear to have accumulated particularly disturbing material (e.g., aggression, chronically reinforced ecclesiogenic anxiety, obsessive-compulsive dynamics associated with consequences of many years of heteroaffective and sexual deprivation, chronically reinforced inadequate identifications) which requires many repetitions over long series of autogenic abreactions to arrive at brain-desired levels of neutralization, the brain-designed program of neutralization keeps repeating a distinctive pattern of thematic release. Unless acutely disturbing material from interim episodes are given thematic priority, a considerable part of the abreactive period is devoted to repetitions of familiar thematic elements which are already known as time-consuming subjects from previous autogenic abreactions. Only during advanced phases of neutralization of this layer of "old" material, more recent or *relatively new* thematic elements are occasionally released. As the brain is given ample time to continue its work, the initially dominating dynamics related to "old" material subside progressively, and thematic shifts with release of *entirely new* material occur. This brain-programmed procedure which follows the sequence: old material–relatively new material–entirely new material, is distinguished as the *stratifunctional pattern of neutralization* (see Case 105, Case 106, Table 42, p. 256; Table 43, p. 257).

*Case 105:* A 24-year-old graduate student (hypothyroidism, sexual deviation, anxiety reaction, multiple psychophysiologic reactions, ecclesiogenic syndrome). Only after a period of 65 minutes, entirely devoted to neutralization of dynamics which were already subject to neutralization during previous autogenic abreactions (e.g., aggressive, homosexual, heterosexual) and which were not neutralized during a 6-week interim, did the processes of neutralization shift to new, thematically related material, which was accumulated at the age of 10 while the patient spent his vacation in a summer camp.

*Case 106:* A 39-year-old priest (sexual deviation, obsessive-compulsive reaction, anxiety reaction, ecclesiogenic syndrome). During the first 58 minutes of this supervised autogenic abreaction, the brain-programmed dynamics of neutralization emphasized repetitions of well known "old" themes of obsessive-compulsive nature (e.g., looking at naked children, engaging in homosexual activities with adolescents and small boys). At the end of this period, *the patient felt tired and proposed to terminate* (patient-directed premature termination). Suspecting *thematic avoidance*, it was suggested that he continue to describe while remaining passive and delegating all initiative to his brain. Subsequently the brain guided the development toward his family and a confrontation with two of his sisters. After 71 minutes *relatively new* dynamics focussing on heteroaffective and heterosexual engagement followed. Ten minutes later (81 minutes) a completely *new* development took place. The patient started cutting his penis and experienced pleasure while doing so. Repetitions of this theme led to association of a childhood episode and a story about a man who badly wanted to smoke a cigarette and who cut off his penis and started smoking it like a cigarette. This also led the patient to remember that he always wanted to be like his sister Elisa because she was preferred by his parents and received more love and affection. He suggested that it was probably for this reason that he was cutting off his penis. While looking at the hole where his penis had been, he transformed into a girl and enjoyed having a vagina. While playing with his vagina, he suddenly started laughing and reported: "Leo [a colleague who frequently was the center of his vivid homosexual projections] *just appeared and we have intercourse.*" Neutralization focussed for about four minutes on this theme. Then brain elaborations shifted back to a normal setting with both men skiing in the mountains. Shortly after, the autogenic abreaction (128 min.) was terminated.

The development of his autogenic abreaction convinced the patient that in his case premature termination (e.g., after 58 min. as he had suggested) was definitely to his disadvantage. Realizing the importance of the developments occurring during the last 30 minutes of the abreactive period, he also decided to get a new tape-recorder, which would permit him automatic recording lasting up to 2 or 3 hours.

The therapeutic management of patients with patterns of stratifunctional neutralization differs in certain respects from that of other patients. To assure adequate treatment progress it is essential to foresee whether the patient's brain needs more time to reach a functional level which permits effective engagement and neutralization of the underlying new material. As it is the therapeutic aim to devote as much treatment time as possible to the neutralization of new material, it is of practical advantage to keep the steadily regenerated upper layer of thematically old material as thin as possible. This can be achieved by shortening the intervals between autogenic abreactions and by encouraging sufficiently advanced and intelligent patients to perform as many prolonged autogenic abreactions as possible at home. When such an intensive treatment program is followed, the time habitually devoted to get through the upper layer of old material tends to get progressively shorter (see Table 43) and a faster treatment response through more effective neutralization of the underlying material is obtained (see Case 105, Table 43). In case such an intensive treatment program is not adopted and the brain is allowed to regenerate and reinforce the disturbing dynamics related to thematically important but old material, difficult, prolonged and frustrating treatment periods may be expected. Such therapeutically unfavorable situations also result in cases where the therapist or the patient makes the technical error of premature termination, thus continuously eliminating the brain-desired possibility of engaging in effective neutralization of the underlying disturbances generating thematic material.

**TABLE 42.** *Duration of Phases with "Old," "Relatively New" and "Entirely New" Material during Stratifunctional Patterns of Neutralization*

| | Stratifunctional Phases of Thematic Neutralization | | | | |
|---|---|---|---|---|---|
| Initials, Sex and Age of Patients | First Phase Almost Entirely Devoted to "Old" Material (min.) | Second Phase Period with Interjected Thematic Shifts to "Relatively New" Material (min.) | Third Phase Period with Thematic Shifts to "Entirely New" Material (min.) | Total Time of Autogenic Abreaction (min.) | Prominent Psychodynamic Manifestations |
| 1. S. L. (m, 24) | 24 | 35 | 21 | 80 | Sex. Dev.; Obs.-Comp.; Anx. |
| 2. A. C. (f, 21) | 79 | 11 | 14 | 104 | Anx.; Hyst. |
| 3. G. B. (m, 32) | 22 | 6 | 18 | 46 | Sex. Dev.; Obs.-Comp.; Anx. |
| 4. M. B. (f, 34) | 81 | 21 | 3 | 105 | Anx.; Depr. R. |
| 5. M. D. (m, 29) | 28 | 11 | 2 | 41 | Sex. Dev.; Obs.-Comp.; Anx. |
| 6. P. L. (m, 38) | 71 | 10 | 47 | 128 | Sex. Dev.; Obs.-Comp.; Anx. |
| 7. F. D. (f, 37) | 28 | 13 | 13 | 54 | Anx.; Hyst. |
| 8. M. D. (m, 27) | 57 | 11 | 63 | 131 | Obs.; Anx. |
| 9. C. D. (m, 43) | 66 | 12 | 22 | 100 | Sex. Dev.; Obs.-Comp.; Anx. |
| 10. A. C. (m, 29) | 21 | 15 | 31 | 67 | Obs.-Comp.; Anx.; Depr. R. |
| 11. B. B. (m, 51) | 40 | 10 | 2 | 52 | Sex. Dev.; Obs.-Comp.; Anx. |
| 12. G. T. (m, 23) | 32 | 3 | 35 | 70 | Sex. Dev.; Anx. |
| 13. Y. S. (m, 28) | 56 | 6 | 7 | 69 | Obs.-Comp.; Anx.; Depr. R. |
| 14. B. M. (f, 33) | 20 | 38 | 16 | 74 | Anx.; Depr. R. |
| 15. M. L. (f, 24) | 55 | 4 | 19 | 78 | Anx.; Depr. R.; Hyst. |
| 16. C. B. (f, 32) | 9 | 38 | 9 | 56 | Post tr. Anx. |
| 17. C. H. (f, 22) | 33 | 15 | 41 | 89 | Anx.; Depr. R.; Hyst. |
| 18. Y. G. (m, 29) | 40 | 13 | 5 | 58 | Obs.-Comp.; Anx. |
| 19. C. L. (m, 28) | 12 | 25 | 27 | 64 | Obs.-Comp.; Anx. |
| 20. L. L. (m, 40) | 59 | 14 | 14 | 87 | Sex. Dev.; Obs.-Comp.; Anx. |

TABLE 43. *Duration of Phases with "Old," "Relatively New" and "Entirely New" Material before and during Intensive use of Prolonged Autogenic Abreactions in a Male Patient with Sexual Deviation, Obsessive-Compulsive and Anxiety Reaction*

| | Stratifunctional Phases of Thematic Neutralization | | | | |
| Date of Autogenic Abreaction | First Phase Almost Entirely Devoted to "Old" Material (min.) | Second Phase Period with Interjected Thematic Shifts to "Relatively New" Material (min.) | Third Phase Period with Thematic Shifts to "Entirely New" Material (min.) | Total Time of Autogenic Abreaction (min.) | Interval Between Last Autogenic Abreaction (days) |
|---|---|---|---|---|---|
| 1. Feb. 20 | 58 | 23 | 17 | 98 | 36 |
| 2. March 15 | 57 | 7 | 25 | 89 | 26 |
| 3. March 29 | 59 | 10 | 18 | 87 | 14 |
| 4. April 20 | 44 | 28 | 11 | 83 | 21 |
| 5. April 22 | 38 | 17 | 45 | 100 | 2 |
| 6. April 24 | 28 | 17 | 60 | 105 | 2 |
| 7. April 26 | 12 | 18 | 46 | 76 | 2 |
| 8. April 28 | 18 | 8 | 84 | 110 | 2 |
| 9. April 30 | 18 | 6 | 84 | 108 | 2 |
| 10. May 2 | 9 | 11 | 92 | 112 | 2 |

*Case 107:* A 39-year-old theologian (sexual deviation, obsessive-compulsive reaction, anxiety reaction, ecclesiogenic syndrome). After it became evident that the patient's stratifunctional pattern of thematic neutralization in combination with unusually long interim periods (see Table 43) did not result in desirable progress in treatment, intensive use of prolonged autogenic abreactions at two-day intervals was applied (see Table 43). This program led to a progressive and significant reduction of time devoted to neutralization of old material. Simultaneously, the brain-directed processes of thematic neutralization engaged with progressively increasing intensity in thematically new material (see Table 43). As this intensive treatment program was continued it became increasingly more difficult to distinguish the previously existing layers of stratifunctional organization. The pattern of neutralization gained progressively in thematic flexibility and speed of productive neutralization. These changes were reflected by an accelerated treatment process and case-specific changes toward desirable normalization (e.g., changes toward readjustment of sexual deviation, decrease of obsessive-compulsive manifestations and significant reduction of anxiety).

## STABILITY OF THEMATIC PROGRAMMING

The psychophysiologic features of brain-designed programming of smaller and and larger sections of thematic neutralization are also characterized by a high degree of functional stability. For example, when technical interruptions (e.g., need to void) occur during the central phase of the abreactive period, and the autogenic abreaction is continued 5 to 15 minutes later, the processes of thematic neutralization tend to continue their program of self-curative work around the same point at which the interruption had occurred (see Case 108). Similar observations have been made during relatively long autogenic abreactions when the dynamics of neutralization are temporarily interrupted by interjected periods of sleep (see Case 109).

*Case 108:* A 42-year-old housewife (anxiety reaction, moderate depression). The following passages permit a comparison between the pattern of thematic neutralization before and after a technical interruption of ten-minutes duration. As in an interrupted showing of a motion picture, the brain continues after the intermission from the point where stopped.

"And I think that the baby is going to die . . . it's still my husband's face, I . . . I see him with that air he has when its' one of his bad days . . . oh . . . [crying] . . . I only think of that . . . [crying] . . . I can't imagine that he's dead . . . his face, I don't want to see it anymore . . . [crying] . . . are you dead? . . . are you dead? . . . what's the matter? . . . I was worried . . . oh, uff . . . and I was afraid . . . oh I was much too scared of that guy . . . [crying] . . . that damn bottle there that's bothering me . . . that's bothering me . . . I don't know . . . I feel like going to the bathroom . . . *[technical termination]*."

Ten minutes later after the patient had visited the bathroom, smoked a cigarette and exchanged a few neutral remarks, the autogenic abreaction was continued. At the end of the introductory heaviness formulas, *"And now you continue to describe"* was added.

"I see my husband looking at me . . . oh . . . [sigh] . . . I just see the head with big eyes . . . [*Can you describe the eyes?*] . . . oh God, yes . . . oh . . . oh . . . [sigh] . . . the malice, oh . . . when he looked at me that it was much better that the baby died . . . it's to pay for that . . . and I think of that . . . and a nurse comes to check my bottle of serum . . . it bothers me . . . I look at the drops falling . . . drop by drop . . . oh . . . I'm in my bed . . . etc. . . ."

*Case 109:* A 51-year-old male teacher, member of a religious community (sexual deviation, anxiety reaction, obsessive-compulsive reaction, ecclesiogenic syndrome). After 40 minutes of cinerama-type neutralization of the devil's realm, the patient was about to leave hell and fell asleep for about 5 minutes. After waking up, the pattern of thematic neutralization continued as if there had been no interruption (see below).

"All the devils . . . as soon as they approach I gun them down . . . then I push a button that stops all the fires, but nonetheless it's black and hot, it's full of soot, it's dull, very hot, very hot . . . and now, I take a pickax and I pierce a hole because there's no way of getting out, while it's hot it's a good time to pierce a hole . . . [patient fell asleep for about 5 min.]. And now I get out of hell through this hole, and I get out of there . . . I have to jump over a ditch . . . and having jumped over the ditch, I come before the Lord. . . ."

Further evidence of the stability of brain-designed programming evolved from studies of longer series of autogenic abreactions which tend to follow a pattern of sequential continuity unless decisively disturbing intervening episodes lead to a modification of the brain-designed sequence of thematic priority. Even in instances when patients discontinued treatment for several weeks or months and autogenic abreactions were resumed, the dynamics of neutralization were observed to continue with about the same themes and the same pattern after brief periods (e.g., several minutes) of initial adjustment.

The impressive functional stability of those brain functions which participate in designing and maintaining the program-related dynamics of autogenic neutralization is of particular importance for the understanding of behavior in general. Of particular clinical interest are the patterns of deviations of psychodynamic and psychophysiologic reactivity which are associated with more specific program-related states of inadequate neutralization and proneness to thematic overmobilization (see p. 152).

## INTERFERENCES WITH BRAIN-DIRECTED THEMATIC PROGRAMMING

For the time it appears practical to distinguish three major categories of variables which may interfere with brain-directed thematic programming: (a) various forms of brain-antagonizing and indirect psychophysiologic resistance (see Vol. VI, Part I), (b) technical errors due to lack of experience, and (c) intervening variables of environmental nature. Since each of these different categories of variables may disturb the brain's program of thematic neutralization and thus result in therapeutically undesirable reactions which require adequate management, a more detailed discussion may be of practical value.

While most interferences with brain-directed thematic programming are due to specific forms of brain-antagonizing and indirect psychophysiologic resistance, and these are elaborated in detail in Part I of Volume VI, the following sections are limited to a discussion of technical errors due to lack of experience and the disturbing significance of certain environmental variables which may intervene during the interim period.

### TECHNICAL ERRORS

Brain-disturbing interferences, with undesirable complications of brain-programmed processes of neutralization can be observed when an inexperienced therapist assumes a directive role by attempting to manipulate the dynamics of the patient's brain, forcing it to follow a direction which is not or is only partly in agreement with the brain's own program of self-curative action. In such instances, manifestations of functional regression of brain elaborations (e.g., increase of symbolic elements, shift from higher levels of visual elaboration to less sophisticated or elementary stages; see Table 33, p. 188), cessation of habitual patterns of dynamics of neutralization can be observed; and *brain-desired* levels of neutralization are not reached or are delayed. Similar brain-disturbing situations with inadequate possibilities of brain-desired neutralization result when patients do not maintain an attitude of passive acceptance toward brain-programmed elaborations, but start "filtering" or permit themselves to direct their brain functions in desired directions. As the positively oriented self-regulatory potentialities of autogenic dynamics cannot unfold under such circumstances, the patient is prone to experience those unfavorable psychodynamic and psychophysiologic reactions which are habitually associated with inadequate levels of neutralization or thematic overmobilization (see Case 113, p. 264; Case 114, p. 264; Case 116, p. 265). Unfavorable interferences in brain-designed programming of thematic neutralization may also result from a therapist's supposedly supportive intervention after failing to make a correct distinction between normal neutralization-promoting dynamics (e.g., brain-facilitating forms of resistance; see Part

I, Vol. VI) and functional phenomena characteristic for brain-antagonizing forms of resistance (see Part I, Vol. VI). The functional disturbances resulting from such technical mistakes are usually of a rather
transitory nature, or the therapist's intervention is simply overruled by
brain-directed maneuvers which indicate that the brain does not wish
to follow the therapist's suggestion. Similar manifestations of sophisticated adaptability in pursuing its own program of curative action are
brain-designed responses (i.e., *brain-designed counter resistance;* see
Vol. VI) to interference from patients who have, for the moment,
adopted an active directive attitude (see Case 110, Case 111, Case 112).

*Case 110:* A 49-year-old teacher, member of a religious community (personality disorder, homosexuality, anxiety reaction, obsessive-compulsive and
depressive reactions, ecclesiogenic syndrome). In the following passages, the
brain overrules the patient's thematically interfering attempt to extinguish the
fire, thus forcing him to continue neutralizing confrontation with thematically
related anxiety material (i.e., burning in hell forever).
"The fire, it's still roasting . . . there's still something in the hot coals . . .
over there are the damned . . . one gets the impression that their ashes won't
disappear . . . they burn constantly . . . and *with the hose full of shit, I spray
the fire . . . but the fire persists . . . the shit changes . . . hardens and turns into
wood . . . and the fire doesn't burn out . . . it stays on . . .* etc. . . ."

*Case 111:* A 52-year-old priest (vocational conflicts, multiple psychophysiologic reactions, ecclesiogenic syndrome). During an unsupervised autogenic
abreaction, the patient became too active by trying to direct his brain toward
engagement in neutralization of aggressive dynamics. Since this patient-directed
interference does not correspond with the brain's own program of neutralization, the brain-directed response indicates repeatedly that the brain does not
wish to engage in these patient-designed maneuvers (i.e., *brain-designed counter-
resistance;* see Part I, Vol. VI).
"I'm thinking again of doing an exercise for the liberation of aggression . . .
I grabbed an ax and I'm taking it out on a big hardwood tree . . . *the ax
doesn't chop:* I keep hacking . . . now . . . *it detaches itself from the handle*
. . . I take another ax . . . *the handle breaks* . . . (would it be that my brain
won't have anything to do with it this morning?) . . . in any case I go into the
house. . . . I'm making plans to put things in better order, to clean up, to make
it more beautiful. . . ."

*Case 112:* A 50-year-old priest (anxiety reaction, multiple psychophysiologic
and phobic reactions, ecclesiogenic syndrome). As the brain-designed program
aims at thematic neutralization (i.e., fear of rats, being bitten by rats, death)
be repeating the process of being devoured by rats, and the patient interferes
by refusing to go along with the brain's program (i.e., *repetition resistance;* see
Part I, Vol. VI) by running away and hoping to find a secure place on top of a
light house, the brain simply overrules the patient's maneuvers (i.e., *brain-*

*designed counter-resistance;* see Part I, Vol. VI) by disintegrating the light house.

"Vermin comes to mind, sewer rats that invade my room and that begin eating me up again . . . I can't think of anything else . . . you could even say that this is extremely unpleasant for me . . . I get out of this room . . . but the rats, this army of rats follows me . . . follows me through the village . . . I take refuge up in the lighthouse tower . . . *this soon tumbles down and breaks my ribs while falling* . . . the rats take advantage of this to continue nibbling at me. . . ."

Brain-directed programming of thematic neutralization is not only confined to a determination of the sequences and combination of thematic elaborations but also includes program-related self-regulatory functions which determine certain quantitative aspects of the material it is prepared to release. For example, attempts to prolong autogenic abreactions beyond the point of brain-directed indications for termination (see Delayed Termination, p. 84 ff.) have not yielded a therapeutically productive performance. This is evidence that certain self-regulatory program-related functions determine the duration of engagement in productive processes of autogenic neutralization and that it is of no therapeutic advantage to force the brain to continue after it has indicated that its own program of thematic neutralization has come to a natural end for the time. Complementary to this program-related aspect are the generally unfavorable psychodynamic and psychophysiologic states of reactivity which tend to follow after premature terminations (see p. 76 ff.; p. 84 ff.). Considering these observations, it appears therapeutically desirable to respect the brain's need for neutralization concerning the duration of productive brain-directed elaborations. It is in this respect that both relatively inexperienced and experienced patients who are permitted to perform autogenic abreactions at home tend to make the technical error of not permitting their brain to continue the brain-designed program of neutralization until a natural self-regulatory limit has been reached. As a consequence these patients do not enjoy the full benefit of their therapeutic work because they continuously leave their brain in a state of incomplete neutralization with disturbing interferences from effects of residual mobilization.

This undesirable effect of inadequate duration of autogenic abreactions is of particular concern during the treatment of patients with obsessive-compulsive dynamics, the neutralization of which usually requires relatively monotonous and long series of thematic repetitions as, for example, encountered in patterns of stratifunctional neutralization (see p. 253).

tralization of two cranial accidents which the patient had suffered a number of years before.

*Case 116:* A 41-year-old career woman (hysterical personality, anxiety reaction, moderate depresive reaction, multiple psychophysiologic and phobic reactions). Seven days after her last autogenic abreaction (AA 15) and 38 hours after she came back from an exhausting business trip to various cities in the United States, this patient called the therapist's home at 9:30 P.M. In a shaky and sobbing voice she explained that she felt panicky and had been crying for some time without knowing why. After some exploratory questioning it was suggested that she perform an autogenic abreaction at home and to call the therapist after termination or in case of unforeseen difficulties.

About two hours later the patient called back reporting that she felt well and calm, and that she now knew why she had felt so disturbed. The dynamics of her autogenic abreaction (AA 16) had revealed that her "unexplained reaction" was related to thematic over-mobilization resulting from a confrontation with a combination of stimuli which fell into specific categories of disturbing material which was undergoing progressive neutralization during the current treatment phase.

During one part of her business trip, she had traveled in a plane which was largely occupied by soldiers returning from Viet Nam. Sitting between two soldiers the conversation had emphasized guerilla warfare and other descriptions of acts of violence which in a number of respects appeared to be similar to her own experience during World War II. Of particularly mobilizing nature (as revealed by AA 16) was the fact that one of the young soldiers who stated that he had earned his plane ticket home by killing 40 of the enemy in action, looked strikingly similar to her own brother (to whom the patient had been very closely attached, who had reported similar stories, and who had died toward the end of WW II). The mobilizing stimuli: (a) acts of violence during warfare, (b) killing and being killed, sudden death by shooting, in combination with (c) the unexpected confrontation with a "brother image" where all closely related to dynamics of thematic neutralization which dominated the central phases of the patient's last four autogenic abreactions. The following passages of AA 16 are generally following the same program-related pattern on neutralization observed during the patient's preceding autogenic abreactions (e.g., violence, death, WW II episodes, inadequate identifications), but new thematic elements clearly reflect the thematic over-mobilization which resulted from the interim episode:

"There are bodies lying all over. One body beside the other. Twisted bodies . . . bodies one on top of the other. The whole meadow is covered with skeletons . . . and bodies. Some are already rotting . . . some are just dying. Some of them are just skeletons . . . I look at them, I walk all across, I step over them . . . sometimes I have to step on them . . . I can't avoid it . . . there are some black bodies . . . Negroes . . . I look at a child's body: stomach all swollen up. He is naked . . . he has huge black eyes looking straight at me . . . he must have died of starvation . . . lots of white bodies . . . stomach bloated

. . . I look at one . . . he is almost a midget, small yellow body and a huge head . . . I look at his eyes, they are blue, bulging eyes . . . vicious eyes . . . his mouth is open . . . he has long pointed teeth sticking out . . . how did they get killed? . . . [crying] . . . I killed them all . . . I just killed every single one of them . . . [crying]. . . . How could I kill them all . . . the meadow is covered with bodies . . . I go back to the edge of the meadow . . . I will have to go step-by-step to see who they are . . . I have a uniform, it is gray . . . I have a gray skirt and blouse with epaulettes . . . I have a gray cap . . . and I have boots . . . I start walking again and look down at the bodies . . . I sit there and try to remember what happened . . . [crying] . . . I look around and then I see him (the G. I. I met in the plane) . . . I see a body not far from Jack lying quietly. I get up and I walk to him . . . I sit down and look at him . . . he is young . . . he looks 18 or 19 . . . he is very thin and he wears an American uniform. He is an American G. I. dead . . . I look at his face . . . he has blond eyebrows and blue eyes, laughing eyes . . . he is dead but his eyes are still laughing . . . he has a stubby nose . . . his lips are open also laughing . . . his teeth are small and white . . . very even . . . his hair is blond and wavy . . . he must have died recently, because beads of sweat show on his forehead . . . his blond hair is sticky with sweat . . . a lock of hair hangs into his forehead and sticks there with sweat . . . [crying] . . . he is like my brother . . . he is exactly like my brother . . . [crying] . . . so awfully young . . . and I look at him and I remember. I didn't kill the people lying around. He did. He got a reward for killing 40 people in Vietnam . . . he got a leave . . . I look around him . . . he has a duffel bag beside him . . . his boots are tied to the suitcase . . . I keep looking at him: his blue eyes, his blond wavy hair and even his ears are like my brother's . . . small . . . a little bit standing away from the face . . . not quite flat . . . I keep looking at the young American . . . he smiles at me . . . I touch his forehead . . . it is still warm . . . and then I also remembered who else he was like . . . the young German with the radio . . . we were in the bunker . . . and so were a few Germans left behind until the Russians were only about a kilometer away . . . we had no more food . . . the young German had potato sugar . . . he gave me a chunk and I sat beside him all the time looking at him because he was so much like my brother . . . I stayed until they left and then I cried for a long time . . . I know now that I am on the front . . . the young American killed a lot of people . . . and so did I because it is war . . . my brother disappeared and told me to take his place . . . I have the same uniform he had . . . only I have a skirt . . . I am the only one who survived . . . and maybe my brother . . . I must look again at the American . . . he is still smiling . . . I hold his hand and it is warm . . . now his face looks a bit chubbier . . . [crying] . . . I don't know anymore if it is my brother or the young German or the G. I. . . . I feel very dizzy . . . I must repeat it from the beginning . . . the meadow is full of dead bodies . . . some are skeletons ugly flies are feeding on them . . . I walk around straight . . . I am ruthless, I step over bodies . . . I step on some . . . I have strong boots and I have a uniform, it is gray . . . it looks like a German uniform . . . I kick some bodies aside . . . and then I see the young man . . . I get up and walk closer to him

. . . he also has a gray uniform . . . I don't know uniforms very well . . . it could be American or it could be German . . . all I know is that he is terribly young . . . , [crying] . . . his blue eyes sparkle . . . they are full of laughter . . . his mouth is open . . . soft and laughing [crying] . . . he has blond hair with a small gray cap on it . . . his hair is soaked with sweat . . . locks of his hair stick to his forehead and face . . . I feel dizzy . . . the face changes . . . it is my brother and then it is the young German . . . but he is exactly like my brother . . . [crying] . . . because the German always had earphones on his head . . . but the same fair skin, blue eyes full of laughter, snub nose, lips that did not cover his upper teeth completely when he laughed . . . slim . . . and looks like a young person who is still growing because his jacket sleeves did not reach down to his wrist . . . and he got a holiday because he killed forty. . . ."

## ADAPTATIONAL ASPECTS OF THEMATIC PROGRAMMING

The biologic forces and brain functions which participate in elaborating and maintaining the thematic organization of programmed processes of neutralization are necessarily subject to adaptational exigencies arising from conditions within their own system. To proceed with a high degree of self-curative efficiency, the organization of thematic programming has to follow a self-facilitating pattern of activity which (a) avoids, circumvents and progressively reduces and eliminates inhibitory forces existing in its own system, (b) avoids and eliminates undesirable side-effects which could result in inhibitory counter reactions and thus compromise the successful pursuit of programmed self-regulatory neutralization, and (c) avoids and eliminates the risk of eliciting damages to its own system through the coordinated control of selective release of well-adapted quantities of neuronal material and simultaneous inhibition of thematically and functionally undesirable dynamics (e.g., undue spreading of excitation). Furthermore, to achieve a high degree of self-curative efficiency it appears desirable that (d) the program of thematic neutralization is designed in such a manner that as many brain-disturbing elements as possible are included in each phase of neutralization activity.

Detailed pattern analyses of autogenic abreactions provide ample evidence which support the assumption that brain-designed programming is carefully adapted to the exigencies mentioned above (see a, b, c, d). For example, during autogenic abreactions it can be observed that the brain-designed program of neutralization never engages in elaborations of unprepared direct repetition or presentation of severely traumatic material. The program of thematic neutralization is invariably composed of sophisticated preparatory phases which ensure

that the disturbing material undergoes a gradual process of neutralization before the reality elements of the original traumatic situation are
released in a recognizable and complex manner as they were recorded
at the time of a given event. In certain instances it may take a long
series of autogenic abreactions which in various respects contain preparatory phases of neutralization of elements of specific material which
the brain wishes to release at a later point. In other instances the
phases of preparatory neutralization are much shorter and perhaps
limited to a few minutes (see Case 117).

*Case 117:* A 28-year-old male teacher (sexual deviation, anxiety reaction,
multiple phobic and psychophysiologic reaction, ecclesiogenic syndrome). During an interim period the patient was involved in a car collision from which he
escaped with only minor injuries. One hour later on the second floor of a garage
while trying to remove some of his belongings from the trunk of his wrecked
car, he slipped and fell head first into an insufficiently protected stairway onto
a pile of boxes one story below and from there onto the cement floor (concussion). About ten days later, during an autogenic abreaction, the brain-programmed sequences of thematic neutralization proceeded in a characteristic
manner. The first 28 minutes of the abreactive period were devoted to dynamics
of largely known, rather innocuous and "easy" themes, and only sporadically
were certain well-camouflaged elements of the accidents interjected. Then followed a 12-minute period containing an increasing number of relatively new
thematic elements which appeared to be more closely related to the recent
accumulated accident material (e.g., sensations of falling, spinning, dizziness,
sudden death, hell). After this thematic preparatory period, about 40 minutes
after the beginning of the autogenic abreaction, the brain-designed program
focussed more directly on (a) the garage accident with concussion, and later
(b) the car collision which had happened earlier the same afternoon. As the
dynamics of neutralization went through many repetitions for another period
of 47 minutes, waves of massive motor discharges kept coming for about 37
minutes. In addition, feelings of nausea, need to vomit, crying spells, various
aches and pains, dizziness, feeling of being about to lose consciousness and
thematic repetitions of dying were quite disagreeable for the patient. Fortunately he was already familiar with the technical implications of the method
and was able to maintain adequate levels of passive acceptance, thus greatly
facilitating efficient neutralization of the accident material.

Program-related functions also provide sufficient integrative flexibility to absorb disturbing material which was accumulated during
interim periods without abandoning its original pattern of programmed
sections of thematic neutralization. This program-related adaptational
facility is largely brought about by thematic modification (i.e., thematic disintegration, distortion, dissociation; see p. 292 ff.). Other program-related adaptational functions involve a "strategic" interjection of

"encouraging" or "particularly pleasing" antithematic elaborations, which sometimes appear to be brain-designed efforts to coax a frustrated and tired patient to continue to go along with the brain's program of thematic neutralization.

## PREDICTABILITY OF THEMATIC PROGRAMMING

Certain data of a patient's history, such as accidents, periods of sexual and heteroaffective deprivation, negatively oriented anxiety-promoting religious education, inadequate identifications, traumatic medical procedures, brain-disturbing professional activities, phobic reactions, depressive reactions (e.g., loss of persons to whom the patient was attached), chronic accumulation of aggressive material, self-imposed inhibition of biologically normal functions (e.g., blocking of crying, vomiting) permit a prediction in a very general sense that brain-programmed processes of neutralization eventually are going to focus on those topics.

However, the possibility of predicting the nature of, for example, the first autogenic abreaction is very low. It is also very difficult to predict when the brain is going to engage in neutralization of severely traumatic events, unless it is evident that the thematic pattern of preceding autogenic abreactions requires further neutralization of the same type of disturbing material. Thematic changes from symbolic to realistic elaborations can only be predicted in a general sense on the basis of the progressive trend of the overall pattern of neutralization. The number of thematic repetitions which the brain needs to arrive at brain-desired levels of neutralization cannot be predicted. It is also impossible to predict when, under which circumstances and how often thematic processes of regressive nature (e.g., to childhood) will occur. The number and intensity of motor and sensory modalities of discharges are unpredictable. Only in cases with established patterns of thematic repetitions (e.g., obsessive, aggressive-depressive) is there a somewhat higher degree of predictability concerning the general nature of content and pattern. In other words, new material and unexpected developments may be expected to occur in each autogenic abreaction the patient and the therapist are going to confront.

# 20. Thematic Determination, Selective Release and Inhibition

How, and according to what principles a brain proceeds to determine the material it wishes to release for thematically programmed neutralization is unknown. Although it is evident that the participating self-regulatory brain functions emphasize neutralization of accumulated disturbing material and that antithematic agreeable elaborations do only occur at "strategic" points which require thematic contrast or specific facilitating "encouragement," it is not clear how these highly sophisticated functions are brought about.

How thematic priorities are determined requires further investigation. It is now hypothesized that a physiologically oriented *pressure principle* participates in determining the material to be released and the order in which sections of this material enter into the brain-designed program of self-regulatory neutralization. This tentative assumption is based on impressions from clinical observations which indicate that progressively oriented thematic shifts appear to occur when the "pressure" in one thematic area has been "lowered" to an extent that other areas with previously somewhat lower levels of pressure now evolve as areas with pressure levels which are higher than the pressure of the area which just had been lowered through processes of thematic neutralization. As relevant brain mechanisms attempt a progressive lowering of pressure in different areas of disturbing material, the brain appears to advance from one area to the next. The hypothesis of the pressure principle is applicable to rotational, sequential, stratifunctional and other forms of brain-designed thematic neutralizations (see p. 251 ff.). Furthermore, it is assumed that physiologic changes related to fatigue of certain neuronal systems also participate but appear to be of a secondary nature concerning the brain-designed structure of thematic programming. Another category of functional variables which is assumed to participate in the program-related determination of thematic release appears to be related to functional changes which are associated with various types of resistance, which may or may not have played a decisive role of self-protection during certain periods of the patient's life.

Closely related to the functions which determine the material to be released for neutralization are other functions which participate in facilitating the coordinated elaboration of the brain-selected thematic elements and which also guarantee through functions of protective inhibition that undesired material is not activated, and phenomena of the brain-disturbing spread of excitation does not occur. How such physiologically highly differentiated and complex tasks are achieved remains to be investigated. Of therapeutically practical interest however, is the fact that no untoward or dangerous developments have been noted (in over 10,000 AAs) as long as the technical implications and the case-adapted application of the method were correctly observed.

The brain's own autoselective self-regulatory mechanisms of thematic release are of biologic nature and, as such, endowed with functional possibilities which are assumed to lose essential features of natural efficiency under relatively artificial circumstances. This appears to be the case when, for example, patient-directed or therapist-directed maneuvers of thematic selection with subsequent dictation of brain dynamics according to their concepts or theories are applied in an attempt to perform a therapeutically better job than the brain could supposedly do.

# 21. Thematic Repetition

The functionally most consistent feature encountered in all varieties of autogenic processes of autogenic neutralization is the phenomenon of self-starting, self-propelling and self-terminating thematic repetition. The great variety of functional improvement which can be observed as being closely associated with the progressively oriented self-regulatory dynamics of repetition (and confrontation) led to the view that brain-directed thematic repetition may be considered as the "vehicle of autogenic neutralization." This view is closely linked to the clinical observation that no undesirable consequences have been noted after what may be considered as too many thematic repetitions, but that therapeutically undesirable emotional and psychophysiologic reactions have frequently occured when the brain has not been permitted to engage in a sufficient number of thematic repetitions (see *Repetition Resistance,* Part I, Vol. VI).

Processes of thematic repetition are not restricted to a particular type or a specific category of brain-directed elaborations but may involve many varieties of physiologic and psychodynamic combinations of brain-disturbing material and may occur at various levels of functional integration (e.g., motor discharges, pain; thematic repetitions aiming at neutralization of a negatively loaded mother image and subsequent facilitation of heterosexual differentiation). As with other phenomena of processes of autogenic neutralization, the timing of repetitions, their intensity, their level of thematic disintegration of functional complexity, their adaptation to various thresholds of systemic or individual tolerance, their symbolic or realistic elaboration, their degree of dissociation and interjected thematic associations appear to be elaborated and co-ordinated with the degree of precision characteristic for biologic self-regulatory mechanisms.

In a very general sense, permitting many exceptions, it may be said that the number of brain-desired repetitions increases with the patho-functional potency of the thematic material in question and the intensity of thematically related brain-antagonizing forms of resistance. Inversely, relatively lower frequencies of thematic repetitions are usually observed when (a) the disturbing potency of relevant material is low, (b) when there is little or no brain-antagonizing resistance, (c) during advanced phases of thematic neutralization, and (d) when brain-antagonizing forms of resistance (see Part I, Vol. VI) do not permit a brain-desired number of thematic repetitions. Repetitions of specific thematic elements subside and stop after a brain-desired degree of thematic neutralization has been achieved. Therapeutically each thematic repetition may be regarded as another step toward better functional adjustment and normalization.

To facilitate the brain's own program of thematic neutralization, it is important that both the therapist and the patient adopt a supportive attitude toward any kind of brain-desired thematic repetition. As a general rule of therapeutic management, it is recommended to tolerate passively and, in case of intervening brain-antagonizing forms of resistance (see Part I, Vol. VI), to support the brain's need to achieve thematic neutralization through an adequate number of thematic repetitions (i.e., until brain-directed elaborations of self-regulatory termination are described or evident; see p. 76 ff.; p. 79 ff.).

Since the therapist's technically oriented explanations of the therapeutic value of thematic repetitions require a case-specific adaptation which is in agreement with the progressively changing nature of temporarily prevailing patterns of thematic repetitions, it is necessary to be familiar with the dynamic nature of different categories of thematic repetition. It has seemed unwise to present the reader with long and possibly confusing discussions of tentative conclusions based on analyses of a variety of patterns of thematic repetition. Instead a simplified but generally valid presentation of three major categories of patterns of thematic repetition are presented. The reader may find it particularly instructive to study the phenomena of thematic repetition by devoting more time to passages concerning various autogenic abreactions presented in this volume, Volume VI and Volume I, p. 201 ff.

## SERIAL MONOTHEMATIC REPETITION

Sequences of repetition of the same thematic material are one of the most characteristic phenomena of the various categories or brain-programmed processes of neutralization. Depending on the predominate level of psychophysiologic complexity of the nature of the thematic material, the sequences of monothematic repetition may be composed of *small thematic units* as, for example, a series of muscular twitches (see p. 292 ff.), repetitions of short intellectual ideomotor or intersensory elaborations (see Case 118, Case 119, Case 120, p. 277). In other instances the sequences of monothematic repetitions are composed of thematically more *complex units* (e.g., being run over by cars) which may comprise larger sections of more complex thematic material. The degree of thematic complexity and the number of repetitions of a given monothematic unit appear to be closely related to (a) the brain-

disturbing potency of the thematic material, (b) the nature and intensity of certain forms of brain-antagonizing resistance (see Part I, Vol.
VI), and (c) other quantitative variables which participate in the accumulation of specific categories of brain-disturbing material (e.g.,
aggression; see Case 118, p. 274). Clinically oriented studies led to the
assumption that there exists a proportional relationship between the
anxiety-generating potency of thematic material and the "size" and
number of monothematic repetitions required for progressive thematic
neutralization. The monothematic units tend to be smaller (e.g., more
elementary, less differentiated, less complex, more symbolic) and seem
to require a higher number of repetitions as the anxiety-generating
material is more forceful (e.g., life-threatenting accidents). Complementary to this are observations indicating that monothematic patterns
of serial repetitions involving brain-disturbing material associated with
relatively low levels of anxiety tend to be composed of larger units
(e.g., more differentiated, dynamically more complex, more reality-
related) which, however, depending on the quantity of the accumulated
material, or the thematically related need (e.g., affective and sexual
deprivation) for neutralization, tend to require comparatively lower
numbers of repetitions.

As brain-directed processes of monothematic repetitions are given
ample opportunity to continue their self-curative work, numerically
increasing thematic modifications or flash-like interjections of related
material indicate a gain in thematic flexibility. Such progressive improvements in thematic flexibility are usually associated with increasing degrees of reality-related differentiation and dynamic complexity.
It is assumed that such brain-desired functional changes are related to
the successful advance in neutralization of the disturbing potency of
the monothematic material.

Case 118: A 35-year-old salesman (moderate depressive reaction). After
attractive and uneventful antithematic cinerama elaboration during the
patient's first autogenic abreaction, there were progressively more indications
of massive resistance antagonizing a brain-desired neutralization of accumulated
aggression. In AA 6 this resistance was overcome and a monothematic pattern
of neutralization of aggressive material followed.

The pattern of this AA began with an antithematic phase (4 min.) focussing
on a peaceful, serene country atmosphere. Then, beginning with a childhood
episode (see passages below) a very dynamic pattern of violent aggression
continues for 133 minutes. During the last 40 minutes of the abreactive period,
occasionally interjected thematic references concerning specific situations of
the persons being attacked (father, bosses, a friend, three girl friends, two
other men; see relevant passages of the patient's commentary, p. 277), reflect a

characteristic increase in thematic flexibility which is usually observable when advanced levels of neutralization are reached in the course of monothematic repetitions (see *Stratifunctional Programming,* p. 253 ff.).

Since the pattern of monothematic repetitions indicated that many more AAs would be needed to neutralize the accumulated aggression, a technical termination was applied when the patient appeared to be tired (see terminal phase). To save space, only brief passages taken from the tape-recorded material at ten-minute intervals, are given below.

"The scene seems to be disappearing with a sort of a gray, with a building or something trying to make its appearance, but nothing very definite or anything I can describe . . . yes, I guess the tenements or three-story flat we used to live in, supposed to be one year that we had stayed there. . . . I guess there comes the scene of a kid that who was much younger than I was . . . oh! he had been bugging me one day and I told him to bugger off, because I would beat the hell out of him, but the kids had egged him on, and I said go away I could beat you with one hand behind my back. One of the guys that had been egging him on, was this other guy that I had a fight with on Eighteenth Avenue. . . . Well this fight had taken place on the street in a lane in and around there I guess I did not want to hurt the kid, but I had to slug him in the face and I pushed him very hard in the body and to make him double up and cower, beneath his arms, I had been using a right arm, and I would stand back some of the time, and the other times I would just go in and let him have it . . . he was too scared really to do anything against me . . . [*well just go ahead*] . . . well I guess it would be a good time to use both fists, it really feels a good sensation of hitting him, in the chest and make him back and around the arms and in the stomach to make him double up, and to slam in the forehead. . . ."

*15 minutes after beginning:*

"I jump up and down on him again . . . just keep jumping up and down . . . just go on bouncing up and down as he tries to throw you off—let him turn over and jump up and down on his chest and his arms, his legs, his midsection, when you are tired of that, just kick and kick. . . ."

*25 minutes after beginning:*

"Grab his arms and force him to the ground, jump up and down on him with your knees, force his face into the dirt, into the hard rock . . . just keep up and down with your knees, then get up and just keep jumping up and up and up and down . . . slam your full weight against his back . . . his ribs and . . . scrape his face against the rocks. . . ."

*35 minutes after the beginning:*

"Hitting and hitting and hitting . . . just keep slugging and hitting . . . and hitting and hitting . . . keep hitting him on the face, make him more bloody . . . keep hitting and hitting. . . ."

*45 minutes after the beginning:*

"Just keep squeezing and twisting his neck . . . [yawn] . . . just get up and start jumping and jumping and jumping again . . . and boot him in the ribs again . . . slam him at the back of the neck, boot and kick . . . jump on his back with your knee again. . . ."

*65 minutes after the beginning:*

"Still squeezing, hitting and squeezing again . . . still grabbing, slapping, slapping, hitting . . . hitting very hard . . . hitting in the ribs and kicking again in the shins and the legs . . . hit him right in the face. . . ."

*75 minutes after the beginning:*

"Just keep hitting and hitting in his ribs . . . face all over his body . . . harder and harder . . . just keep slugging and hitting . . . smash him right in the nose again . . . harder . . . [yawn] . . . keep hitting harder and harder. . . ."

*85 minutes after the beginning:*

"Really squeeze hard . . . really squeeze and squeeze and squeeze, squeeze harder and harder . . . hit him right in the face . . . harder and harder . . . hit him right in the face . . harder and harder . . . really slug . . . harder . . . [yawn] . . . really belt . . . harder and harder. . . ."

*95 minutes after the beginning:*

"Hit him in the face . . . hit him in the face . . . again and again . . . give him a couple of good ones right in the eye . . . really beat the hell out of him . . . again and again and again. . . ."

*105 minutes after the beginning:*

"(Shortly before this I mention that I have beaten up about eight guys and they are quite bloody) . . . squeezing and squeezing . . . still harder and harder . . . just keep hitting and hitting him and hitting . . . hitting and hitting harder . . . really slug him in the body and face again. . . ."

*115 minutes after the beginning:*

"Harder and harder . . . slug him in the face and around the body again and kick him and stamp on him . . . slug her, really hit her again and again. . . ."

*125 minutes after the beginning:*

"Kick and kick and kick hard . . . kick and kick and kick . . . just kick kick and kick . . . just kicking him in the head, blood is pouring out now, just keep kicking him. . . ."

*135 minutes after the beginning:*

"Face again and again . . . just keep hitting and hitting . . . just keep kicking him harder and harder. . . ."

*From 137 minutes to end as follows:*

"Harder and harder . . . just keep hitting him and hitting him. . . [*Well, how many are there still around there?*] . . . they are unconscious by this time . . . [*Do you have the last one now?*] . . . I'm just going to chop his head off . . . the blood squirting all over the place . . . [*Can you bury the whole bunch of them?*] . . . Yep, get a big bulldozer and shove them all into a big common grave . . . they are all just nicely in the grave now and you can't see anything on the ground . . . [*Well how does everything look now?*] . . . It's the black of night . . . I guess you should always bury people that you murder in the dead of the night . . . [*How do you feel now?*] . . . Very good right now, exhausted . . . [*So then we are going to terminate here*] . . . (termination procedure).

*Passages from the patient's commentary:*

"From the first to the last, the trip appears to be a résumé of me fighting with a fellow I knew as a child. After a while I started to get bored with hitting the one poor fellow, so I changed to people who I have a grudge against, disliked or for any reason. During the trip, there was definite indication that after a while I felt occasionally like changing but I somehow persisted. I wasn't sure whether I was deliberately doing it or not. Occasionally, there were brief flashes onto another subject, such as an open arm invitation with Lucie to start love-making. However, this was only a brief flash and I was back to the punching (she frustrated me quite a bit on many occasions). I think that the move to other subjects was spontaneous by the brain rather than forced. I am pretty sure that some of these distractions lasted about 15 seconds at times. At the end, I was itchy and restless all over. I wanted either to terminate or to stop the fighting. One of the after-effects of the trip was a curious sense of well-being the next day and the following day."

*Case 119:* A 52-year-old priest (vicational conflicts, multiple psychophysiologic reactions, anxiety reaction, moderate depression, ecclesiogenic syndrome). During the neutralization of material related to many years of affective deprivation, the following pattern of thematic repetitions occurred.

"Let me caress you, let me caress you, hold you against me, press your naked body against me . . . ah, ah . . . ah . . . you are clinging to me, and I'm holding you, I'm holding you . . . let me press your arms against your body once more, let me press your two arms against your body once more . . . I desire you, I desire you, I desire you, I desire you, I desire you . . . my body desires you . . . my body desires you, my body desires you, come nearer . . . come nearer . . . your womanly body, your womanly body . . . I feel my body trembling . . . ah, I'm trembling as I hold you, I'm trembling as I hold you . . . my love . . . my whole body is erotic . . . oh . . . the joy, the joy, the pleasure, the pleasure, the pleasure of feeling your flesh . . . oh, my flesh, the pleasure of feeling your flesh against mine . . . [sigh] . . . how soft it is, what fun it is, how good it is, how good it is, oh, oh, oh, oh . . . I desire flesh, I desire flesh, I desire your flesh . . . how I desire your flesh, I desire your flesh, my flesh, how I desire your flesh, how I desire your flesh . . . ah, ah, how good your flesh is, how good your flesh is, how good your flesh is, how good your flesh is, how good it is . . . my body needs your flesh . . . ah, give me your body, give me your body, give me your body . . . my body needs your flesh . . . my body needs your flesh . . . I desire your flesh. . . ."

*Case 120:* A 51-year-old male teacher, member of a religious order (sexual deviation, anxiety reaction, obsessive-compulsive reactions, ecclesiogenic syndrome).

"I'm afraid . . . I'm afraid . . . I'm afraid . . . I'm afraid to appear before God . . . to begin with we were told that God would judge us as we judged . . . I judged others severely, therefore I'll be judged severely . . . that's why I'm afraid . . . then to have constantly searched for myself instead of having searching for God's will . . . I'm searching for myself . . . I'm searching for myself . . . that's why I'm afraid . . I'm afraid . . . I'm afraid of dying . . . I'm afraid of dying . . . I'm afraid of dying . . . I'm afraid of dying. . . ."

*Case 121:* A 36-year-old business man (anxiety reaction). During earlier autogenic abreactions (AA 7-11), brief and vague images of animals' heads (e.g., "Like a fox head," "Like a wolf's head") had occurred repeatedly. In all these instances there was no further development of these thematic elements. It was assumed that these images were related to (a) a traumatic incident which had occurred at the age of five, when the unsuspecting patient was bitten by a dog in the right thigh, and (b) aggression with associated anxiety material in a more general sense.

In AA 12, after 28 minutes of alternating multithematic engagements, a wolf's head appeared again. This time the visual presentation was followed by more differentiated sequences of images and characteristic dynamics of thematic repetition. Considering the patient's previous pattern of resistance (i.e., thematic evasion, abortive engagement; see Vol. VI) and to help the patient's brain to proceed in a repeatedly indicated thematic direction, specific technical support (i.e., *"Can you go over and pat the dog?"*) was given after indications of impending *abortive engagement* became evident (see below). A little later, after the brain had clearly indicated that it wished to continue this course of thematic neutralization, further thematically adapted technical support was applied (i.e., *"Can you give the dog permission to bite you?"*). As the patient's brain-antagonizing resistance was overcome, the brain-desired processes of thematic neutralization of the childhood trauma and certain interjected phases of thematically related elements unfolded in a progressive manner with many thematic repetitions. Of particular interest are repetitions of thematically associated motor discharges involving only the shoulders and arms [m] and repeatedly occurring waves of more generalized motor discharges [M] involving shoulders, arms, trunk and legs simultaneously. As the brain is given ample opportunity to go through a variety of maneuvers of thematic repetitions (note technical support to overcome *repetition resistance;* see Part I, Vol. VI), there is a decrease of motor discharges which finally disappear.

Of further interest are the following dynamic aspects which are typical for processes of neutralization of similar material:

(a) A progressive trend toward dynamic facilitation with decrease of disagreeable effects.

(b) Periodic interjection of relatively neutral phases or transitory thematic changes (permitting recuperation of systems which are directly involved in this intensive process of neutralization; see *Facilitating Forms of Resistance,* Part I, Vol. VI) with subsequent continuation of thematic repetitions.

(c) Diminutive variations of thematic repetition, followed by reversal of aggressive dynamics from a masochistic, self-destructive orientation to outwardly directed expression (see p. 280 ff.).

(d) Elaborations indicating brain-desired termination.

"Hmm, I see a wolf's head or a fox's head, but it looks more like a wolf's head or a wolfdog. . . . Oh yes, it has its paw up on a fence, its head is up . . . I'm sort . . . sort of looking at it from the bottom up . . . it's got very pointed ears . . . its muzzle is sort of slightly opened, the tongue is sort of hanging out . . . it's dark . . . and, it well, it's like what a wolf looks . . . like a German sheep dog looks . . . like a wolf dog looks . . . I guess it could be like that dog that was next door to us on Bridge Street . . . it's got a collar on and I'm trying to see it . . . it has a tag on . . . yes, it's got a tag on and I'm trying to make up my mind if it's a rectangular or a round tag . . . it seems to be sort of flipping back and forth, between rectangular and round. . . . [*Can you go over and pat the dog?*] . . . Yes, I'm patting it on the head, sort of lifting his muzzle a bit . . . I try scratching him under the chin, they like that . . . I get the impression that the dog bit me, I scratched him under the chin . . . yes, he's snapping away at me . . . well I'm feeling . . . I'm getting very, very . . . most unusual . . . [*Can you give the dog permission to bite you?*] . . . I'm holding out my hand to him . . . now he's taking a bite out of my . . . yeah . . . aha . . . that's just like it was when that big dog bit, when I was a child . . . he took a real snap at me and I . . . amazing . . . ah yes, it was a wolf dog too . . . a German shepherd that took a bite out of my rump . . . well that's what I did that time when I was a child, I just walked up to him and he took one lunge at me and . . . yes, I sort of remember . . . he was staying in front of the garage and he had a chain around him, and I just walked right up, and he went snap, up . . . yes, I can see him lunging at me . . . I'm sort of twitching around to avoid the dog . . . *strangely enough I've never been afraid of dogs.* . . . Well, that's gone . . . now I see myself in one of those swings . . . I think I was . . . I remember going into that thing and getting thoroughly sick to my stomach . . . [m] . . . I can see myself swinging up and down, up and down . . . I remember I got sick in the car . . . they had to stop so I could vomit . . . [M] . . . ah, another twitch . . . [m . . . m . . .] . . . . I see the dog again . . . [m] . . . he seems to be more distant from me now . . . [*Can you go over to the dog?*] . . . I'll try . . . try to go over . . . yes, he is standing over there [m] and I'm going to walk over there . . . and I'm walking over . . . I'm walking very slowly . . . I seem to be very reluctant to walk over there . . . [*Can you give permission to the dog to eat you?*] . . . It seems hard to realize that . . . yes, I can feel . . . [m,M,M,M] . . . yes, [M] . . . I can [M] . . . yes, he's [M] . . . he's taking some nice [m,M] . . . nice chunks out of my buttocks . . . [m] . . . hmm . . . [M] . . . [m,m,m] . . . well . . . [M] . . . he's [m,M] working away at my leg . . . [m] . . . that [M] . . . feels most [m,M] . . . uncomfortable . . . [M] . . . and my right leg . . . [m] . . . is nearly . . . [M] . . . all gone . . . I just don't seem to have any bones in there . . . [M] . . . [m] . . . he just . . . [M] . . . like if I were a drawing and you were erasing me, more than anything else . . . well, goes my leg up to the knee . . . [M] . . . the buttocks pretty well . . . [M] . . . [m] . . . gone . . . [M] . . . hmm . . . [M] . . . there goes my stomach . . . [M] . . . [m] . . . there goes the left leg . . . [m] . . . it went in one big gulp . . . well there is . . . [M] . . . not

ribs of beef again . . . like I saw in one of the earlier trips, except I don't
think they are ribs of beef . . . its my own chest . . . I don't know, something
looks like a big cat eating through them . . . ripping them, chomping through
them . . . looks like a black panther . . . yes, he's eating me up again, except
this time he's biting, and not swallowing me as a whole like the others . . . the
left shoulder, my head, my right shoulder, right arm, there's only my left
are hanging there . . . by nothing, he took it in one snap . . . now he's going
down on the right side . . . going down . . . yes, a black panther . . . he's
slowing down considerably . . . he's sort of chomping away . . . going down
my right foot . . . down to my ankle, there goes my foot . . . Now I see a
goose . . . now I got gobbled up like a worm again. Whew! I'm just seeing some
concentric circles . . . I don't know, I'm seeing some abstract shapes that
don't mean anything . . . looks perhaps like a door handle, European
style. . . . Now I see a little frog . . . I guess I'm a fly and he's just taking a
snap at me . . . I felt about three times like that, like a fly . . . sort of light
violet color, a little bit of shimmering. . . . I get the impression of being
under water. . . . Now I can't see anything . . . that looks like a duck, or
something . . . he's chasing after me . . . I'm a little bug skittering along, and
I'm trying to get away, and he's chasing me . . . ah, there I go, he snapped me
up . . . ah, I don't know, I got mad all of a sudden, I said I'm not a bug, I
turned around and I took the duck, and I just swung him around and flung
him away . . . I got very aggressive or independent . . . I felt I didn't want to
get eaten up any more . . . I see sort of a texture, like sharkskin, or something
like that . . . I seem to have a different sort of shape it isn't really me . . . I
don't know . . . I'm sort of a shapeless blob . . . a tiny miniature thing, a bug
or something. . . . Now there is a robin . . . he's pecking at me . . . yeah, I feel
his beak going into me . . . ah, that's funny, I took the robin by the beak and
sort of threw him over my shoulder, in a sort of judo hold, or I just flipped him
over me . . . I don't want to get pecked to death . . . I can see the bird sort
of lying there, he's much bigger than me, but I just sort of threw him over me
and he crashed down on his back. . . . Now I'm walking away from him . . .
I seem to be walking on a beach or something . . . it's sort of mud colored. . . .
Ahh, I seem to see a snake . . . hmm . . . the snake had wide-open jaws and
I just walked up and put my foot up and my other hand on the other
jaw, and reached in, and turned the snake inside out. . . . That's a good
trick. . . . Now I feel very calm. . . . [*Can you describe the visual field?*] . . .
Sort of stripes, wavy stripes, and sort of monochromatic colors in shades of
light gray . . ." (termination).

## SYNCHRONIZED THEMATIC MULTIPLICATION

A specific brain-designed maneuver of thematic repetition involving
visual elaborations (e.g., stages III-VI; see Table 33, p. 188) consists
of a synchronized repetition of the same thematic elements (see Case
73, p. 168; Case 122). Depending on the prevailing level of differentiation of visual elaborations, synchronized thematic multiplication may

"Hmm, I see a wolf's head or a fox's head, but it looks more like a wolf's head or a wolfdog. . . . Oh yes, it has its paw up on a fence, its head is up . . . I'm sort . . . sort of looking at it from the bottom up . . . it's got very pointed ears . . . its muzzle is sort of slightly opened, the tongue is sort of hanging out . . . it's dark . . . and, it well, it's like what a wolf looks . . . like a German sheep dog looks . . . like a wolf dog looks . . . I guess it could be like that dog that was next door to us on Bridge Street . . . it's got a collar on and I'm trying to see it . . . it has a tag on . . . yes, it's got a tag on and I'm trying to make up my mind if it's a rectangular or a round tag . . . it seems to be sort of flipping back and forth, between rectangular and round. . . . [*Can you go over and pat the dog?*] . . . Yes, I'm patting it on the head, sort of lifting his muzzle a bit . . . I try scratching him under the chin, they like that . . . I get the impression that the dog bit me, I scratched him under the chin . . . yes, he's snapping away at me . . . well I'm feeling . . . I'm getting very, very . . . most unusual . . . [*Can you give the dog permission to bite you?*] . . . I'm holding out my hand to him . . . now he's taking a bite out of my . . . yeah . . . aha . . . that's just like it was when that big dog bit, when I was a child . . . he took a real snap at me and I . . . amazing . . . ah yes, it was a wolf dog too . . . a German shepherd that took a bite out of my rump . . . well that's what I did that time when I was a child, I just walked up to him and he took one lunge at me and . . . yes, I sort of remember . . . he was staying in front of the garage and he had a chain around him, and I just walked right up, and he went snap, up . . . yes, I can see him lunging at me . . . I'm sort of twitching around to avoid the dog . . . *strangely enough I've never been afraid of dogs.* . . . Well, that's gone . . . now I see myself in one of those swings . . . I think I was . . . I remember going into that thing and getting thoroughly sick to my stomach . . . [m] . . . I can see myself swinging up and down, up and down . . . I remember I got sick in the car . . . they had to stop so I could vomit . . . [M] . . . ah, another twitch . . . [m . . . m . . .] . . . . I see the dog again . . . [m] . . . he seems to be more distant from me now . . . [*Can you go over to the dog?*] . . . I'll try . . . try to go over . . . yes, he is standing over there [m] and I'm going to walk over there . . . and I'm walking over . . . I'm walking very slowly . . . I seem to be very reluctant to walk over there . . . [*Can you give permission to the dog to eat you?*] . . . It seems hard to realize that . . . yes, I can feel . . . [m,M,M,M] . . . yes, [M] . . . I can [M] . . . yes, he's [M] . . . he's taking some nice [m,M] . . . nice chunks out of my buttocks . . . [m] . . . hmm . . . [M] . . . [m,m,m] . . . well . . . [M] . . . he's [m,M] working away at my leg . . . [m] . . . that [M] . . . feels most [m,M] . . . uncomfortable . . . [M] . . . and my right leg . . . [m] . . . is nearly . . . [M] . . . all gone . . . I just don't seem to have any bones in there . . . [M] . . . [m] . . . he just . . . [M] . . . like if I were a drawing and you were erasing me, more than anything else . . . well, goes my leg up to the knee . . . [M] . . . the buttocks pretty well . . . [M] . . . [m] . . . gone . . . [M] . . . hmm . . . [M] . . . there goes my stomach . . . [M] . . . [m] . . . there goes the left leg . . . [m] . . . it went in one big gulp . . . well there is . . . [M] . . . not much left below the waist . . . [M] . . . now nothing . . . ah . . . I'm seeing mustard yellow . . . there's just my chest now, I feel as if I'm still there . . . see sort of greenish . . . I don't know, I couldn't bring it up to the top . . . I could't get myself eaten up to the top . . . the diaphragm . . . [m] . . . I still sort of feel as if I'm half there and half not there . . . [Can you keep describing?] . . . As I say I feel half present and half absent . . . [Is the dog still around?] . . . Yes, he's still sort of roaming around . . . all right . . . [M] . . . he's . . . [M] . . . starting at my head now . . . [m,M,M] . . . he's got . . . [M,M] . . . [M] . . . well my head is gone . . . [m,m] . . . my right shoulder, my right arm, that's [M] . . . [m] . . . I'm seeing different colors . . . there's only my left shoulder and my left arm . . . [M] . . . yes . . . [m,M] . . . there goes the left shoulder . . . [m] . . . its sort of a greenish light color . . . and he is down to my hand . . . [M] . . . I guess there goes the . . . [M] . . . rest of me . . . [m,m] . . . I guess I'm all gone. . . . I feel sort of exhausted, sort of shook. . . . I see the dog again . . . he is coming after me again . . . [m] . . . [M] . . . he's taken my whole top in one gulp . . . [m] . . . now down to the waist . . . [M] . . . he's taking another . . . [m] . . . and now only down to the knees and the rest of me . . . [m] . . . I'm all gone again . . . [Can you repeat again?] . . . Yes, he's getting smaller and farther away . . . but now he's getting near my feet . . . [m] . . . there . . . [m] . . . goes my right leg . . . [m] . . . up to the hip . . . my abdomen, my left leg . . . [m] . . . that's all gone . . . my . . . [M] . . . up to the chest, my head . . . my arm . . . my left and my right arm . . . [M] . . . still . . . [m] . . . my hand . . . ah . . . [m] . . . I still feel my head . . . [M] . . . he took my head off at a bite . . . my left shoulder, my left arm and hand . . . [M] . . . my chest . . . I don't know, it seems to be very calm . . . I got down as far as my chest and my abdomen, and things sort of stopped . . . I tried to imagine him doing any more, but things became very calm. I just couldn't go any farther with it . . . I see sort of my field of vision, it is sort of gray . . . a fairly medium gray . . . I'm still trying to see if I can find the dog . . . Yes, now he's nibbling away at my left toe . . . it doesn't bother me . . . he's sort of nibbling it up, up to the knee . . . up to the hip . . . going all the way up one side . . . my chest, my shoulder . . . down my left arm . . . there's just half of me here . . . [m] . . . there he's starting on my right leg . . . just half of me here . . . up to the knee, the hip, up to the shoulder . . . [m] . . . the arms gone in one snap . . . now just the head . . . [M] . . . and now he's . . . [M] . . . and I'm all gone . . . [m] . . . he took the head in one snap. . . . It seems like if I'm lying in some feather cushion . . . things are very soft and comfortable. . . . I see the dog again . . . [m] . . . he took a bite out of my side, but he didn't like that . . . now he's taking out of me . . . going down on the left waist, all the way down . . . he is nibbling away at me . . . [m] . . . my left leg is all nibbled away . . . now he's nibbling away the right leg . . . all the way up and down the other side . . . now he's chomping away at my midsection . . . he's going faster and faster and faster . . . and down to the waist and the chest . . . my arms . . . now my head is gone . . . only my shoulders and my two arms . . . my right arm and shoulder are gone . . . now my left, and I'm just all gone again. Well that

conclusion *after* he has already arrived at it. On the contrary, he must proceed surely, step by step, advancing to the next step only after thoroughly checking the last.

Even a very talented musician cannot become a real artist except by long practice and training. Similarly, to be intuitively sensitive and, at the same time, objectively critical of one's own insights is an art that requires practice and long training. It requires, above all, a happy synthesis of intuitive imagination and self-discipline.

CHAPTER

# III

## INTERPRETATIONS AS
## WORKING HYPOTHESES

In this chapter, we shall study the first dream in the analysis of the patient discussed in Chapter II. The patient reported this dream (of the night before) in Hour 5, immediately after his analyst had completed his initial anamnestic survey, in Hour 4.

DREAM, HOUR 5.

Riding in a car—I was driving. One of my business accounts was in the car with his wife. There was also another couple in the car. I didn't recognize them. They were criticizing me for driving on rocks, then going down an incline. They said, "Never been a car down here before."

Cave down below—car backing—.* It turned out to be a huge animal, something like a dinosaur. They said, "Now look what you got us into!"

---

* The patient's report of his dream is not clear at this point. The authors' guess is that a vague impression of something startling was followed by the patient's recognizing it as a huge animal.

(E *) Like Dream 100, this one is at first unintelligible—until we guess that the trip that this patient is making in a car represents his anticipation of what his psychoanalytic treatment will be like. This suspicion seems to be confirmed when we read his associations during the rest of the hour.

ASSOCIATIONS.

Everyone was excited when we were on the rocks. I couldn't see any way to get out of it. The businessman is a critical man—difficult to please. (The patient recalls a conversation in which the businessman's wife said, "You never know what he's thinking or whether he's satisfied." Somebody told the patient, "If this man doesn't say anything, he's satisfied.")

(Then the patient begins to recall his application to the Psychoanalytic Institute for treatment and his being called by the social worker at the institute, who told him that he had been accepted for analysis. He next talks about his attitude toward treatment. He had doubts; maybe he shouldn't go. There might be unpleasant things to face. Maybe he's not willing to divulge enough. He didn't know what might come up. At this point, the analyst begins to make extended explanations to the patient about free association, etc. In response, the patient smiles. He has a hard enough time saying anything, he explains. He was surprised that he was able to talk for an hour the other day.)

(After more explanations, the patient says that the ana-

---

* In the following discussion we shall alternate between elaborating a working hypothesis (see below) and checking it. To facilitate the reader's attempts to follow our argument, we shall designate elaboration by "E" before the relevant passage, checking by "C."

lyst resembles his brother, the one just ahead of the patient. He resembles him mainly in appearance.)

(He remembers his brother coming in drunk, turning on the lights, and saying: "Everybody get up and piss, the world's on fire." The patient's brother and sister used to give Christmas presents, but his parents did not. The parents gave only oranges, money, and coal—as reminder of a bad year. The patient next says that he wants to keep his analytic material to himself. He answers his wife briefly when she asks, and she accepts his reticence.)

(The patient has talked over his analysis with a friend who has been in analysis for three years and is better. The friend asked him about the start. The friend was particularly interested in whether the patient was lying on the couch.)

(C) Thus, after telling his dream, the patient has spent most of the hour talking about his feelings about starting analysis. This confirms our suspicion that the dream, too, may be giving expression to the patient's reactions to starting analysis.

### FIRST ELABORATING,
### THEN CHECKING, A WORKING HYPOTHESIS

As a preliminary to checking this working hypothesis, we shall first elaborate it by interpreting what the details of the dream would mean, in case the hypothesis were correct. Our hypothesis is that the trip that the patient is taking represents his psychoanalytic treatment. If so, the patient in the driver's seat must represent the patient's own ego. Also, if the trip is his treatment, the others in the car, who are criticizing him, must be his own resistance, based on fear. (E) Later in the dream, the "car backing" gives more energetic expression to the patient's resistance. "Driving on rocks," "going down" into something unknown ("Never been a car down here before") are dangers he expects to encounter. The "cave down below" and the "dinosaur" seem to be symbols of the patient's unconscious—which is dangerous and somehow related to the patient's unknown past (a prehistoric animal). At the end of the dream, the critics who are giving voice to the patient's unconscious resistance protest more vigorously. "Now look what you got us into!"

What we have just been doing is elaborating a working hypothesis. Our hypothesis was that, in the dream, the patient's trip represents his treatment. We have used this hypothesis as a key for interpreting, or translating, the manifest dream as though it were a text in another language. When thus interpreted, the manifest dream gives us a *focal-conflict hypothesis.* (E) According to this hypothesis, the conflict with which the patient was preoccupied at the moment of dreaming was:

| The conscious purpose to continue with his psychoanalytic treatment | *versus* | Fear of reactivating disturbing conflicts from his "prehistoric" past |
|---|---|---|

Our next task is to check this hypothesis against other evidence. If the patient really is developing resistance to his treatment, we should expect to find some evidence of such resistance in his associations later in the hour. Actually, the patient does recall doubts when he first applied to the Institute for treatment. (C) "Maybe I shouldn't go," he thought. "Might be unpleasant things to face. Maybe I'm not willing to divulge enough. I don't know what might come up." When the analyst starts to explain free association, the patient also says that he has "a hard enough time saying anything." He was surprised that he was "able to talk for an hour the other day." In other words, we actually do find in the patient's associations evidence of the resistance that our dream interpretation led us to predict.

Thus encouraged, we continue with our procedure of alternately elaborating our hypothesis (E) and then checking it (C) repeatedly. We turn back first to our task of translating the manifest dream. This time our attempt to translate yields only a question. (E) The dream has pictured the patient's resistance as motivated by fear of a dinosaur. What does this dinosaur represent? we ask next.

We turn back to reality for an answer. In the patient's actual situation in the analysis, what has he to fear? We have already suggested a partial answer to this question. (C) He is afraid of reactivating disturbing conflicts from his "prehistoric" past. This answer is suggested by our clinical experience with other patients.

Does the dinosaur in the dream give us any hint as to the nature of this prehistoric conflict? Yes. (E) The dinosaur was an aggressive animal that might be expected to attack. We ask next: Why should this patient have fantasied and feared being attacked by a huge animal? In order to find an appropriate answer to this question, we draw again on our clinical experience with other patients. (C) The dinosaur probably represents some aggressive urge of the patient, dating from a "prehistoric" period of the patient's life.

(E) Since, in the manifest dream, the patient was not aware of any such aggressive impulse, we infer that this impulse must have been repressed. Because, in the dream text, he is not attacking but being attacked, we must conclude that his aggressive impulse has been turned back against himself. Analysis of the dream text also permits and requires another inference. In the manifest dream, the "prehistoric animal" is not yet attacking the patient, but may be expected to do so if he approaches closer. (E) "Translating" this detail, we infer that in the past the patient's aggressive impulse and fear were not only repressed, but also deactivated, robbed of their cathexis. At the time of dreaming, they were still latent. If the patient continues in treatment, however, he fears that they will be reactivated. (C) Our clinical experience tells us that such fears are probably well-grounded.

We ask next: How will such reactivation of disturbing impulses take place? The dream and its associations suggest an answer to this question. One of those in the car with the patient is a man with whom the patient does business. (E) Since the analyst also does business with the patient (i.e., is in a professional relationship with him), we now suspect that this man represents the analyst.

(C) The dream associations about this man seem to confirm this inference, since they apply equally well to the analyst. The analyst, too, is silent much of the time.

We conclude, accordingly, that the patient fears that the analyst, too, is "difficult to please." (E) Another association about this man probably also refers to the analyst. As this man's wife said recently: "You never know what he's thinking or whether he's satisfied." "Somebody told him," the patient adds, " 'If this man doesn't say anything, he's satisfied.' "

When we elaborate our hypothesis further, these details give us a tentative answer to our question. (E) One reason for the patient's avoidance of disturbing topics in the analysis is his fear of displeasing the analyst. As long as he can keep from thinking about his infantile disturbing impulses, they may remain latent. Nevertheless, the patient has secret hopes. So long as the analyst says nothing, perhaps he is satisfied.

Perhaps the analyst will be permissive of disturbing thoughts, is the implied hope.

This interpretation is confirmed later in the hour by an association in which the same hope seems to emerge much more vividly. The patient thinks that the analyst resembles his brother. (C) Then he remembers this brother coming in drunk, turning on the lights and saying: "Everybody get up and piss, the world's on fire." Back of this memory, we now conclude, is the secret hope that the analyst will release him, too, from his inhibitions.

This hope is very seductive; it is also very dangerous. Why has the patient had to inhibit his disturbing impulses ever since his "prehistoric" past?

(E) The answer is that the patient probably inhibited his disturbing impulses in this "prehistoric" past because at that time they stirred up equally intense fears. Now, if he lets the analyst encourage him to "go down" into his unconscious and reactivate his inhibited impulses, then he will reactivate also the consequences, his associated fears.

(C) This conclusion, too, corresponds to our clinical experience with other patients.

## DIFFICULTIES AND PITFALLS IN THE
## USE OF WORKING HYPOTHESES

We have spelled out in seemingly pedantic detail our interpretive reasoning in this case. We have done so in order to illustrate our procedure of formulating explicitly and precisely the evidence on which our intuitive insights are based. Such explicit spelling out of our "interpretive reasoning" is particularly desirable and also particularly difficult whenever we have to elaborate extensively the implications of a working hypothesis before we can check it against evidence. In such a case, it is easy to mistake elaborating a hypothesis for proving it. Elaborating a hypothesis is essentially a deductive procedure. We start with the working hypothesis and then work out its implications deductively. After we have done so, these implications are still only a hypothesis. Our initial hypothesis, now expanded, still needs to be checked against evidence. If we assume that it is already proven, our elaboration of a hypothesis is likely to become a Procrustean-bed technique of interpretation. Instead of checking our hypothesis against other evidence, we are in danger of trying to force the evidence to fit the hypothesis. Our best precaution against this error is to spell out our interpretive reasoning with great care.

Skillful elaboration of a working hypothesis sometimes gives the impression of a highly intuitive, even speculative, procedure. Quite the contrary is true. Given a well-chosen working hypothesis, the elaboration of this hypothesis becomes a precise deductive process whose conclusions follow inexorably from the details of the "text" that we are "translating."

Thus, in our example, given the working hypothesis that the patient is picturing his treatment as an automobile trip into an unknown terrain, it requires no speculative imagination to conclude that the patient in the driver's seat is the patient's ego, that those who are protesting are his own resistance, and that the area into which they are penetrating is the patient's own unconscious. On the contrary, all this follows from our initial hypothesis plus our clinical knowledge of what psychoanalytic treatment involves for a patient.

What is intuitive, on the other hand, is what precedes and what follows the elaboration of a working hypothesis. Choice of a promising working hypothesis is an act of intuitive imagination; checking the hypothesis after it has been elaborated is an act of critical judgment, also intuitive.

If our imagination has led us along a false trail, then conscientious deductive elaboration should make it more and more evident that our working hypothesis is only a bad guess. It is at this point that we run into the danger of a Procrustean-bed technique. If we are too fascinated with our hypothesis, we will not be strict enough in our deductions, but will force the evidence to fit the hypothesis. We will not discover that it is a bad guess.

## TWO INTERPRETIVE APPROACHES COMPARED

We next propose to compare our interpretive approach to Dream 5 in this chapter with our approach to Dream 100 in Chapter II. In principle, our interpretive method is the same in both cases. In both, we have concentrated first on that part of the evidence whose significance we were most certain that we could intuitively grasp. Then, step by step, we have checked our first insights against other parts of the evidence, revising and expanding our understanding as we proceed.

Our approaches differ, in the two cases, as to the nature of the clues that we selected as starting points. In the case of Dream 100, we started with a bit of evidence that promptly led us back to the situation, reported in Hour 98, which had served as precipitating stimulus for the dream. Then, after we had found it, we could proceed straightforwardly to analyze the patient's reactions to this precipitating stimulus.

In the case of Dream 5, it was not possible at first to determine the precipitating stimulus * so precisely. Our first clue was the thought that the automobile trip in the manifest dream might be a metaphorical description of the patient's reactions to his beginning treatment. This thought could not be immediately and directly checked against evidence. It was necessary first to elaborate it as a working hypothesis, to use it tentatively as a key for interpreting (translating) the manifest dream content. Only after we had thus elaborated our working hypothesis deductively could we proceed to check our hypothesis (now expanded) against other evidence.

### THE CONCEPT OF COGNITIVE STRUCTURE

Elaborating a working hypothesis has one advantage to compensate for the difficulties and subtle pitfalls of this interpretive method: it introduces us immediately to the complex network of interrelated meanings that underlies every dream. Every dream has many meanings. This is the most important reason why intuitive analysts will often give differing interpretations of the same dream. Each analyst, starting with the bit of evidence to which he is intuitively most sensitive, will find another one of the dream's "overdetermined" meanings. Thus, in the case of the dream presented in this chapter, one analyst might try first to find a meaning for the dinosaur. Another might try to interpret "driving on the rocks." Still another might be impressed with the story of the patient's brother coming in drunk and saying, "Everybody get up and piss, the

---

* We did suspect early that the dream was a reaction to beginning treatment. What was not clear was why this dream was not dreamed until just after the patient's fourth hour. Basing their inference on clinical experience with other patients, the authors now suspect that completion of the anamnestic survey was the precipitating stimulus for this dream. Giving a history under guidance from the analyst tends to protect a patient from free association. When free association begins, the danger of reactivating "prehistoric" conflicts is much greater.

world's on fire." In the end, if we were willing to accept each analyst's intuition, we would have only a list of some of the overdetermined meanings of the dream.

In our objectively critical approach to interpretation, we are not content to accept a mere list of meanings. Rather, we expect the different meanings of a dream to fit together intelligibly. We also expect each dream to fit intelligibly into the context of the dreamer's real life at the time of dreaming. In fact, these expectations are our only real checks on the correctness of our interpretations. If our interpretations do not fit together intelligibly, then we regard this fact as a discrepancy to be bridged. We are even less willing to accept an interpretation as valid until we can discover how it fits into the context of the dreamer's emotional situation in real life.

We shall use the term "cognitive structure" to designate the way that the meanings of a dream fit together and fit into the context of the dreamer's emotional situation in real life. In our attempts to interpret Dream 5, we have been guided by both these criteria for the reconstruction of an intelligible cognitive structure. Our attempts to elaborate our initial working hypothesis have been guided in the main by the criterion that the meanings of a dream should fit together intelligibly. Our attempts to check our expanded hypothesis against other evidence have, then, been based on the principle that our interpretations, if valid, must fit intelligibly into the context of the dreamer's emotional situation in real life.

## THE CONCEPT OF AN INVOLVEMENT CONFLICT
### OR OF A COMMITMENT CONFLICT

Let us now examine the cognitive structure that we have begun to reconstruct. What impresses us first is that the cognitive structure of Dream 5 is somewhat unusual. In this dream, the dreamer is not preoccupied directly either with his own impulses or with external reality, present or past. The patient's ego in this dream is more detached. In this dream, he is not dealing directly with his conflicts, but rather with a choice whether to allow his underlying conflicts to be reactivated. Until recently, these underlying conflicts were latent. The problem that is now focal for the patient (the problem with which he is *pre*occupied) is to choose whether to allow these deeper conflicts to be reactivated or to divert attention from them so that they will remain latent. This kind of conflict about whether to allow a deeper conflict to be reactivated we shall call an "involvement conflict" or a "commitment conflict." *

The concept of degree of involvement in, or of commitment to, a deeper conflict is one that can be fairly precisely measured (subjectively estimated) by a simple comparison. For example, if this patient should vividly imagine himself attacked by a dinosaur, we would expect him to be in a panic. In the manifest dream, the patient is not in a panic. This is evidence that he is not intensely involved. On the other hand, the car's backing away is evidence of some degree of involvement (i.e., he would not feel the need to back away if he were not somewhat involved). The car's backing away is also evidence of the dreamer's effort to diminish involvement in the "dinosaur conflict" by withdrawal of cathexis.

* By "involvement" in a conflict, we mean reactivation that is still reversible. When involvement becomes *irreversible*, we call it "commitment." For example, in the dream, the car is able to back away from the dinosaur. This is a sign that the patient has begun to be involved, but is not yet committed to the conflict symbolized by the dinosaur.

### ONE FOCAL CONFLICT AND
### A CONSTELLATION OF SUBFOCAL CONFLICTS

When we now re-examine this dream and the associations that follow it, we are reminded of the fact that the dinosaur is not the only symbol of a deeper conflict in the dreamer's latent thoughts. There are still many unexplained details, both in the dream and in the associations. For example, why are there two couples in the car with the patient? The fact that the patient does not recognize one of the couples is probably a sign that they are closely related to the deeper conflicts whose reactivation he is resisting. "Driving on the rocks," too, probably symbolizes another conflict, the content of which we cannot yet guess. In the associations, we do not yet know why the dream work chose a memory in which "pissing" and "fire" played such prominent roles. From all this, we infer tentatively that there are many conflicts, not just one, whose reactivation the patient fears.

In this respect, this dream is like most dreams. We often succeed in recognizing the focal conflict on which the dreamer's interest is for the moment centered, but underneath this focal conflict there is always a whole *constellation* of "subfocal" conflicts, some of them dating back to the "prehistory" of the patient's infancy. We speak of a constellation because we expect to find that these conflicts are closely related to one another. At the time of our first interpretation, we can usually only dimly grasp what these subfocal conflicts are and how they are related. Often we have to wait until, in later dreams, some of these subfocal conflicts rise, one by one, into a focal position.

It is of interest that, already in the associations of this patient's fifth hour, one such conflict seems about ready to emerge into focus. When the patient expresses reticence about telling his wife about his analysis, we have good reason to expect that a triangular conflict involving both his analyst and his wife may be the next conflict to become focal.

We shall reserve for Chapter XVII our discussion of how, by analysis of the dream symbolism and of recurring patterns, subfocal as well as focal, we are often able to reconstruct much of a patient's prehistory long before it has emerged into focus.

### A NEW INTERPRETIVE INSIGHT

In the meantime, we have learned something new about dream interpretation. We have learned how we can *estimate* a dreamer's *degree of commitment* to an emerging conflict.

CHAPTER

IV

## *FURTHER EXAMPLES: RECONSTRUCTING THE COGNITIVE STRUCTURE OF INTERPERSONAL RELATIONS*

As an example of another kind of cognitive structure, we shall study a dream reported by our patient in his fifteenth hour.

DREAM, HOUR 15.

(He remembers only a *fragment of a dream* from a few nights ago:) Mixing cement.

(Immediately on awakening, he felt as though he really knew exactly how to mix it, but really he does not.)

(Only spontaneous association: recent tuckpointing. The patient was going to do it himself, but did not know how to mix concrete, so he hired somebody.)

Again we suspect that it is the analyst who is hired to do an expert job that the patient cannot do himself. If so, why should the patient compare his treatment to mixing cement or to tuckpointing?

### SYMBOLIC SIGNIFICANCE OF TUCKPOINTING

We shall try again to guess the significance of the dream symbolism. Tuckpointing is done to hold the bricks of a house together more firmly. A house is often a symbol for a woman. Perhaps this patient fears (or wishes) that some woman will fall apart and is reacting to this fear with a fantasy of putting her together again.

To test this hypothesis, we report this patient's associations both before and after telling his dream:

HOUR 15.

> [The analyst is twenty minutes late.]
> PATIENT: Very fuckin' mad at this hospital last night [about a matter concerning business dealings of the patient with the hospital]. My dear wife went to a bingo game last night. (The patient was late starting his work and did not finish until 3:30 A.M.)
>
> Thursday, a three-year-old boy was killed by a hit-and-run driver. I don't see how people can leave the scene of an accident. I could not.
>
> I was also pissed off while waiting for you. I thought that you were in your office. But two doctors came looking for you. Then I realized that you were not there and felt better; I assumed that you had some emergency, and so it was understandable.

After reporting his dream fragment at this point, the patient continues:

> I told my wife that I wanted to get rid of our dog. The dog is a nuisance. My wife says that I want to get rid of everything. She says that I don't enjoy my family—just tolerate them.

I know that I don't show my feelings much, but I have been getting along much better with the children lately. I don't know what she expects sometimes. [Seems genuinely perplexed.]

She says that I don't enjoy my family—just tolerate them. This is one of her worst statements. But she makes other similar ones. Sometimes I feel that she is confined too much. When she sees other people, she appreciates me more. She may be more irritable now because of her pregnancy and because I am doing much night work.

I find it difficult to satisfy her—no matter whether she goes out or stays home. She feels that I should take care of the family more closely. She is in a bad mood.

We were affectionate one night recently. We had intercourse for the first time in over two weeks; but I lose pleasure because it is too much trouble for her.

Crazy idea about colored people. Always enjoying themselves. Eat, sleep, drink, and fuck. (He pictures 90 per cent of colored women as prostitutes.)

Almost any time I see an attractive girl, I imagine myself having intercourse with her.

When having intercourse the other night with my wife, I did not reach climax; the phone rang.

We shall skip over a few intervening associations and quote only the last few sentences in this hour:

My wife says I only help around the house when she nags. I say that I would do it anyway—later. Nagging only aggravates. She leaves projects unfinished, too, e.g., curtains for basement windows.

In these associations, we find several points that might con-

firm and give more precise content to our interpretive hypothesis. First, we learn that the patient's wife is pregnant. The
notion of a woman's falling apart might be giving expression
to a hostile wish against his wife's pregnancy.

The patient's reference to, and condemnation of, a hit-and-
run driver now does suggest a hostile wish toward a child.
Then, immediately after telling the dream, the patient remembers having told his wife that he wanted to "get rid of their
dog; the dog is a nuisance." The patient's wife seems to have
quickly suspected that he was (preconsciously) thinking of
his family. She reproached him with wanting "to get rid
of everything," then accused him of not enjoying his family, of
just tolerating them.

At this point, we must confess that we have been playing the
role of Devil's advocate. Intuitively, we are skeptical of this
hypothesis. Our next duty is to spell out the reasons for this
intuitive judgment. First we must make explicit just what it is
that we doubt. We do not question (the possibility, at least)
that a hostile wish toward his wife's pregnancy may be one of
the overdetermined meanings of this dream. What we do question is whether such a wish is focal at this time.

We define the focal conflict of a dream as the conflict which
is the most intensely cathected of all the dream's overdetermined meanings. Thus, the question at issue is one of the intensity of the patient's involvement in the hostile wish that we
postulated. To test this we make the same kind of comparison
that we did in the case of the patient's fear of the dinosaur: we
appraise the manifest dream. Is the patient as disturbed as we
should expect him to be if he were taking such a hostile wish
really seriously? Our intuitive judgment is that he is not. We
conclude, accordingly, as in the dinosaur dream, that if such

a hostile wish has been activated, it has been activated only slightly, that some less disturbing conflict nearer the surface is just now in the focus of the patient's interest.

## "POETIC" SIGNIFICANCE OF "HOME"

In search of this focal conflict, we shall turn next to the possibility of interpreting the dream symbolism at another level. The "universal symbolism," from which psychoanalysis has learned so much, dates from a time when a child's thinking is very concrete, when his curiosity is directed toward understanding the behavior and relationships among other people in anatomical and physiological terms. At later stages in his intellectual development, a child becomes capable of understanding more abstract relationships. In particular, he becomes capable of understanding his own emotional responses and those of others in terms that need not be reduced to concrete physical acts. In these later stages of intellectual development, there develops a symbolism which we sometimes call "functional," sometimes "metaphorical." It is a kind of symbolism for which artists often have a more sensitive understanding than do psychoanalysts. For this reason, the authors like to call it "poetic" symbolism.

Let us now try to understand the significance of "tuck-pointing" at this level. A house, a home, is symbolic of family life. Perhaps the problem with which the patient is just now concerned in his treatment is holding his family together. The patient's associations seem to confirm this hypothesis. The patient's sarcastic remark about his "dear wife's" going off to a bingo game is followed immediately by his condemnation of a hit-and-run driver. The (preconscious) implication is that she is neglecting her children, leaving them unprotected on the

very night when the patient had to be away working until
3:30 A.M. Immediately after the dream, he quotes a similar
reproach by his wife to him—that he wants to "get rid of
everything," that he "just tolerates" his family. Thus, the
patient's associations imply that both parents resent their responsibility for their children. Each is reproaching the other
for not taking better care of the family. The patient senses
also that this conflict is being aggravated for both of them by
his wife's pregnancy (another child) and by his own need to
do so much night work.

### SOURCE IN CHILDHOOD
### OF WISH TO HOLD FAMILY TOGETHER

This interpretation leaves an important question unanswered.
Why has this patient reacted to his resentment of his responsibilities with a fantasy of mixing cement, of trying to hold his
family together? The usual answer to such a question is
"guilt." This answer is not satisfactory because it is not sufficiently specific. Many kinds of reaction are attributed to
guilt. For example, if guilt is the reactive motive in this
dream, why has he not dreamed of being punished? To answer
such a question, we should always turn back to the patient's
own fantasy or thoughts, to his own words.

The patient's dream thoughts suggest a simple and direct
answer to our question: the patient loves his family; the integrity of his family is important to him; the prospect of his
family's falling apart is disturbing to him. This answer leaves
us with another unanswered question. What is the source of
this love of his family? The patient was not born with a wife
and children. From what earlier roots does his need to hold
his family together derive?

### A FANTASY WITH SIMILAR IMPLICATIONS

In search for an answer, we turn back to Hour 12. The patient did not tell us *when* he had the dream of "mixing cement," only that it was "a few nights ago." His twelfth hour had also been a few days ago. We select this hour for study because it contains a fantasy of strikingly similar content, one of "fixing a house up."

HOUR 12.

(The analyst is twenty-five minutes late; he apologizes. The patient says, O.K.; his schedule is also unpredictable.)

PATIENT: I worked until 3:30 A.M.

I have been fixing a drain at home.

After the last hour, I was very busy. I was irritated with my wife. She tried to pin me down on time. "Will you be back at 5:00 P.M.?" This is tough because of rush-hour traffic.

(More friction with wife. The patient tells an incident of conflicting wishes.)

On the way down, I had crazy thoughts about my parents' home.

FANTASY.

My brothers and I were at the old house.

When I was a child, I would think: When I grow up, I'll fix the house up.

In actuality, I was glad to get out.

[Fantasy continued:] I was talking with two of my brothers about how much each does around the house. I said: "I give up. . . . What did you do? I can't see it." Then we fought.

ASSOCIATIONS.

(His route here takes him near his parents' home. He is uneasy with his brothers. His older brother is loud, cocky, destructive. The two brothers in the daydream are the second oldest and the youngest of six siblings.)

ANALYST: These two aggravate you the most?

PATIENT: These two are the only ones in Chicago.

The youngest one never bothered me much, but we never did things with others' being present. I was surprised to see brothers who really supported one another. Also, one of my brothers threw a rock at me and hurt me (age ten) just because another fellow told him to. I have often thought about that.

I also envied my youngest brother because he was a better ball-player. I was a "butterfingers."

I dreamed a lot on the ball field—about growing up—great things in the future.

Oddly, I still feel this way. I feel that my present life is temporary—a fill-in for something better later.

[Pause.] My wife went to school last night. The nun at school says that Dominick [the patient's son] is intelligent but not good in spelling. We have not been practicing spelling with him at home. Dominick daydreams in class.

My wife promptly made arrangements to get help with this. [Some guidance set-up—the patient is uncertain.]

On Sunday afternoon, I watched a television show, *Crime without Motive*. The father [*sic*] was crying, blaming himself. I thought of myself and Dominick—felt that I had not done enough.

I feel that I neglect the boy. But I have admonished him about crimes and sin; sometimes I wonder whether this only stimulates curiosity. Maybe ignorance is bliss; for example, should you tell kids about masturbating?

Dominick "loves" a girl classmate. He tells my wife [i.e., Dominick's mother] a "secret." He usually doesn't tell me. He wishes that he was in the park with his love. Giggling—he wanted his mother to tell me that he wants to marry her.

Dominick said to me, "Mommy loves you." He was excited when I said that I love Mommy, too.

I have been reading about "puppy love." The worst thing is to discourage puppy love.

My brother once asked me what I thought of his girl. I objected to my brother's marrying her. I often wondered whether my remarks had anything to do with their breaking up. My brother married somebody else, later divorced.

I felt that I may have "loused him up" and that the girl was not bad. This was my next older brother. I was dating more; perhaps this brother looked to me for guidance.

She [the girl his brother married] told me later that she really only married him because she felt sorry for him. I almost pushed her over the railing when she said that. I told her that I did not like it. They argued all the time.

All these people bring back unpleasant memories. The whole damn thing is rotten to the core. I don't like all these people from my past. (He speaks very harshly, swearing at them—unpleasant memories of a bunch of related people—a vicious circle.) [Real disgust.]

All unpleasantries in childhood. [His tone of voice expresses distaste.] I want it different for my children.

About the daydream: My mother always tells me how much I do for my parents. She has not mentioned it lately. Perhaps I wanted to reassure myself about it. I feel this is somehow connected with reassuring myself about slow work at home. My wife "rides" me about this.

Perhaps I am reassuring myself that at least I do something for somebody.

In this hour, as in Hour 15, both the patient and his wife are concerned with their responsibility as parents and with friction between themselves. What is different in this hour is that feelings dating back to his childhood are being reactivated. He is reliving his past. In his fantasy he thinks, "When I grow up." Later in the hour, he remarks that, "oddly," he still feels this way, i.e., as though he were still a child, looking forward to growing up. As he puts it, he feels "present life is temporary—a fill-in for something better later."

In this Hour 12, he is even more vividly preoccupied than in Hour 15 with the theme of disharmony and the longing for harmony within the family. He repeats this theme in relation to one family after another—his own wife and children, sibling competition in his family in childhood, his fantasy of fixing up the parental home, his son's and his brother's "puppy love," and his horror at the disharmony in his brother's marriage. Finally, his repudiation of strife within the family comes to intense expression: "The whole damn thing is rotten to the core." He does not like all those people from the past. He swears at them, speaking very harshly— "a vicious circle." Then the longing for harmony in his own family emerges: he wants it different for his children.

## A HISTORICAL RECONSTRUCTION

The last few comments in Hour 12 finally give us the clue to the answer we are seeking. "Mother always tells me how much I do for them. Maybe I wanted to reassure myself about them. Maybe I am reassuring myself that at least I do something for somebody."

These attempts at reassuring himself contain the hypothesis that we seek: The childhood source of this patient's longing for a harmonious family was his longing for harmony with his mother. In childhood, his brothers intruded between him and his mother. She could not give all her love to him, and his rivalrous hostility toward his brothers threatened to estrange him still further from his mother. There was only one way that he could hope to get back a harmonious relationship with mother: his brothers must be included in the harmonious circle and become one happy family.

This was an ideal that he could not achieve as a child. He postponed it into the future and fantasied "fixing the house up"—"when I grow up." He still feels himself a child incapable of including a whole family in his longing for harmony with mother. So he still fantasies "fixing the house up" "when he grows up" and dreams of "mixing cement."

## HOW CAN HISTORICAL RECONSTRUCTIONS BE CHECKED?

To the authors, this reconstruction carries a sense of conviction. Yet, if we are to continue our objectively critical approach, we must interrupt our "thrill of omniscient satisfaction." We must ask again: How can it be checked?

For purposes of checking (to counterbalance other difficulties), historical reconstructions have one great advantage. If a particular conflict in the past has been important enough to influence a patient's behavior once, it will do so many times. Our best policy, therefore, will often be to wait. If our reconstruction has been correct or nearly so, other dreams or behavior of the same patient will sooner or later lead us back to it or even, in most cases, suggest revisions or expansions of it.

### ANOTHER DREAM OF A HOUSE

We shall next turn to a dream reported by our patient in Hour 16, immediately after the session in which he had reported the cement dream. The dream that we shall study was the second one reported in Hour 16.

SECOND DREAM, HOUR 16.

> I was at my mother-in-law's house. We used to live there, five years ago. She was talking to lady next door, an attractive woman about my age. She was dressed in rags, her hair wasn't fixed. My mother-in-law was talking about the people next door—how awful it was they didn't take care of their lawn. While looking at this house, it suddenly changed—became a very beautiful mansion (like a governor's house) with fine lawns, etc.
>
> Then the scene shifted. I was taking out garbage, got a lawn chair. A man came along and sat in a chair. I mixed him a drink. Then somebody mentioned time, and I woke up. This person was a girl—can't identify her.

In our first approach to this dream, we shall start again with the "poetic" symbolism of house, home, and family. Then we shall try to follow where the imagery and ideology of this particular dream lead us.

A home, for this patient, is, we think, symbol of a family living together in love and harmony. In this dream, we find this symbol contrasted with another kind of symbol—a lady dressed in rags, her hair not fixed. Later: "how awful it was" that people did not take care of their lawn. Next, attention is abruptly focused on this contrast. The house "suddenly changed—became a very beautiful mansion . . . with fine lawns, etc." Taken together with our hypothesis that a house represents his family, the "beautiful mansion with fine lawns, etc." must represent the patient's ideal of a loving, harmonious family. If so, the people's failure to take care of their lawn would represent his own failure to realize this ideal. Then, the sudden change of the house with a poorly kept lawn into a beautiful mansion would probably be giving expression to the patient's hope that he will "suddenly" become an ideal husband and father. As a result of his treatment, he hopes that his family will become an ideally loving and harmonious one. Again, we have been elaborating a working hypothesis. To check this hypothesis, we report next the associations to this dream.

ASSOCIATIONS.

PATIENT: I heard on the radio that Governor D. of Iowa was killed in a car crash.

The lady next door to my mother-in-law appealed to me sexually.

ANALYST: Ever make a pass?

PATIENT [surprised]: Oh, yes, yes. Several years ago. One night, this woman locked herself out. I got in through the window. She asked me to have a bottle of beer. I remember the details. Kissing and "feeling her up." But she wouldn't let me have intercourse with her. (There were similar incidents later. Also, he took her dancing once. There was mutual masturbation on this occasion. The patient finally got disgusted.)

I wonder whether I dreamed of her as unappealing because I couldn't have her.

ANALYST: As if to say, "Oh, I don't really want her; she's not pretty?"

PATIENT: Yes, that's it.

ANALYST: Why dream of her now?

PATIENT: Don't know.

Mother-in-law said something about hot water—her husband takes a bath, etc. Yet her husband wasn't there; [in reality] they are divorced.

ANALYST: Has anything like this occurred recently?

PATIENT [embarrassed]: Yeah, I haven't been taking enough baths. Can't figure why the guy was sprawled out on the lawn chair. I was unhappy about my mother-in-law. My first year of marriage was generally unhappy. Guess I'd expected something different. I never felt comfortable with mother-in-law. [Scratching now.]

I was disappointed in my wife. There wasn't the warmness I had hoped for. She was cold, matter-of-fact. I thought that other girls I knew might have made me more comfortable. I felt almost like an outsider; often felt not wanted.

My wife has been talking about covering the rose bushes lately. I got some stuff, but a friend told me that they grow better if you *do not* cover them. My wife disagreed. Problem about what to use. I would have preferred clearing them alone. I haven't picked up the stuff yet. If they are so much trouble, it isn't worth it. If they can't stand the winter, that is too bad. [The analyst gets the feeling that there is a childish impatience here.]

My wife was criticizing me yesterday about the whole issue of housework.

ANALYST: This dream seems to have something to do with your concern about her criticism of your work around the house, e.g., mother-in-law's criticism of neighbor's lawn.

[The patient laughs almost explosively.]

ANALYST: Then you change it into a beautiful lawn. You are angry with your wife. You feel that you do your duty, that her criticisms are largely unjustified.

PATIENT: Lately, she asks me about *times,* e.g., when I will be home. This bothers me. I don't like being pinned down. If I give her a time, then it will be hanging over my head. Then, if I am late, there is trouble.

She also asked me to call if I am going to be late. I started doing this. Then she complains about my being late. So I stopped calling.

Lately, it is not pleasant at all with her. Maybe it's her pregnancy.

There has been pressure from the church for a contribution of $10 for fifteen months, for an addition to the school. My wife wanted to give more. I held to the minimum. All went well; the church people were cordial. But afterward my wife was ashamed. She did not want other people to know that we had given so little.

Thus, in his associations to this dream, as in Hour 15, the patient gives evidence of continuing preoccupation with his wife's criticisms of him and with his own dissatisfaction with his wife. Like any other sudden emotional outburst, the patient's explosive laughter is probably highly significant. It was provoked by the analyst's comment comparing the patient's mother-in-law's criticism (about people not taking care of their lawns) to the patient's wife's criticism of the patient's work around the house. In this context, the patient's explosive laughter pointedly suggests two conclusions: first, the patient is exceedingly sensitive about his wife's criticisms of his work around the house (probably as a symbol of his feelings of inadequacy as head of the family), and second, in the dream, his mother-in-law's criticism of the next door neighbor's lawn is actually an allusion to this disturbing theme.

### GAPS IN OUR EVIDENCE

We based this interpretation on one small episode in this patient's dream. Then we found confirmation for it in the patient's explosive laughter when the analyst suggested a relationship between this episode and the wife's criticisms of his work around the house. So far, so good, but there are big gaps in our evidence. There are still many details in both dream and associations that we have not yet accounted for.

As our next clue we shall examine one of these unexplained details. We have recognized a contrast between a "beautiful mansion . . . with fine lawns" and people who "didn't take care of their lawn." In this case, the significant contrast seemed to be between taking care and not taking care of one's lawn, one's house, one's family. The relationship between taking care of one's family and the lady in rags, "her hair not fixed," does not seem so clear.

### ADAPTATION TO LIVING TOGETHER IN A GROUP

On reflection, there does seem to be another similarity. Taking care of one's lawn, of one's clothes, and of one's hair—are all ways of making oneself acceptable and attractive to other people. (E) Perhaps the problem with which the patient is preoccupied in this dream is that of socialization of behavior. This is a process which must begin early in childhood with training in cleanliness and order. It continues progressively into normal adult life. It culminates, if successful, in the assumption of responsibilities in the family, at work, and in the community. All this suggests the hypothesis that the focal problem in this dream is one of *adaptation to living together in a group.*

(C) In confirmation of this interpretation, we find that other details in both the associations and the dream fit it well. Comparable to the lady "in rags," "hair not fixed," is the patient's own embarrassment about "not taking enough baths." The "guy sprawled out on the lawn chair" implies a similar disregard of what is expected in company. (C) Then, in his many references to the first year of his marriage, the patient is reactivating the memory of a time when his attempts to start a new family with his wife were complicated by the presence of her mother. Next come the centrally important associations about working around the house and about his conflict over being "pinned down" by his wife's wishes. Finally, the hour ends with an account of his reluctance to adapt to a larger community, the church.

## THE BASIC PROBLEMS OF EACH INDIVIDUAL ARE THE PROBLEMS IN MUTUAL ADAPTATION OF THE GROUPS TO WHICH HE HAS BELONGED

We promised to follow where the imagery of this dream would lead us. It has led us in an unexpected direction. First we found that the patient was preoccupied with the problem of maintaining the integrity of his family. Then many other details of the dream made it necessary to broaden the hypothesis. In Hour 16 as a whole, the patient seems to be preoccupied with his own and other people's problems of making their behavior acceptable and pleasing to others. The basic problem seems to be one of how groups or pairs of people can live together in some degree of harmony or accord. The latent thoughts of this dream seem to have led us away from individual psychology and into the psychology of groups.

The authors believe that this trend in our patient's thoughts is not so extraordinary as it may at first appear. In fact, most of the problems that our patients bring to us *are* problems of interpersonal adaptation. Most exceptions to this statement are only apparent. For example, a patient may be struggling with his conscience, but we know (from clinical or from everyday experience) that what is now a conflict with his conscience was once a conflict with one or both parents.

In our role as psychoanalytic therapists, we are treating individual patients. Our role as individual therapists has caused us to be interested primarily in the emotional development of one individual and only secondarily in the dynamic problems which inevitably arise when a family or other group tries to live together in some kind of accord. We may forget that man is a "social animal." Almost all the problems that our patients bring to us have arisen out of difficulties or failures in their attempts to find satisfying ways of fitting into some group. In other words, individual psychology is only one indissoluble part of the psychology of groups.

It is now gratifying to discover that our interest in the group facilitates our understanding of the individual. By focusing our attention on the problems of mutual adaptation within groups to which a patient has belonged, we can greatly simplify our attempts to understand a single individual's responses at a particular time. Stated simply, the principle involved is: the patient's problems in fitting into one group today are sometimes identical with, and *always* derivatives of, problems in adaptation to the same or other groups in his past. Even when the problems of today are not identical with those of the past, it is often easy to recognize how the recent problems have been derived from those in the past. In this chapter, we have already made one such attempt. We have shown how our patient's present preoccupation with holding his family together may well have arisen as a derivative of his longing to be at one with his mother in childhood. In childhood, his relationship to his mother was disturbed by sibling rivalry. If he had been able to include his brothers in the harmonious circle, they could have become one happy family. He continues to long for one happy family.

As psychoanalysts, we have one major difficulty in trying to apply these principles. Our tradition is to focus our interest on the disturbing infantile wish that has played an important motivating role somewhere in the historical background of every dream. This tradition tends to deflect us at two points from our task of recognizing the dreamer's present problem. In the first place, it directs our attention prematurely toward the past and away from the problem with which the patient is preoccupied now. The other disturbing influence of our tradition is that it causes us to be too narrowly interested in a disturbing wish, rather than in the problem to which this disturbing wish has given rise. Discovering a disturbing wish should be only a first step. Next we should ask: Why is this wish disturbing? What consequences does the dreamer expect if it should be fulfilled? When we have recognized both the wish and its anticipated disturbing consequences, then we are well on the way to understanding the problem with which the dreamer is struggling.

We are too often careless in our attempts to formulate the nature of a patient's "reactive motive." We are content to call every reactive motive either "guilt" or "shame." Sometimes we do not even take the trouble to distinguish between "guilt" and "shame" (Alexander, 1938; Piers & Singer, 1953). At this point, we should listen more carefully to the patient's own words. We should let the patient's thoughts and behavior tell us precisely the nature of his reactive motives. If we do this, the patient, without himself knowing consciously exactly what he is saying, will often tell us something very specific (about the nature of his early relationship to his mother, for example). All that is necessary is that we really listen.

We return now to the main thesis of this chapter and our last. The goal of our interpretive art is to get an increasingly comprehensive grasp of the cognitive structure of our patient's behavior. A cognitive structure is a constellation of related problems. Usually the problems with which our patients are most deeply concerned are those of mutual adaptation, of fitting into groups (pairs).

Both the personality structure of an individual and the structure of his neurosis are cognitive structures. They are both *precipitates* of his successive *attempts to fit into the groups* to which he has belonged. In general, his personality structure, insofar as it has not been disturbed by neurosis, has been built around the patterns of his successful adaptations to groups. His failures in adaptation to groups constitute the nucleus about which his neuroses have been organized.

The simplest and surest procedure for trying to understand both a patient's neurosis and his personality structure involves two steps. First, we reconstruct, as precisely as possible, the nature of the problem with which he is preoccupied now. Then we trace this problem back, step by step, to the earlier problems in fitting into groups from which his present problem is derived. If our reconstruction of a significant early problem has been correct, then the analysis of other problems that emerge into focus in the course of treatment should sooner or later lead us back to this earlier problem.

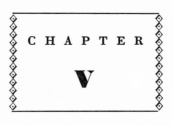

CHAPTER

V

# RECONSTRUCTING THE

# DREAMER'S THOUGHT PROCESSES

The most thorough check possible on the interpretation of a single dream is to reverse the procedure by which we have arrived at our focal conflict hypothesis. Starting with the focal conflict that we have postulated, we try to reconstruct the actual thought processes by which the dreamer arrived at the manifest dream content.

Our first assumption is that *every substitution* in the dream work was *intelligibly motivated*. For example, in the cement dream of Hour 15, we have concluded that the patient was preoccupied with the problem of how to hold his family together. If so, we can now reverse the question. Why did he choose tuckpointing and mixing cement as symbols for trying to restore harmony in his family?

To account for the choice of a particular symbol, we must ask first what is the difference between the symbol and what is being symbolized. In this case, what is the difference between a house and a family? The bricks of a house are inanimate; a family is composed of people. This is the most obvious difference between them. We shall use the term "deanimation" to denote such a substitution of a conflict concerning inanimate objects for one involving people.

We ask next what motivated this particular substitution. In this case, what purpose was served by deanimation of the dreamer's conflict? The answer to this question is not difficult to guess. We tend automatically to identify empathically with other people, especially with those we love. This is why it is so painful to be in conflict with someone we love. By substituting an inanimate object, however, we diminish our sympathic resonance * with the loved person. In this way, we make thinking about our conflict with him much less painful.

## THE DREAMER'S THOUGHT PROCESSES

Our goal is to reconstruct the thought processes of which the manifest dream was a momentary end product.

In the case of the cement dream, after the dreamer has substituted tuckpointing as a symbol for holding his family together, he seems to be trying to solve the problem that he has substituted. In the manifest dream, he is mixing cement as a preparation for tuckpointing. We shall call this kind of substitution an "end–means substitution."

After this, he awakens with the illusion that he knows how to mix cement. Then he recalls that he had recently thought that he would do his tuckpointing himself. But he "didn't know how to mix concrete," he adds, so he "hired somebody."

Now we recognize that, without admitting it to himself, he is

* By "sympathic resonance" with another person we mean our tendency to identify with what he feels, to feel as he does. See chapters VIII and XIII for a more detailed discussion of this mechanism.

still thinking of his original problem. Masking his thoughts by the house symbolism, he has first recognized (preconsciously) that he does not know * how to hold his family together. So he has decided to "hire" the analyst to do the job for him.

This is an entirely rational and valid train of thought. Why, then, can this patient not allow himself to think it through consciously? Actually, we have already given the answer to this question. It would be excessively painful for the patient to become frankly conscious of both his intense desire to hold his family together and his inability to do so. The patient has spared himself this pain by substituting his house as a symbol for his family. The dream work has substituted a problem that is analogous, but also easier and much less painful. Instead of being overwhelmed by pain, the patient's ego has been able to continue with its effort to solve its problem. Actually, behind the mask of the house symbolism, the patient has been able to think his way through to a valid conclusion.

### ALTERNATION OF WITHDRAWAL AND PROBLEM-SOLVING

In our reconstruction, we have made a theoretical and a methodological innovation. Our theoretical working hypothesis is that the substitutions in the dream work are substitutions of one problem for another. Each of these substitutions, we postulate, is intelligibly motivated. If we do not succeed in

* The words "know" and "decided" give expression to the authors' belief, based on many dream analyses, that the essential acts in problem-solving thought (such as knowledge, decision, deliberate choice) usually occur preconsciously, without the thinker's or dreamer's necessarily becoming conscious of them. Sometimes consciousness merely registers acts of thought that have already been performed preconsciously. Perhaps the essential function of conscious awareness is to review critically (and perhaps revise) thinking that has already occurred preconsciously.

finding an intelligible motivation for each substitution, then we regard this as a discrepancy to be accounted for. In the case of Dream 15, at least, these working assumptions have enabled us to reach an understanding of the underlying thought processes. As we have reconstructed them, these thought processes make good sense from beginning to end. This is our check on the validity of our reconstruction.

When we now examine and compare the substitutions in the dream work in this case, we find that they are of two kinds. First, deanimation of the patient's conflict was a "defensive substitution." It was motivated by the dreamer's need to protect himself from the too-great impact of his conflict. He achieved this by withdrawing from his conflict, by deflecting his interest and focusing it on a similar but less disturbing problem. Second, two other substitutions were end–means substitutions. These were the substitution of (1) mixing cement for tuckpointing and (2) "hiring" the analyst to solve for him his underlying conflict about holding his family together.

These two kinds of substitution are signs of two opposing trends between which the dreamer alternates throughout the dream work. Part of the time he is trying to find a solution for his conflict. When the problem threatens to become too difficult or disturbing, he withdraws from it and focuses his interest on a similar but less disturbing problem. Even after he has withdrawn in this way, however, he continues his problem-solving effort, trying to find a solution for the problem that has been substituted.

### COORDINATION OF PROBLEM-SOLVING AND WITHDRAWAL

Sometimes, instead of alternating, these two trends are coordinated in one or another way. Our patient's cement dream and his fantasy of fixing his house are both examples of such coordination. Both tuckpointing and fixing up the house are symbolic attempts to solve the patient's problem; but in each case the attempt at solution has been preceded by a defensive maneuver. In each case, the defensive maneuver has been to substitute an analogous but less disturbing problem. Tuckpointing and fixing up a house are both mechanical problems. These mechanical problems are nowhere near so disturbing to this patient as is the problem which is focal for him at this time—the interpersonal one of trying to hold his family together.

In this dream and this fantasy, the manner of combining a defense with an attempt at problem-solving is a distinctive one. In each case, the *defensive maneuver* has been *subordinated* to the attempt at *problem-solving*. The dream work has substituted an easier problem and then continued with its problem-solving effort. By substituting an analogous but easier problem, the dream work has made it possible to continue with its effort to solve its problem.

Such subordination of a withdrawal maneuver to continued efforts to solve a problem is a device that is not peculiar to the dream work. It is also a very valuable device in rational thinking. If we become too involved emotionally in a problem of intimate personal relations, it is often helpful to try to think in more abstract, less personal, terms. In this way, we can free our thinking from disturbing emotional overtones. For example, if one is involved in an emotional conflict with a close friend, it may be impossible for him to think clearly and objectively about it. He may be able to clarify his thinking greatly, on the other hand, by thinking of the conflict first in abstract, general terms as one between two otherwise-unidentified persons, A and B.

Similarly, the essential difficulty in our patient's problem of trying to hold his family together is the fact that he is too intensely emotionally involved in it. The resentments and the strong sense of failure that have been stirred up, especially in relation to his wife, are too strong. They interfere with his ability to think clearly. Substituting a mechanical problem from which disturbing interpersonal relationships have been eliminated has made it possible for him to envisage his problem more clearly. Behind the protective screen of an impersonal symbolism, he has been able to sense preconsciously that his problem is essentially one of fixing up his "house," of holding it together.

When we think of the cement dream (15) in these terms, we realize that the problem which *more immediately* preoccupied the patient was not the fundamental one of how to hold his family together. This problem was still insoluble. His more immediate concern was whether to "hire" the analyst to help him solve this fundamental problem. As we have already recognized, it was still too disturbing for him to face his conflict directly and admit to himself that he needed help from the analyst. So, in the dream, after substituting the less disturbing problem of "mixing cement," he entertained the illusion that he was able to do it himself. He did not get any further with his problem until he awakened from his dream. Then he realized (preconsciously) that the problem with which he was struggling was one that he could not solve by himself, that he needed to "hire somebody" to help him. Even in his thoughts on awakening he did not quite succeed in getting back to this problem with which he was really preoccupied. Had he finally succeeded in realizing that his thoughts about his house really had reference to his family, then the train of thought that began with his dream would have been completely equivalent to the rational device of withdrawing temporarily from a problem in which one is too intensely involved in order to think more clearly about it.*

At this point, the analyst could probably have helped him complete his train of thought. He could have told the patient that what he was really thinking of was his analysis and his need for help in holding his family together.

DEFENSES AS DEVICES FOR

DELAYING COMMITMENT TO A CONFLICT

The role played by deanimation of the patient's focal conflict in this dream of Hour 15 suggests a somewhat new concept of the function of defense. Our theoretical assumption is that wish-fulfillment has definite limits, even in the dream work. To the extent that a dreamer has become committed to a conflict, it is impossible to "wish it away." This is the principle that Zeigarnik (1927) proved years ago for "intentions."

The dreamer's ego has only one defense with which to protect itself against disturbing conflicts. This defense is to delay or prevent these conflicts from being activated or to postpone or forestall further involvement in or commitment to them. The success of such a defense depends greatly on its timing. The best defenses are prophylactic,† diverting the dreamer

---

* Arnold Toynbee (1934) has used the phrase, "withdrawal and return" to describe this mechanism in the case of prophets who retire into solitude (wilderness, desert) for a time before they start on their prophetic missions. Such a period of retirement is probably one of "incubation," during which the prophet reaches some sort of resolution of underlying conflicts. His "prophetic message" takes form as a solution to these conflicts before he returns with his message to the world. Boisen (1936) has discussed this phenomenon at length. See also Kasanin and French (1941) for a discussion of two clinically psychotic cases illustrating the same principle.

† French (1958) called such a prophylactic defense a "successful defense."

from his potentially disturbing conflict at a time when it is only slightly activated.* The deanimation of the patient's conflict in the cement dream is such a prophylactic defense. Evidence for this conclusion is the fact that there is no sign in the manifest dream of the patient's being disturbed.† In fact, he is even able to maintain the illusion that he knows how to mix cement. Even when he wakes up and decides (preconsciously) that he will "hire somebody" to mix the concrete, our patient can reassure himself about this decision. He was earlier able to admit to himself that he could not mix concrete. It did not disturb him at that time, so why should he be disturbed now? This is the implication.

In Chapter VI, we shall discuss a dream in which the defensive substitutions were made later—only after the underlying disturbing conflict had been activated to a considerable degree. Such defenses are necessarily much less successful. All that the dreamer's ego can then accomplish is to prevent *further* activation of his conflict.

* When such a prophylactic defense is used, Freud (1926) spoke of "anxiety" as a "warning signal."

† Our methodological assumption is that implied by our concept of "commitment." Once one has been committed to it, a disturbing affect cannot be "wished away" for long. An ideational content can be repressed, and the quality of the affect can be transformed. Anger may be replaced by fear. Either anger or fear can be given outlet in energetic activity, either physical or mental. Even impulses to violent activity can be replaced by intense absorption in motionless looking or in deep sleep. Quantitatively, however, once one has been committed to it, an affective charge must be discharged in overt activity, appear in consciousness, or find outlet in the activation of physiological functions (e.g., psychosomatic symptoms, muscular tension, deep sleep). In accordance with this methodological assumption, we can usually make a subjective estimate of the degree of a dreamer's commitment to a conflict by scanning the manifest dream and the dreamer's thoughts immediately after awakening (French, 1952, Ch. XLI, esp. pp. 202–203).

## *RUDIMENTARY PROBLEM-SOLVING*
## *AND COMPLEX DEFENSES*

The patient could remember only a fragment of the cement dream. This was probably, in part, why the problem-solving function of this dream was much easier to recognize than usual. To balance this oversimplified impression, we shall next study a dream in which the patient's defenses were less successful and his problem-solving efforts much more rudimentary.

We suggested in Chapter I that sometimes a dream and its associations offer such abundant evidence that the dream's significance cannot be grasped all at once. In order to make full use of such abundant evidence, the interpreter must proceed as he would with a jigsaw puzzle, trying to piece together first one part of it and then another until he finally gets a glimpse of the whole picture.

Our patient's sixteenth hour is a good example of the necessity for such a procedure. We have already suggested two focal conflicts for the dream of the beautiful mansion in Hour

16. We do not yet know how these two conflicts are related, and we do not yet have an adequate grasp of the thought processes underlying this dream. We shall, accordingly, make use of a "jigsaw-puzzle" technique. First concentrating our attention on a number of questions about parts of this dream, we shall try to answer these questions one at a time. At the end of the chapter, we shall try to assemble what we have learned from these detailed inquiries.

## EVIDENCE POINTING TO THE
## PRECIPITATING STIMULUS OF THIS DREAM

Our first question is: How does the patient's mother-in-law fit into the cognitive structure of this dream? In search for an answer, we shall first consider two facts. First, in the dream text, the criticisms (which are really criticisms of the patient as head of his family) come from his mother-in-law, and, second, the patient's associations lead back to the first year of his marriage, when he and his wife were living in her mother's home. The picture that he gives of this year is not a happy one. It is not the picture of a man who feels adequate as a young husband. When we put this picture together with the mother-in-law's critical remarks in the dream text, we conclude that, in his first year of marriage, the patient must have felt very inadequate in his mother-in-law's eyes.

We ask next: What is causing these unhappy memories to be reactivated now? To be sure, his wife is critical of him. But why bring in his mother-in-law again, several years later, to reinforce his wife's present criticisms? Another fact suggests the answer to this question. This patient is now in analysis. He is again in a situation in which his inadequacy as a husband must be exposed to another person's view. As recently as his last hour (15), he was coming to the realization that he needed the analyst's help in trying to hold his family together. Now, in order to get the analyst's help, he must expose his distressing inadequacy to the view of the analyst. He shrinks from thus exposing himself. He recalls, instead, how he used to feel exposed to his mother-in-law's critical scrutiny when he and his wife were living in her house. It is less painful to recall his unhappiness in the past than to face the prospect of the same kind of humiliation now.

Now we also discover the answer to a question that we have not yet asked. What was the precipitating stimulus of this dream? It was, we now suspect, the dreamer's first *realization that he would have to expose to the analyst the inadequacy* which he felt so keenly.*

To check this working hypothesis, we look for other possible references to the analyst in this dream. One such reference now takes on new meaning in the light of our present hypotheses. In the dream text, the house with a poorly kept lawn suddenly changes into a beautiful mansion. We suspected that this dream detail was expressing the patient's hopes of what might happen as a result of treatment. As a result of treatment, he hopes that he will "suddenly" become an ideal husband and father. Yet the dream at this point does not even mention the analyst. The dream text gives no credit to the analyst for the sudden transformation of the house. Now we

* Recognition of this precipitating stimulus now requires a slight revision of one of the focal-conflict hypotheses proposed in Chapter IV. The patient's focal problem is more superficial and more specific than we thought. His immediate cause of concern is not so much his own sense of inadequacy in trying to hold his family together, but rather his reluctance to reveal this inadequacy to the analyst. Accordingly, we should now formulate his focal conflict as:

| Desire for the analyst's therapeutic help in the patient's effort to become an adequate head of his family | *versus* | Great reluctance to reveal his distressing inadequacy to the analyst |
|---|:---:|---|

realize that this fact corresponds exactly to our hypothesis. The patient would like to believe that he can be cured without having to reveal to the analyst his painful inadequacy. He prefers to fantasy that he can be cured without the analyst's help.

Still looking for references to the analyst, we turn next to the second part of his dream. Does the man in this part of the dream represent the analyst? In this part of the dream, the patient "got a lawn chair," and a "man came along and sat" in it. Then, in the dream, somebody interrupted the patient's entertaining this man by "mentioning time." At this point, the patient awoke. A psychoanalytic session, too, is often terminated by "mentioning time." This parallel offers suggestive confirmation of our hypothesis that the man in the dream represents the analyst.

If so, then certain implications follow. In the dream, the patient is not in treatment. The situation is only a casual social one. He is entertaining the analyst, not in his home, but outside, in a lawn chair. This implies that the patient does not want the analyst to come into his house. Again we get an unexpected confirmation of our hypothesis that the patient is reluctant to expose to the analyst's view his painful inadequacy as a family man.

### FLIGHT NEXT DOOR

We turn now to another question: In our first suggested interpretation in Chapter IV, we thought of the neighbor's unkept lawn as a symbol of the patient's failure to realize his ideal of a loving, harmonious family. We paid no attention to the fact that the house whose lawn was poorly kept was not the patient's own house; it was the house next door. Why?

In order to account for this fact, we must infer that the dream work has substituted the house next door for the patient's own. To check this suggestion, we ask whether there is an understandable motive why the dream work should have made this substitution. Such a motive is not difficult to find. The patient would prefer not to recognize as his own his problem about holding his family together. He would rather focus his attention on the house next door.

The patient's associations to the lady in "rags" next door even suggests an urge to act on his need to escape from his problems at home. This "attractive woman," next door to his mother-in-law, is one whom the patient had once been able to help effectively. She is also one to whom the patient had made sexual advances on a number of occasions. In the context of what we already know of this patient, his motive for occasionally transferring his affections next door is not difficult to guess. He is turning away from his own home, where he feels so painfully inadequate, to the memory of a lady whom he once helped, adequately. In his thoughts, he is also escaping, at least temporarily, from the responsibility for taking care of a family, which is the source of so much conflict for him. In brief, this patient not only looks next door in order to avoid looking at the problem in his own house; he also has a need in real life to escape from his conflict at home by going next door to another woman.

### DEFENSIVE STRUCTURE OF THIS DREAM

In Chapter V, we studied another pattern of defensive substitution. We recognize that this patient's substitution of a house for his family had served the purpose of protecting him from feeling the emotional impact of a painful conflict involving his relations to people. This pattern of deanimation of the patient's conflict has also played an important role in the dream of the beautiful mansion.

Now that our attention has been called to them, we find evidence also of other substitutions in Hour 16, all with similar motives. The dream has substituted not only a house for the patient's family, but also a lawn for a house, as well as the house next door for his own house. Another set of substitutions is even more radical. There is no mention of the patient's children in this hour. Instead of taking care of children, the talk is of dressing acceptably (lady in rags, hair not fixed, not taking baths), of working about the house, of taking out garbage, and the like.

In our interpretive discussion in Chapter IV, we successively suggested two focal conflicts for this dream. First, we thought of his conflict as similar to the one that was focal in the earlier dream (Hour 15) and in the fantasy of Hour 12:

| | | Painful incapacity to |
| Wish for a loving and | *versus* | realize this ideal (based |
| harmonious family | | on inability to master |
| | | underlying resentments) |

Later, after paying attention to other details of the dream and associations, we thought of the patient's problem as a more general one, as one of adaptation to living together in a group.

In our earlier discussion, we did not inquire how these two conflicts were related. We did not attempt to decide which was focal. Now, our survey of the defensive substitutions in this dream is beginning to make it possible to answer these two questions. Now it becomes clearer that the focal problem in this dream is closer to the one that we first recognized (see

Page 76). It seems to be closely related to the one in the earlier dream of Hour 15 and to the fantasy of Hour 12:

| Intense longing for a harmonious family | *versus* | Painful incapacity to realize this ideal |

The patient's generalized problem of trying to fit into groups has emerged as a consequence of a series of attempts to escape from the circumscribed problem of trying to hold together his own family. This is excessively difficult for him. To succeed as head of a family in holding his family together would be a last and most difficult achievement in adapting to living in a group. Reacting to the patient's incapacity to achieve this goal, the dream has tried to make his failure less painful by turning back to memories of less important failures in achieving harmonious relationships to other people.

### TWO PATTERNS OF DEFENSIVE SUBSTITUTION

In the attempts of this dream to reduce the patient's own problem to more elementary, less painful terms, we can recognize two main principles. One is the principle that we have just discussed briefly, that of *deanimating* the patient's *conflict*, of substituting problems in which painful sympathic resonance * with other people is not necessary.

The other principle is illustrated by the patient's going next door to another woman. The defensive principle involved in this case is one of *shifting* one's interest *from one group to another*. If attempts to adapt to one group fail, one tries to escape by turning to another group.†

---

* See note, Page 64.

† For the purpose of the present discussion, we are not distinguishing between "groups" and "pairs." A "pair" is a "group" of two.

### COMPLICATIONS RESULTING FROM ATTEMPTS
### TO TURN FROM ONE GROUP TO ANOTHER

Complications often occur when a person tries to turn from one group to another. One complication is that difficulties arise in the new group similar to those from which the patient is fleeing in the old group. Even more frequently, complications result from the fact that one does not really become detached from the first group, but remains suspended between the two.

As examples, we shall first discuss briefly the outcome of our patient's flight to the lady next door. Then, at greater length, we shall consider complications that are to be expected and seem to be threatening to develop in his relationship to his analyst.

### THE LADY NEXT DOOR

The patient's attempt to turn to the "attractive" lady next door was not long successful. In real life, it ended in "disgust." In the dream, he finds her "in rags," with her "hair not fixed." In the dream, the patient has protected himself from disgust with himself by focusing his attention on the unkempt appearance of the woman.

### COMPLICATIONS TO BE EXPECTED IN
### THE PSYCHOANALYTIC SITUATION

We should expect that this patient's pattern of trying to escape from one group to another would have important consequences for his psychoanalytic treatment. If the patient really has a need to escape from his disturbing family situation to a new group, then his relationship to his analyst in therapy should offer him an ideal opportunity for such an escape.

Let us now further elaborate the implications of this possibility. There are certain inevitable complications involved in trying to escape from one group to another. Either one must keep the two groups insulated from each other, or one runs the danger of stirring up intense jealousies of each group for the other. In the case of the analysis, our therapeutic policy is to try to keep such jealousies at a minimum. We encourage the patient to keep his family insulated from knowledge of what is happening in the analysis. On the other hand, in the interests of therapy, it is impossible to maintain insulation in the opposite direction. The rule of free association requires the patient to tell the analyst of his emotional relations to his family. Sooner or later, in his fantasies at least, the patient's transference will bring the analyst into intimate relationship with the family.

In this patient's case, it is not difficult to guess at least two things that are likely to happen. Sooner or later, the analyst may be felt to be an intruder between the patient and his wife. In view of what we know about the relationship between the patient and his brothers and mother, still another development seems probable. The analyst will become a mother to the patient, and the patient will tend to develop a sibling rivalry conflict, with his wife as the rival.

We return now to the patient's dream. Are there any hints in this dream of a tendency for the patient to try to escape from his family by turning to the analyst? Actually, we have already found such a hint. If the man in the second part of his dream represents the analyst, then we can recognize another motive for the patient's not wanting the analyst to come into his home. He probably does not want the analyst to intrude on his relationship to his wife. Perhaps, also, he does not want his wife to intrude on his own relationship to the analyst. In confirmation of this inference, we recall the patient's reticence, reported in Hour 5, in talking to his wife about his analysis. When we discussed this hour, we suspected that he needed to protect himself against reactivation of a triangular conflict. To this end, he must try to keep his wife and his analyst apart.

In the second part of his dream (Hour 16), he has succeeded for the moment in keeping the analyst and his wife apart. Earlier in the dream, he had warned himself of the impending danger by reactivating the memory of another triangular situation. Instead of allowing his triangular conflict to be lived out in the analysis, he had revived the memory of the first year of his marriage. At that time, he and his wife and her mother were all living together. In his associations, he has described some of his difficulties in trying to fit into this group of three. He "never felt comfortable with his mother-in-law," he says. He "was disappointed in his wife's lack of warmness," "almost felt like an outsider," and "often felt not wanted." Something like this is what the patient (preconsciously) now fears would develop if, even in fantasy, he should allow the analyst to become too intimately associated with his family.

## SUMMARY OF THOUGHT PROCESSES
### UNDERLYING THIS DREAM

We shall now try to view in perspective the picture that we have been building up of the thought processes of which the "beautiful-mansion" dream was a product. The situation which served as precipitating stimulus for this dream can be described as follows: Ever since Hour 12, at least, the patient had been struggling (preconsciously) with the problem of trying to "hold his family together" and with the realization of his inadequacy to perform this function as "head of the family." In Hour 15, he came close * to the realization that he needed therapeutic help from the analyst in order to become capable of performing this function. Some time after Hour 15, he came to the further (preconscious) realization that, in order to get therapeutic help, he would have to reveal to the analyst his distressing inadequacy as head of his family. This realization of the need to reveal the inadequacy which was so painful to him became the precipitating stimulus for the dream which he reported in his next hour (16). His conflict over revealing his inadequacy became the focal conflict of this dream.

His first step in trying to deal with this conflict was to shrink from it. However, it was not possible merely to "wish away" his conflict.† All that he was able to do was to reactivate, as a substitute, the memory of an analogous conflict in the past. In the first year of his marriage, he was painfully aware of his mother-in-law's realization of his inadequacy as a young husband. In his dream thoughts, instead of dealing directly with his present conflict in relation to the analyst, he began to relive the memory of his analogous conflicts over starting his married life in his mother-in-law's home.

At that time, neither, could he solve his conflict. He consoles himself by recalling that once he was able to momentarily escape from his painful sense of inadequacy at home. He rescued the lady next door when she found herself locked

---

* This could also be phrased: "He came for a moment to the preconscious realization, from which he then shrank."

† See note, Page 70.

out of her house. Then and later, he tried to escape further from his problems at home by sexual play with the woman, but this attempt gave him no enduring relief. It ended in "disgust."

In spite of his attempts to run away next door, he still cannot get out of his mind the memory of his mother-in-law's critical attitude toward his inadequacy as a husband. Again, all he can do is to recall, as a substitute, her criticisms of the neighbor's poorly kept lawn. There follows next a real attempt to "wish away" his problem. The house with a poorly kept lawn becomes a "beautiful mansion." This beautiful dream fantasy had its real basis in the dreamer's hopes for therapeutic help. Yet it is a conspicuous fact that the dream text does not even mention the analyst. This omission can be recognized as a "deliberate attempt" on the patient's part to "wish away" the necessity of seeking help from the analyst. In this beautiful dream fantasy, the dreamer is playing with the wish * that he might be cured without having to suffer the

---

* By using the words, "deliberate attempt" and "playing with the wish," the authors are again expressing their belief that it is often possible to read from the manifest dream the attitude of the dreamer's "preconscious ego" toward the wishes and fantasies that are emerging. In this case, the authors were at first puzzled by the "beautiful mansion" fantasy because it seemed to run counter to our methodological assumption that a dream cannot "wish away" unsolved problems. Our intuitive impression was that the dream had much too easily achieved fulfillment of the dreamer's wish for a cure without the analyst's help. His dream fantasy gave an impression of magic, of a fairy story, rather than of symbolic expression of a hope based on reality.

Stimulated by this apparent discrepancy, we were next even more impressed with the extravagant unreality of this wish-fulfilling fantasy. Not only does this dream incident have the magical atmosphere of a fairy story, but the dreamer also describes the beautiful mansion as "like a governor's house," much beyond anything that the patient could realistically hope for in actual life. Then we began to sense that the extravagant unreality of this fantasy was overcompensatory, that this extravagant unreality was actually a sign of the dreamer's underlying preconscious realization that it was impossible for him to be cured without

pain of revealing to the analyst his intense longing and distressing inability to hold his family together.

This attempt to wish away his conflict does not last long. In the second part of his dream, the patient is no longer playing with unreality. He has returned to his focal conflict about turning to the analyst for help. Now a new danger has begun to emerge—that he will become really attached to the analyst and thus activate a triangular conflict involving himself, the analyst, and his wife. He tries to forestall this danger by entertaining the analyst on the lawn and not inviting him into his home.

### APPRAISAL OF THE DREAMER'S THOUGHT PROCESSES

We began this chapter with the working assumption that the dreamer's thought processes would make good sense—if only we could penetrate their disguise. Our reconstruction of the cognitive structure of this dream has now confirmed this expectation. It is true that this dream is struggling with a problem for which the dreamer can find no satisfactory solution. He wants therapeutic help from the analyst, but cannot overcome his reluctance to reveal to the analyst the nature of his conflict in relation to his family. Yet, once we have studied the relationships among the problems touched on in the dream thoughts, we find nothing strange or essentially irrational in the way that he has turned from one problem to another in his search for a solution. As in the cement dream, his defenses

---

the analyst's help. For the moment, he was deliberately and playfully indulging himself in a fantasy that he knew (preconsciously) to be unrealistic.

This impression was confirmed by the fact that, in the second part of the dream, the patient was no longer playing with unreality, but had returned to his focal conflict about turning to the analyst for help.

involve in each case the substitution of a less disturbing but analogous problem whenever the immediately preceding problem proves too difficult.

Thus, in this dream, as in the cement dream of Hour 15, we get the impression that the thought processes in dreaming have a much greater similarity to the thought processes underlying rational behavior than they appear to have. In the beautiful-mansion dream, however, we have been able to recognize this similarity only after we have taken the trouble to reconstruct the dream's cognitive structure with great care.

### OUR BEST CHECK ON OUR INTERPRETATIONS

We should now like to suggest that our best check on the essential correctness of our interpretation of a dream is the criterion that the underlying thought processes make good sense. We began this chapter with some doubts about the possibility of being certain of the validity of our interpretations. We answered that the interpreter should ask himself more questions before giving up to skepticism. He should try to make full use of the evidence actually available. Now we have illustrated this procedure by further study of a dream in which the underlying dream thoughts seemed very complex.

The results of our careful study of this dream now suggest a more precise answer to our skepticism. The only really trustworthy check on the validity of a dream interpretation is a thorough reconstruction of the dream's cognitive structure. This answer seems surprising at first. The underlying dream thoughts are usually complexly interwoven. Will not attempts to piece them together only lead us into totally untrustworthy speculations?

To answer this new doubt, we make use of Freud's analogy

of a jigsaw puzzle. The more numerous and the more irregular the pieces are, the more certain we can be of our solution when we finally succeed in piecing them together. In many jigsaw puzzles, we also have another criterion which only the correct solution can meet. The picture that we reconstruct must make sense.

We have the same two criteria to guide us when we attempt to piece together the cognitive structure of a dream. The stranger and the more incomprehensible the fragments of a manifest dream and its associations are, the more certain we can be of our understanding when we can finally piece them together into an intelligible cognitive structure.

CHAPTER

# VII

## FURTHER DISCUSSION OF
## OUR INTERPRETIVE APPROACH

### Our Thesis and Some Objections to It

An indispensable requirement for an objectively critical interpretive method is the working assumption that the dreamer's
thought processes make good sense—if only we can penetrate
their disguise. This is our only really adequate check on the
validity of our interpretations. If we are content to assume that
the thought processes in dreams are strange and unaccountable, we have no basis for distinguishing between one interpretation and another. Unless we insist that the dreamer's
thinking makes sense, we shall be too easily satisfied with
interpretations that may have no merit except that they fit our
preconceptions or even our individual whims.

Let us spell out our working assumption more carefully.
Our thesis is that the really significant thought processes in
the dream work involve practical thinking, rather than verbal
thinking. In most cases, the dreamer's thinking is struggling
with concrete, practical problems involving his relationship
to other people. This kind of thinking we call "empathic."

When we carefully reconstruct this empathic thinking, the impression grows on us that the thought processes in dreaming have a much greater similarity than they seem to have to the thought processes underlying rational waking behavior.

Before elaborating this thesis further, we shall consider some objections to it. The most obvious one is based on the fact that many dreams are at first incomprehensible. If the thought processes in dreaming are really intelligible, why should it take us so long to come to an understanding of them? In answer to this question, two thoughts suggest themselves:

(1) While he was dreaming, the dreamer had no need to put his thoughts in a form that could be communicated. He was struggling, often unsuccessfully, for a solution to a practical emotional problem of his own. When he describes the dream, he is not trying to explain to the analyst or to anyone else what he was thinking about. Usually he did not even know consciously what his problem was. Therefore, the analyst must listen empathically, sometimes for a long time, before the nature of a problem with which the dreamer is struggling begins to dawn on him.

(2) Our initial impression is that the dreamer's thinking does not make logical sense. This is an impression that we gain before we know what he is really thinking. Before we have discovered the problem that the dreamer is trying to solve, we cannot judge whether his thinking about it makes sense.

This answer reminds us again that the dreamer is thinking about a practical problem. Our initial impression was *not* that dreaming resembles *rational thinking*. It was, rather, that the thought processes in dreams resemble *those underlying rational behavior*. What we call "rational thinking" is usually *verbal thinking*.

Freud, as is well known, had a much more comprehensive answer to our question, an answer which he documented by detailed analysis of many dreams. In the manifest content of dreams, he pointed out (Freud, 1900), the latent dream thoughts seem to have undergone distortion. Freud attributed this distortion to a dream censor. Like a political censor, Freud believed, the dream censor finds certain thoughts unacceptable and excludes them from consciousness. The censor permits other thoughts to enter consciousness, provided that they first submit to distortion; they are permitted to enter consciousness in disguised form.

### FREUD'S CONCEPT OF "THE PRIMARY PROCESS"

Up to this point, we are in full agreement with Freud's account of the dream work. But Freud went further. He denied that problem-solving ever plays more than an incidental, completely unessential role in the dream work. He thought of the dream work as dominated by a need to achieve hallucinatory fulfillment of an infantile wish. To this end, he believed, the dream work uses the dreamer's rational waking thoughts (either conscious or preconscious) merely as material. In the dream work, he postulated, the dreamer's rational thoughts are subjected to highly irrational processes, which he called "the primary process." The basic principle of this primary process, he believed, is free and massive displacement of energy from one psychic element to another along any available associative pathway, without regard for reality or logical relations. When the dream work is studied by the technique that Freud used, the thought processes in dreams do indeed seem highly irrational, even bizarre at times.

How, then, can we account for the difference between

Freud's view and our own? This difference must be a result of differences between Freud's and our own way of studying the dream work. These differences can be reduced to two. One is Freud's one-sided interest in the infantile wish, which he regarded as the essential "motor" of the dream work. As a result of this one-sided interest, he tended to think of the process of elaboration of this infantile wish as merely "resistance," as an obstacle to our discovering the roots in the past of the conflict with which the dreamer was struggling. For this reason, he neglected to take what we believe should be the next step in dream interpretation—to inquire carefully into the *motives* for the dreamer's "resistance." In each particular case, why did the dreamer have to repress and to react in opposition to his infantile wish? Why was this wish disturbing to him? Trying to answer this question precisely is the next step in the interpretive approach that we propose.

There was another reason, we believe, for Freud's failure to recognize the dreamer's persisting attempts to solve his problem. Freud's technique of reconstructing the dream work was by tracing chains of association. This technique seems to imply that rational thinking involves some kind of subordination of chains of association to a goal and to rules of logic (Freud's "secondary process"). The authors' thesis is that thought processes are not built up atomistically out of chains of associations. On the contrary, all concrete, practical thinking, whether rational or seemingly irrational, is in terms of total *Gestalten,* in terms of what we call "practical grasp" * of situations, in terms of "practical understanding" of concrete problems to be solved.

There remains another possibility—even probability. Per-

---

*For several good examples of this principle in the thinking of schizophrenics, see Fromm-Reichmann (1942).

haps the "problem-solving" that Freud is talking about is *not* the same thing that we mean by "problem-solving." Perhaps the problem-solving efforts, which we seem to find so regularly in the dream work, have been recognized by Freud under another name.

This suspicion is confirmed when we read some of Freud's examples of dream interpretation.* In some of these dreams, the interplay between the dream censorship and the dreamer's disturbing wishes gives evidence of practical intelligence of a high order. The task of permitting unrecognized and indirect wish-fulfillment while acceding to the demands of censorship is what we call a "practical problem." When we have once discovered the "reactive motive" responsible for the censorship, it becomes even easier for us to recognize that the dreamer's ego is struggling to find a way of reconciling two conflicting motives. This task of reconciling conflicting motives is a "practical problem" in the sense that we are using these words.

Freud's description of the "primary process" seems to the authors to undervalue the thought processes involved in dreaming. "Free and massive displacement of energy along any available associative pathway," sounds like an automatic and mechanical process, not guided by any directing intelligence. Freud's next phrase, "without regard for reality or logical relations," confirms this impression. When we make a careful study of the dream work, either in our own or in Freud's examples, we discover that the dreamer's ego's attempts to solve its practical problem are guided by an alert and often adroit intelligence.

* See especially the first two examples in Chap. IV (on "Dream Distortion") in Freud (1900).

Indeed, Freud was not consistent in his devaluation of the "primary process." Sometimes he recognized the high degree of intelligence of which unconscious thinking is capable. For example, in Chapter I we quoted Freud's advice to the analyst —to use his own unconscious as a tool for understanding his patient's unconscious. This implies an intuitive understanding on the part of the analyst which is far superior to anything of which verbal thinking would be capable. It is impossible to conceive how thought processes based only on "free and massive displacement of energy along any available associative pathway" could give rise to the sensitive intuitive understanding that gifted artists possess and that psychoanalysts require for their work.

### DIFFERENCES BETWEEN FREUD'S METHOD AND OURS

We return now to the differences between Freud's way of studying the dream work and our own. Our impression is that the reason Freud did not find the dreamer's practical problem was that he was not interested in it. He was content if he could find the dreamer's disturbing infantile wish and was willing to dismiss the dreamer's reactive motives as "resistance."

What is new in our technique of interpretation begins after the dreamer's disturbing wish has been discovered. Our next step is to inquire why this particular wish was disturbing to the dreamer. With this question in mind, we compare the disturbing wish with the manifest dream. There are many possible ways that a particular disturbing wish might find expression in a dream. By comparing the manifest dream to this wish, we try to deduce the dreamer's "reactive motive." For example, if the manifest dream detail that we are studying seems an appropriate punishment, we may conclude that guilt is the reactive motive. Even so, we should be cautious. It may not be his conscience that is disturbing this dreamer. Perhaps it is fear of estrangement from some parental figure. *Careful study of the dreamer's own words* and of the context should tell us whether the dreamer has substituted an internalized "conscience" for the parent he once feared he would offend.

We know, of course, that Freud did not completely ignore the dreamer's reactive motive. In the early years,* he deliberately postponed questions about reactive motives and took account of them provisionally by his concept of the dream censor. He postponed inquiring in detail into the motives for dream censorship. Freud later identified the dream censor with the superego. This would seem to imply that the dreamer's reactive motive is always guilt. Actually, guilt is the reactive motive in some dreams, but not in others. In other dreams, the disturbing motive may be incompatible with the dreamer's pride or in conflict with fear of estrangement from a loved person, or with fear of loss of a dependent relation to another person, or with fear of some kind of retaliation, etc. In each case, the patient's reactive motive should be deduced from the patient's actual words, viewed in the actual context. It is easy to be too stereotyped in our inferences about reactive motives.

### Our Interpretive Approach

Piecing together suggestions that we have made earlier, we shall now try to spell out in more careful detail how we go about trying to understand the thought processes underlying

* See the Introduction to Freud (1923).

the dream work. For convenience of presentation, we can divide our procedure into two stages.

### FIRST STAGE. TRYING TO
### FIND THE DREAMER'S PROBLEM

Our first task is to discover the dreamer's problem. We start by "scanning" the manifest dream and the dreamer's associations. We shall often not be able to find immediately the dreamer's focal problem. The dream as a whole may at first be incomprehensible. In such a case, we try to sensitize * ourselves to some problem that is recognizable from some part of the dreamer's material. Even better, we may try to catch some significant *parallels* between various parts of the material. Often, we do not even succeed in finding a problem. We find only strongly suggestive evidence of a disturbing wish. This is where the classical approach to dream interpretation often ends. For the authors, this is only a beginning.

As already indicated, our next step is to find out why the particular wish that we have found was disturbing to the dreamer. When we have found the dreamer's reactive motive, we have made a good beginning toward finding one of the dreamer's problems. The dreamer's problem is to find a way of reconciling a disturbing wish with the reactive motive to which it has given rise. This problem of reconciliation is a concrete one. It can be understood only in the context of other relevant facts concerning the dreamer's actual emotional situation at the time.

---

* This is close to what Freud (1912) calls "evenly suspended attention." The important point is that we are not looking for some particular problem in which we ourselves are already interested. We are trying to be impartially sensitive to what is emerging in the patient's material. In any case, we should seek the answer, not in loose or stereotyped interpretive habits of our own, but out of the patient's own words.

## SECOND STAGE. ATTEMPTS TO RECONSTRUCT
### THE DREAMER'S ACTUAL THOUGHT PROCESSES

Our next task or series of tasks is to inquire how this problem is related to other parts of the dream and of the associations. In particular, we want to know what precipitating situation has served as a stimulus to activate the disturbing wish. In the end, we shall find ourselves reconstructing, not just one problem, but a constellation of problems. This constellation of intimately related problems is what we call the cognitive structure of the dream. In this cognitive structure, we expect to find one problem on which deeper problems converge and from which more superficial problems radiate. This is the dreamer's focal problem at the moment of dreaming.

To reconstruct the cognitive structure of the dream is the second stage in our interpretive procedure. This task, too, requires empathic identification with the dreamer. As soon as we become involved in this task, we discover that the processes that we are trying to understand are much less rigid than the word "structure" seems to imply. What we are trying to understand is the dreamer's actual thinking, the thinking of which the manifest dream is a temporary end product. Thinking is a dynamic, living process, comparable to the biochemical and physiological processes involved in the growth and functioning of a living organism. It is a much more dynamic process than the building of such a stable "structure" as a house.

When we begin to study practical thinking, we discover that the functional units in this living process are problems, not wishes or fantasies. Wishes are the dynamic stimuli that activate problems. Wish-fulfilling fantasies are attempts— often fleeting attempts—to solve problems. Both wishes and wish-fulfilling fantasies are only parts or phases of a more comprehensive problem-solving effort.

The thought processes underlying dreams differ considerably from one dream to the next. It is impossible to prescribe in advance a rigid procedure for reconstructing them. Putting together a jigsaw puzzle is our best analogy.

In assembling our jigsaw puzzle, we are guided by two working assumptions: (1) The dream work consists of and can be resolved into a series or hierarchy of substitutions of one problem for another; (2) each of these *substitutions* is *intelligibly motivated*.

Our task of reconstruction, accordingly, involves: (1) finding the dreamer's focal problem (focal conflict); (2) finding the derivative problems that lead, by intelligibly motivated substitutions, to various parts of the manifest dream; and (3) tracing the dreamer's focal conflict and his patterns for responding to it to their sources in the dreamer's past.

# PART 2

---

# AN OPERATIONAL APPROACH TO INTER-PRETATION AND THEORY

# CHAPTER VIII

## EMPATHIC UNDERSTANDING
## AND CONCEPTUAL ANALYSIS

### ARTISTIC AND SCIENTIFIC USES OF LANGUAGE

In Chapter I, we called "intuitive" thinking "nonverbal." This statement may have seemed perplexing, since both the patient's dream and our whole discussion of it were expressed in words. What was "nonverbal" was, of course, the meaning expressed by the words. The distinction can be approached from another direction. Words can be used in two ways in order to communicate to others our understanding of what we ourselves or some other person feels. We shall call these the "artistic" and the "scientific" uses of language.

The "artistic" use of language is evocative. A gifted artist can evoke in us a vivid sense of another person's emotional experiences without formulating in direct statements the impressions that he is trying to convey to us. He does not—perhaps he cannot—describe or explain to us what he is trying to say. His words are intended rather to evoke in us an empathic understanding of what the other person is feeling, fantasying, hoping, fearing, and so on. A scientist's ideal is different. His use of language is not evocative, but expository. He tries to define his terms precisely and then to formulate what he has to say in propositions that are either true or false and that can be checked against evidence.*

What we have called "the language of the unconscious" is an evocative language. It differs from the language of the artist only in the fact that its meaning has been disguised by the psychic censor.† When we have once penetrated their masks, dreams (and other seemingly irrational products of the mind) can express a patient's unconscious feelings and thought with a vividness and accuracy that a more technical language cannot even approximate. This kind of communication is what Freud has in mind when he compares the analyst's unconscious to a telephone receiver. The patient cannot describe or explain to the analyst what he is unconsciously feeling or fantasying. Nevertheless, the patient's words are able to evoke in the analyst an empathic sense of what is going on in his unconscious. This evocation in the analyst of feelings and fantasies similar to the patient's own is what Freud thinks of as resonance between the analyst's unconscious and the patient's. This evocative effect of the patient's words makes it possible for the analyst to "understand" the language of the unconscious.

---

* This distinction is an old one, dating back to Bacon, Hobbes, and Locke. In recent years (1942, 1957), Susanne K. Langer has made use of a somewhat similar distinction in her attempts to explain how words are used in poetry. She distinguishes between the "discursive" use of language and the "creative speech" of a poet. Poetry, she says, "is not discourse at all." The poet is not trying to tell us something. He is seeking, rather, to construct an emotionally charged "poetic image" "for his and our imaginative perception."

† This difference is far from absolute, since artists, too, often take delight in disguising their meaning.

### THE DIFFICULT ART OF TRANSLATION

We pointed out in Chapter I that an objectively critical approach to interpretation involves two steps. First, we must understand the language of the unconscious. This we shall call "empathic understanding." The second step is even more difficult. We must translate what we have "understood" into a language suitable for scientific analysis. This we call "conceptual analysis." * This art of translation is indeed a difficult one.

The interpretations in Chapter II were mostly couched in the patient's own words. In this way, without fully realizing what we were doing, we were trying to preserve the evocative (artistic) character of the language of the unconscious. The words that we borrowed from the patient have a precise meaning which we can understand empathically.

We encounter difficulties when we try to define in words just what we have "understood." For example, at the end of Hour 98, the patient characterized his new-found feelings for his wife as "like falling in love all over again—maybe better than the first time." In our interpretation, we concluded that he was unconsciously "in love" with the analyst also. By empathic identification with the patient, we "understood" what he meant by "falling in love." Yet, we cannot define in words what being "in love" meant to him.

We now encounter the essential task involved in "conceptual analysis." Our task is to translate the evocative (artistic) language of the unconscious into a language of carefully defined terms and of propositions that can be tested against evidence. When we try to do this, we run the risk of losing the

---

* This procedure as a whole—"empathic understanding" followed by "conceptual analysis"—we call "interpretive analysis."

vividness and even much of the precision implicit in our intuitive "understanding." A good translation must aim, rather, to preserve the subtle shades of meaning in the "language of the unconscious" and to make them explicit.

The dream that we discussed in Chapter II will serve to illustrate this problem. We have an intuitive sense that we "understand" this dream. We have an even surer feeling that we "understand" the patient's responses in Hour 98. Yet, when we try to formulate it carefully, this sense of "understanding" is strangely elusive.

To point up the difficulty, we ask: What was the focal conflict in this dream? What was the problem that was most intensely cathected? If we were content to use familiar stereotypes, we might formulate the patient's conflict as one between "dependence" and "shame." This formulation is suggested vividly by the patient's analogy of a puppy's love for his master.

Yet, "dependence" is a colorless and vague concept when compared to the impression conveyed by this patient's analogy. The analogy of the puppy is not only more vivid, but also more accurate than the notion of dependence. On the other hand, "the love of a puppy for his master" is only an analogy. What does the patient mean by it? What does a puppy feel when he follows his master around?

### NEED FOR A PRECISE SCIENTIFIC LANGUAGE

When we seriously undertake the task of conceptual analysis, we come upon a disconcerting fact. In psychodynamics, we do not yet have an adequate scientific language. When we try to formulate what we have understood, we are often content to use formulas that are more-or-less current. This proves to be a "Procrustean bed" technique. These formulas are stereotyped and poorly defined. They do not even approximate the sensitive (artistic) precision of which our intuitive understanding of the unconscious is capable.

Our next task is to devise a language that is adequate for the conceptual analysis of our intuitive understanding. In our next few chapters, we shall discuss and illustrate principles that should guide us in such an attempt.

### "DEPENDENCE" AND "SHAME" AS EXAMPLES

We return now to our characterization of the patient's conflict as one between "dependence" and "shame." There are many kinds of dependence. One may be dependent on another person for help or for money, or one may long to be loved or need moral support or reassurance. Can we characterize more accurately the nature of the "dependence" that this patient feels for the analyst?

"Shame" is the name that we have given to the patient's reactive motive. The word "shame" is more vivid and seems to characterize rather adequately many of this patient's reactions to his "dependence." Still, in this case, the word "shame" is not quite accurate, either. In the patient's associations, there are several hints of a reactive motive that does not fit our usual concept of "shame." For example:

(1) "Sometimes people will first give you a medal, then lay the egg"; (2) "being chased" out of the hospital; (3) "Why doesn't he [Jack Benny] help out?"; (4) "One brother should help another." We cannot understand what these dream details have to do with "shame."

"SYMPATHIC RESONANCE" AND FEAR OF ESTRANGEMENT

Let us now re-examine the patient's own words and our analysis of them. We first began to understand the nature of the patient's feelings when we studied the first part of his ninety-eighth hour.

> (The patient talks about a movie he saw Friday, *A Man Called Peter*. He was deeply moved by it. Death seems especially moving. The hero's wife reminded him of his wife. He felt an acute sense of appreciating his wife. He thought of how much he would miss her if she were to die.)
>
> (The patient had tears in his eyes when telling her this. He found it very difficult to tell her. Almost gave it up.)
>
> ANALYST: Why was it so hard?
>
> PATIENT: I don't know. . . . Perhaps I feel that nobody wants to listen to it. . . . Also feel that these things are understood, but not expressed.
>
> This is the first time I've felt it so deeply. I know she felt it too; I could feel her increased heartbeat. [Chuckles.]
>
> Strange that I should feel so deeply moved. It's a new experience for me. [Scratching.]
>
> I was very glad I told her.

When we reread this part of the patient's report, we immediately become aware of the inadequacy of the word "dependence." We are impressed, rather, by two contrasting features of his account. The first is that he was so reluctant to tell his wife of his warm, "appreciative" feelings for her. He "almost gave up" telling her. His "deeply moving" experience occurred after he had overcome his reluctance. Then he and his wife embraced, and he could "feel" her "increased heartbeat." He knew that "she felt it, too." He was very glad he told her.

When the analyst presses his inquiry, he learns something further about the reason for the patient's initial reluctance and also about the "deeply moving" experience that followed.

> PATIENT: I am afraid of not being accepted; for example, by Bertha (a girl whom he had loved before marriage). Afraid I might stick my neck out and find that she didn't care much for me. Hadn't intended to have intercourse, but my telling her what I felt naturally led to it. [The patient is now again talking about his wife.]
> Will this feeling always be so intense? It seemed tremendous; I had goose-pimples, etc.

We can now recognize the essential feature of this experience. Perhaps we should call it "reunion after (overcoming fear of) estrangement." On closer scrutiny, we notice further that the "reunion" of which we speak is only incidentally a physical reunion. Physical reunion is rather an evidence of, a means of recognizing, an emotional reunion. When the patient felt his wife's "increased heartbeat," he "knew" that she was "feeling it, too." We shall give the name of "sympathic resonance" to this kind of emotional reunion.

We now realize again how inadequate the concept of "dependence" is to characterize this emotional experience between the patient and his wife. In order to characterize it properly, we have had to invent a new term, a term that emerges directly and precisely when we sensitize ourselves to the patient's own description of what occurred.

### PARALLELS, CONTRASTS, AND AXIS OF POLARIZATION

Our method of finding and defining a new term is an adaptation of John Stuart Mill's (1843) "joint method of agreement and difference." We shall speak of "parallels" and "contrasts." The patient's telling his wife of his warm, appreciative feelings; his embracing her; and, later, his intercourse with her—all involve reunion with her. In two of these cases, the reunion is a close physical one. Talking involves a less close physical contact. What the three acts all have in common is the achievement of an emotional reunion, to which we now have given the name of "sympathic resonance."

In direct contrast to this goal of sympathic resonance is the patient's fear of estrangement. For our purposes, a "contrast" may be thought of as a "negative parallel." A contrasting element is one that reverses just those features that are common to a number of "parallel" elements. Two contrasting sets of mental contents may be thought of as an "axis of polarization." In these first associations of our patient's ninety-eighth hour, his thoughts and feelings are "polarized" between desire for sympathic resonance and a fear of estrangement from his wife.

### ENLARGEMENT OF THE CIRCLE OF
### SYMPATHIC RESONANCE

We can check the significance of a particular axis of polarization by comparing it to the patient's succeeding associations. In the simplest case, a significant polarization will persist with easily understandable modifications in the thoughts that immediately follow. In our patient's ninety-eighth hour, his

polarization between desire for sympathic resonance with his
wife and fear of estrangement from her is followed by a similar polarization in relation to the analyst.

> ANALYST: Your attitude seems to be that there's some-
> thing wrong about being emotionally excited.
> [After this remark there is a long pause.]
> (Later the patient remarks:) Seems like a long hour
> after telling you what I had done.
> It was hard to tell you. I thought you might think it
> irrelevant or silly. Really childish or like a woman.
> (Then the analyst concludes a long interpretation with
> the comment that he regards the patient's expression of
> feeling as natural and healthy. The patient responds
> gratefully to this encouragement, but also with embar-
> rassment.)
> PATIENT [at door, embarrassed]: It's like falling in love
> all over again . . . maybe better than the first time.

In this sequence of associations, polarization continues to
be between desire for sympathic resonance and fear of estrangement. What is new is that (preconsciously) the analyst
is being drawn into this axis. Evidence of this is the patient's
long pause followed by his confession of reluctance to tell
the analyst; his fear that the analyst might think that what he
had to tell was "irrelevant," "silly," "childish," "like a
woman"; his thrilled feeling of "being in love all over again";
and his embarrassment at telling the analyst about it. In
Chapter II, we recognized that his release of affection for his
wife had been followed by a preconscious intensification of
his admiring affection for the analyst. In other words, the
patient has now drawn the analyst into his circle of sympathic

resonance. As earlier, in the case of his wife, he now fears that his reaching out for sympathic resonance with the analyst will result in his being rejected.

### A NEW AXIS

The fate of this patient's love for the analyst was different, however. In the case of his wife, the patient's fear of being rejected was temporarily quieted when he felt her heart beat and realized that she "felt it, too." In the case of the analyst, he did not permit his love to become conscious. Consequently, he could not overcome his fear of rejection by putting this fear to the test. He could not tell the analyst about his love and thus win the reassurance that the analyst would accept instead of reject him.

Still, there has been a change in the quality of his fear. Instead of being rejected, the patient fears that he will be thought "silly," "childish," "like a woman." At the end of the hour, he is "embarrassed." There has also been a change in the quality of his love. Especially after Hour 98 and in the dream of Hour 100, he and the analyst no longer love each other as equals. The patient's love is like that of a "puppy" for his master, of a little boy for an idealized older brother. Thus, in this period, there has been a fundamental change in the patient's "polarization"—not just a change in object but a change in the nature of his conflict.

### ANALYSIS OF CHANGE IN PATIENT'S CONFLICT

To analyze this change, we return again to Mill's "joint method of agreement and difference." * By this method, we

* French (1952) has called this method "analysis by comparison."

can analyze a complex phenomenon into simpler components. "Being in love" (in the sense that this phrase was used at the end of Hour 98) and the love of a puppy for his master have one feature in common. They both involve sympathic resonance. In another feature, they differ. "Being in love" is love between equals. It involves mutual honor and high evaluation bestowed by each on the other. In the love of a puppy for his master, this kind of equality does not exist. The puppy does not expect to be loved as an equal.

Thus we analyze the patient's feeling of being in love into two components. One component is that which it has in common with a puppy's love—the sense of sympathic resonance between the patient and his wife, between the patient and the analyst. The other component is that in which "being in love" differs from a puppy's love. This other component is mutually high evaluation of each for the other.

By a similar method, we can recognize the patient's embarrassment at the end of Hour 98 as a kind of estrangement. This is the feature that embarrassment and estrangement have in common. The two feelings differ quantitatively. The patient was afraid of complete estrangement from Bertha. His fear of being thought "silly" and "childish" by the analyst involved only a partial estrangement.

By means of this "analysis by comparison," we can now answer a question that recently puzzled us. Earlier in this chapter we were puzzled by hints in the patient's associations (to Dream 100) of a reactive motive that does not fit our usual concept of shame. Two of these hints are: (1) "being chased" out of the hospital; (2) "Why doesn't he [Jack Benny] help out?" and "one brother should help another."

In these passages, total rejection, complete loss of "sympathic resonance," is emerging in a context in which "shame" seems to be the predominant response. Now, by our method of analysis by comparison, we have recognized "embarrassment" as a kind of "estrangement." This parallel resolves the difficulty that puzzled us earlier. The reactive motive that is focal in Dream 100 is fear of estrangement. The shame which we earlier recognized is a mitigated form of this fear of estrangement.*

## ONE ESSENTIAL DIFFERENCE BETWEEN ARTISTIC AND SCIENTIFIC LANGUAGES

The "artistic" and the "scientific" languages differ in structure. When used evocatively, words activate total impressions. In the art of conceptual analysis, we use words analytically. We break down fantasies or even feelings into parts or aspects. Then we use different words to designate each aspect that we have recognized. For example, in Chapter II, we spoke of the patient's "loving overestimation" of the analyst. Neither of these words alone gives us an adequate sense of the patient's feeling for the analyst; each has singled out one aspect of this feeling.

In order to come closer to the impression that the patient's own words have evoked in us, we must put together the two words, "loving" and "overestimation." Even when we have put these words together, we are still far from having reproduced the vivid and precise impression evoked in us by the patient's own phrase, "like falling in love all over again."

* A number of years ago, Gerhart Piers (Piers & Singer, 1953) suggested that shame is closely associated with "fear of abandonment." At the time, the senior author was not able to recognize this relationship. Now, our comparison of this patient's responses to his wife, to Bertha, and to the analyst has led us to recognize just such a parallel as Piers postulated. "Embarrassment" is a mitigated fear of "estrangement," we conclude.

What we try to do is similar to the chemical procedures to which we must resort in order to transport bulky foods in concentrated form. We remove the water from milk and send the milk to its destination in the form of dried powder. Then we try to reconstitute the original milk by mixing the powder with water. Often, the milk thus reconstituted has lost some of the properties of the milk with which we started. It tastes different.

Our procedure is one of analysis and resynthesis. By isolating parts or aspects of total impressions, we are able to study and explicitly formulate the relations between these parts or aspects. This is the advantage we gain by analysis of our empathic understanding.

CHAPTER

IX

## *VALUE OF CONCEPTUAL ANALYSIS*

Conceptual analysis can be used for a number of purposes. One of these is to trace with microscopic precision just what happens dynamically in a sequence of psychoanalytic hours. We can illustrate this procedure in the sequence of hours that we have just been studying. Our analysis of the concepts of love, shame, and estrangement now makes it possible for us to follow intelligently the transformations in the nature of the patient's conflict in the course of two psychoanalytic hours.

First, by analysis of parallels and contrasts, we have been able to recognize sympathic resonance and "mutual appreciation" as two components of "being in love." "Sympathic resonance" we contrast with "estrangement." Then we find a "polarization" between desires for sympathic resonance and fears of estrangement as a common feature, a continuing thread running through both of these interviews (98 and 100). Afterward, recognition of fluctuations in the "mutual-appreciation" component of "being in love" helps us to follow intelligently the patient's successive ways of dealing with this underlying conflict.

ANALYSIS OF THERAPEUTIC PROCESS IN
TWO PSYCHOANALYTIC HOURS

At the end of his ninety-eighth hour, the first change that we note is mitigation of the patient's fear of estrangement from the analyst. As price for this mitigation of his fear of estrangement, he has begun to accept depreciation of the love that he desired. He has had to renounce being loved as an equal. Eventually, he compares his love to that of a puppy for its master.

Then, in the dream, his pride rebels. Rather than accept a depreciated relationship, he will accept estrangement from the analyst. His estrangement first takes an aggressive form. He retaliates by degrading the analyst from a "colonel" to a private. Finally, he attempts a more radical defense. He tries to repudiate love altogether. In his dream, he has substituted the Army and a mess-hall for a really loving relationship. He asks for matter-of-fact satisfaction of physical needs ("just good food") instead of affection. He dreams of the trappings of honor ("serve you like a king, gold plates") instead of the mutual honor and high evaluation that is part of all genuine love.

Unfortunately, such repudiation of love comes close to the complete estrangement that the patient has been fearing. After he has succeeded in debunking love, the underlying conflict becomes intensified. At the end of the dream, his fear emerges plainly in its original form. Brothers no longer love each other. After being "in love," he must be chased out of the hospital.

The dream has, however, found another way of mitigating his sense of rejection. In the dream thoughts, the analyst (Jack Benny's brother) has not rejected him. On the contrary, the estrangement that he dreams of is not between the patient and the analyst but between the analyst and his chief. Both he and the analyst are chased out of the hospital; but he and the analyst remain together in their flight.

This kind of conceptual analysis can be an important first step toward appreciating the full significance of the sequence of events in a psychoanalytic treatment. Only by this kind of microscopic analysis, we believe, will it be ultimately possible to get a really adequate understanding of the therapeutic process.

CHAPTER

X

## AN OPERATIONAL APPROACH

We evaporate the water from milk. Later, we try to reconstitute the original milk by mixing the dried powder with water. This analogy has an important implication for our present purpose. When our purpose is to reconstitute the milk with which we started, we must take care not to mix in extraneous substances. Similarly, a good "interpretive analysis" *will shape itself* without the aid of concepts introduced by the analyst from other sources.

In "interpretive analysis," our basic principle is to build up our scientific concepts directly by analyzing the colorful words and vivid analogies that the patient himself uses to awaken our empathic understanding. The logically articulated system that we seek is already implicit in an unverbalized cognitive structure that underlies all that the patient says and does. Our basic task is to expose this cognitive structure to plain view without destroying it.

In so doing, we must avoid contaminating our picture with

concepts borrowed from current theories or other extraneous sources. If bits of theory are legitimately applicable, we should be able to rediscover them in the material that we are studying. Insofar as our theories are valid, each case will confirm them anew. On the other hand, we must be on our guard against forcing our interpretations to fit preconceived theories, Procrustean-bed fashion. In other words, we are proposing an operational approach to both psychoanalytic interpretation and psychoanalytic theory.

### FREUD'S CONCEPT OF THEORY

With this suggestion in mind, we shall first review briefly Freud's attitudes toward theory. Freud writes:

> We have often heard it maintained that sciences should be built up on clear and sharply defined basic concepts. In actual fact no science, not even the most exact, begins with such definitions.*

In another connection, contrasting science with speculation, Freud emphasizes again that

> . . . a science, erected on empirical interpretation . . . will gladly content itself with nebulous, scarcely imaginable basic concepts, which it hopes to apprehend more clearly in the course of its development, or which it is even prepared to replace by others. For these ideas are not the foundation of science, upon which everything rests: that foundation is observation alone. They are not

---

* Freud (1915), p. 117.

the bottom but the top of the whole structure, and they can be replaced and discarded without damaging it.*

## MISUSE OF THEORY

For our present purpose, we start with this last statement of Freud. Theoretical concepts "are not the foundations of science." We must be ready to replace or modify them whenever such modification is necessary for the understanding of empirical observations. Unfortunately, Freud's admonition is often more honored in the breach than in the observance. The temptation is great to start with theory, usually with a learned discussion of successive changes in Freud's views on a particular subject. When we do turn to empirical observation—if we do so at all—we are set to interpret what we see in terms of what we have already deduced from Freud's views.

We aggravate this error with another one. We love to start our theoretical discussions with just those parts of psychoanalytic theory that are farthest removed from empirical observation. The psychoanalytic theories of the drives, for example, are impossible to check on the basis of work with adult patients. So much has happened in the twenty or more years since a patient's birth that it is impossible to disentangle how much was inherited pattern and how much has been acquired later, either by learning or as a result of disturbance of normal learning by traumatic experiences.

This is one of the most important reasons why, in our own interpretive approach, we recommend starting much closer to the surface. We start with a dreamer's focal conflict, which we try to understand with sensitive empathy and with as little contamination from previously accepted theories as possible.

* Freud (1914), p. 77.

## OUR FIRST OBJECTIVE—
### A TRUSTWORTHY INTERPRETIVE METHOD

For the present, building a system of theoretical concepts is not our primary purpose. We are first concerned with a more circumscribed task. Our task is to devise a trustworthy procedure by which our empathic understanding of a particular patient's behavior can be first checked against the available evidence and then analyzed. Interpreting the behavior of many patients, one at a time, is an essential first step toward building theories with more general validity.

The formulation and checking of interpretations involve two steps. First, we try to formulate in such a way that we, ourselves, can check our conclusions. Then, if possible, we would like to formulate them so that they can be checked by others. In a new science such as ours, there is always danger of attempting the second step in this procedure prematurely, before the first has been thoroughly worked out. First we must develop an interpretive method of which we, ourselves, can be sure. Otherwise, how can we hope to have our conclusions checked by others no more trustworthy than we? In our field in particular, many are impatient to vindicate our science. For this reason, we are tempted to skip the necessary first step of developing a trustworthy interpretive method of our own. We fondly hope to formulate in terms that anybody can understand. We make use of terms that we cannot precisely define (like "oral erotic character," "dependence," "aggression," etc.), terms that anybody can "understand" and define as he will. Then we estimate the probability of our untrustworthy guesses statistically, hoping that we can make them more adequate in this way.

Although we are reluctant to admit it, psychoanalysis has

not yet developed so far that it can be checked in such a mechanical way. The terms that we use are often so vague that it is impossible to check them. "Dependence" and "aggression," for example, are so all-pervasive that it is possible to find them anywhere. We return, accordingly, to what should be our first task—to develop an interpretive method that we, ourselves, can check, one that yields conclusions of which we can be reasonably sure. This is a task that requires more than usual sensitivity for intuitive discernment, refined by practice and self-discipline. We cannot expect others to check our conclusions until they have learned a comparable method.

### DANGER OF BECOMING STEREOTYPED IN OUR THINKING

As already stated (Chapter VIII), our interpretive method involves two steps. The first and crucial step is to understand the language of the unconscious. If the interpreter succeeds in this task of understanding, without contamination from other sources, he discovers that the language of the unconscious is not only vivid, but also has a precision *which we lose* when we try to translate it into a carelessly devised technical language. Our next task is to learn an art of translation that is sensitive to all the nuances of this language of the unconscious.

Our present technical language is not only vague and inaccurate, but is also stereotyped. We see only what we are in the habit of seeing (oral eroticism, oral character, anal eroticism and anal character traits, phallic eroticism and Œdipus complex, guilt, etc.). At its worst, this need to translate our patients' material into stereotyped concepts results in hopeless distortion. In any case, it tends to distract us from the patient's present problems, concerning which our evidence is most adequate. It diverts our interest to stereotyped theories about infantile conflicts for which we usually do not have adequate evidence in the case that we are studying.

Each of us has his characteristic stereotypes and his characteristic blind spots. These stereotypes and blind spots are usually closely associated with the theories that we accept. To counteract these blind spots, we advise the analyst to try to forget his theories while he is interpreting. He should concentrate his attention, rather, on resonating empathically with what is focal in the patient's thoughts. The danger of relapsing into stereotyped thinking is always present. To counteract this danger, we must keep our intuitive imagination always alert and fresh, always sensitive to insights that have not occurred to us before. Theodor Reik's (1937) admonition should be kept constantly in mind: What is most significant in a patient's behavior and associated thoughts usually takes both analyst and patient by surprise.

### AN OPERATIONAL APPROACH TO THEORETICAL CONCEPTS

As already indicated, we are proposing an operational approach, first to psychoanalytic interpretation and then to psychoanalytic theory. We try to use only concepts that we can define in terms of the interpretive procedures by which they were arrived at. This is the only way that we can free ourselves of misleading stereotypes. The "operations" that we use are of two kinds:

*Our initial operations are interpretive.* We make elementary interpretations of promising clues, of clues that are sufficiently simple so that we can be reasonably sure of their meaning. We interpret just those parts of the evidence that we feel most certain that we can grasp intuitively. In other words, our initial operations are elementary intuitive acts, acts of "understanding" language that has been used evocatively.

*Our next operations are also intuitive.* Step by step, we bring other parts of the patient's material into our intuitive picture. From time to time, we also subject this picture or parts of it to intuitive appraisal, trying to sensitize ourselves to gaps and discrepancies in the evidence, as well as to the new perspectives that suddenly arise after our interpretive reconstructions have reached a certain critical point.

This whole system of intuitive operations, taken together, constitutes the phase of "empathic understanding" in our procedure. This is the phase in which we try to understand the language of the unconscious.

Next comes the phase of conceptual analysis. *The operations that belong to this phase are deductive.* They are comparable to the mathematical calculations with which one analyzes and checks "working hypotheses" in other fields (e.g., the careful calculations, based on astronomical observations, which Isaac Newton used to check his gravitational hypothesis). Analyzing out the features that are common to a number of parallel elements is one of the most important of these "mathematical" operations in our "conceptual analysis." In this phase, it is most important that we try to be very strict in our reasoning.

### EXAMPLES OF OUR OPERATIONAL PROCEDURE

We have already given extended illustrations of our operational approach in the phase of empathic understanding. To illustrate the operational principle of the conceptual-analysis phase of our method, we shall first recapitulate how we arrived at and elaborated our concepts of involvement in and commitment to a conflict.

In the dinosaur dream (Hour 5), we noticed that the dreamer was not in a state of panic, as we would expect him to be if he were to vividly imagine himself attacked by the dinosaur. From this we inferred that he was not intensely "involved" in his fear. This inference constituted an operational definition of "involvement." We also noticed that the car was able to back away from the dinosaur. We interpreted this as evidence that the patient was able to diminish his involvement in the dinosaur conflict by withdrawing cathexis. We regarded this as a sign that the patient had begun to be "involved," but was not yet "committed" to the conflict symbolized by the dinosaur. In this inference, we were applying an operational definition of "commitment." Commitment is "involvement" that has become irreversible.

In an operational approach to theoretical concepts, the "principle of parsimony" ("Ockham's razor") is very valuable; we try to clarify our theoretical thinking by reducing it to the simplest possible terms. In particular, we do not permit ourselves to introduce any concepts into our theoretical framework *except such as are necessary to account for all the available and pertinent evidence.*

A good example of this principle is our use of the concepts of "involvement" and "commitment" as basis for an operational definition of a "prophylactic defense." A "prophylactic defense" is one in which defensive substitution of a less disturbing problem occurs *before* the dreamer has become committed to his underlying disturbing problem. This simple definition seems to be all that is necessary to account for a dreamer's being able to avoid being much disturbed by a conflict that is potentially very disturbing.

We distinguish a "prophylactic defense" from a "less successful" defense, in which defensive substitution has occurred *only after* the dreamer has been committed to the underlying conflict. After commitment to a conflict, the dreamer is unable to "wish it away." This is the distinguishing feature that characterizes a "less successful defense."

Of course, the principle of Ockham's razor necessarily gives theoretical thinking a tentative character. A conclusion is good only until new evidence is found to contradict it or to make necessary a further elaboration of it. We must always be alert for new evidence, sensitive to gaps and discrepancies, and ready to modify our theoretical constructs whenever necessary in the light of new evidence. On the other hand, we can also proceed, one step at a time, with a considerable degree of certainty, if we take care to limit ourselves to concepts that we can define operationally and to make use as fully as possible of the evidence actually available at each step. Such a tentative but sure-footed procedure is, in fact, a prerequisite to all sound theoretical thinking. Any procedure that does not have this tentative character is dogma, not science. A procedure that does not try to make systematic use of all available evidence is dogmatic speculation.

# GROUP COLLABORATION IN
# THE INTERPRETIVE PROCESS

We pointed out in Chapter X that the checking of scientific conclusions involves two steps. First, we should develop an interpretive method of which we ourselves can be sure. Until now, we have focused our interest on this first task. Our next task will be to ask how we can get the help of others in checking our interpretations.

Ideally, others can help not only in checking but, much more, in building up our interpretations. We have described how we try to sensitize ourselves to gaps and discrepancies in the evidence. Discrepancies are our best clues for revising and improving our interpretations, for discovering relationships we have not yet suspected. Ideally, this kind of critical scrutiny of our interpretive reasoning can be exercised better by a group of two or more than by a single investigator (interpreter). The thought processes involved in the ever-shifting cognitive structure of a dream are so rich that it is difficult for any one interpreter to catch them all. One investigator will often catch highly significant discrepancies or relationships that another has missed.

In the past twelve years, the authors have made a number of attempts to develop such collaboration. We started with students in seminars on interpretive method. Often, the leader of a group, as well as the others, will at first be at a loss to grasp the meaning of a dream. Then, the group will begin piecing together suggestions offered, first by one and then by another, until finally, often rather suddenly, there emerges a solution that is satisfying to all.

Ideally, in a psychoanalytic interview, analyst and patient can often achieve the same kind of collaboration.* Sometimes an interpretive comment by the analyst will activate fantasies, thoughts, or memories in the patient which unexpectedly "resonate" with what the analyst has said. The patient's new associations may then enable the analyst to elaborate his interpretation further. This kind of interchange may continue for some time. Then, suddenly, the patient says something that does not seem to fit. Such a discrepancy should stimulate both analyst and patient to consider how the interpretation needs to be revised.

Of course, this kind of collaboration of several interpreters is not always successful. Two kinds of difficulties may interfere with successful cooperation. Often a suggested interpretation will be rejected just because it is new, because it runs counter to someone's stereotypes concerning the kind of evidence that is admissible. The answer to such an objection should be to turn back to the patient's material for new evidence, either for or against the interpretation suggested. On

---

* Walter Bonime (1962) has stressed and extensively illustrated the thought that, in psychoanalytic treatment, analyst and patient should cooperate in the interpretation of dreams.

the other hand, the analyst who is offering a possible interpretation may harden his partial or approximate insight prematurely into a proposition to be defended. In this way, he may cause discussion of his suggestion to degenerate into an argument. He will thus destroy the flexibility necessary for impartial examination of gaps and discrepancies.

Such difficulties call attention to the fact that, if collaboration is to be successful, a group of interpreters must first achieve a certain degree of mastery of our objectively critical method. They must also learn how to work together. If these prerequisites can be achieved, then the intuitive imagination and critical scrutiny of a group should be much more creative and trustworthy than that of a single interpreter.

A few samples of discussions between the authors of these essays will illustrate the kind of collaboration which we aim and hope to achieve. The crucial step in our interpretation of the cement dream (Hour 15) resulted from a conversation something like the following:

E.F.: I don't think we should even try to interpret Dream 15. Just "mixing cement" is too little manifest content to do more with than merely speculate.

T.M.F.: Let's not give up that easily. When the patient awoke, he felt as though he really knew exactly how to mix cement. In reality, he says, he does not. He associates that he recently hired someone to tuckpoint his house, i.e., to help him with a problem that he could not solve by himself.

E.F.: There is a parallel here. The patient had this dream just before his fifteenth analytic hour, that is, in the initial stage of his analysis. . . . The hiring of somebody could refer to the analyst whom he has recently "hired" to help him solve his personal problems.

T.M.F.: Correct. But the dream content and the associations must tell us more, namely, what the *specific* problem is with which the patient is preconsciously concerned *right now*.

The patient says that his house recently needed tuckpointing. Let us visualize a house, cement . . . tuckpointing. . . . What is tuckpointing?

E.F.: In tuckpointing, fresh mortar is put between the bricks of a house to keep the bricks from falling apart and the house from crumbling.

T.M.F.: Oh, so the *function* of tuckpointing is to hold the bricks of a house together. . . . A house is a home, a home for a family, a symbol for the family. . . . That's it! The patient's problem may be one of holding his family together.

Our interpretive hypothesis at this point was: The patient must be afraid that his family will fall apart. He wishes to hire the analyst to make the repairs necessary to prevent this.

Such opening of perspective on facts that had seemed incomprehensible is often experienced aesthetically as a sudden illumination. As the authors pointed out in an earlier paper (Fromm & French, 1962), this kind of aesthetic experience is an elementary first step in validating conclusions arrived at intuitively. The confirmatory value of this experience is, of course, greater when it is shared by two or more investigators. Even so, it must be checked. In Chapter IV, we discussed how we proceeded to check this interpretive hypothesis at which we had arrived together.

At one point in our discussion of the beautiful-mansion dream, there was a discrepancy that needed to be resolved.

We were agreed that the sudden transformation of the neighbor's house into a beautiful mansion symbolized the patient's hopes of what might happen as a result of therapy: he hoped that, as a result of therapy, his family might become an ideally loving and harmonious one. At this point, E.F. continued to be impressed, as previously, with the aspiration for social status that seemed to be implied by the "beautiful mansion, like a governor's house with fine lawns," etc. The governor's house, in particular, seemed to imply a longing for social status far beyond anything that the patient could realistically hope for. On the other hand, T.M.F. could not see how such an aspiration for social status could fit into the context of the longing for a loving and harmonious family, which both E.F. and T.M.F. had recognized.

We have already discussed in a footnote how this difficulty could be resolved. This discrepancy could be brought into relation with another one which had caused T.M.F. some discomfort. It had seemed to T.M.F. that the dream had succeeded much too easily in wishing away the patient's distressing sense of being unable to hold his family together. Then it occurred to him that the extravagant unreality of this dream fantasy was itself a clue. This impossible overcompensatory fantasy was giving expression to a (preconscious) realization that what the patient was wishing was indeed impossible. Then E.F. was struck by the fact that the dream fantasy of the patient's beautiful cure did not even mention the analyst. Together the authors arrived at the conclusion that the patient's impossible wish-fulfilling fantasy was one of being cured without the analyst's help.

This dialogue between the authors also illustrates another important fact—the fact that two discrepancies are often easier

to resolve than one. The clue for the solution of one discrepancy is often contained in another.

Finally, another discrepancy had long continued to baffle
both authors. The first association to the dream of the beautiful mansion concerned a radio announcement that the Governor of Iowa had been killed. We were both unable to guess
how this fact could fit into the context of the patient's distress
about betraying to the analyst his inability to hold his family
together. Then, a clue was supplied by several students in a
seminar led by E.F. Perhaps the patient wished for the death
of the analyst in order to rid himself of the need to tell the
analyst about his disturbing conflict.

To this suggestion, T.M.F. suggested a slight emendation.
Perhaps the Governor represented not only the analyst but,
even more, the patient's own ego ideal, his own demand that he
be an ideal husband and father, able to hold his family together. In the dream thoughts, we suggest, this demand has
been symbolized by the Governor of Iowa and attributed to
the analyst. If he could be rid of these ideal figures and of his
own exacting ideal for himself, then he would not need to be
so distressed by the realization of his inadequacy as a family
man.

The last two of these examples, especially, illustrate the
fact that interpretation is a creative art that is never finished.
Even the best interpretation can be improved and refined as
we take into account one bit of evidence after another, the
significance of which had previously escaped us. We approach
a really sensitive empathic grasp of a dream or of other behavior only by successive and never-ending approximations.

# PART 3

---

# PSYCHOLOGY OF DREAMING

CHAPTER

XII

QUESTIONS CONCERNING THE
DEVELOPMENT OF THINKING

Our operational approach to dream interpretation leads us
next to questions of how dreaming is related to the thought
processes underlying rational behavior in waking life. The
thought processes in dreams are usually regarded as regressive, "primitive." This is the implication of Freud's phrase,
"the primary process." The assumption is that "primary-
process thinking" is an earlier stage in the development of
rational, "secondary-process," thinking. This assumption dis-
torts the actual facts concerning the development of thought
processes. Verbal thinking is a specialized refinement of nonverbal thinking. It is more adequate for certain purposes, in
particular, for the communication of thought to others and for
generalization made possible by abstraction. On the other
hand, nonverbal thinking also undergoes development and
continues to be much superior for the practical understanding of other people.

Careful examination of the actual evolution of thought
processes reveals the fact that thinking develops, not along one

single line (Hypothesis 1; see Figure XII-1), but along at least three or four diverging lines (Hypothesis 2; see Figure XII-2).

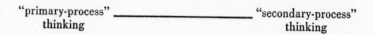

"primary-process"                                           "secondary-process"
thinking                                                    thinking

FIGURE XII-1

For our present purpose, it is important to distinguish between thinking that is not dependent on the understanding of language and thinking that is organized on linguistic patterns. The first of these we call "practical thinking," or "practical problem-solving." The second may be designated as "verbal," "syntactical," or "propositional" thinking.

In our next few chapters, we shall review some of the facts, known from other sources, on which the above statements are based.

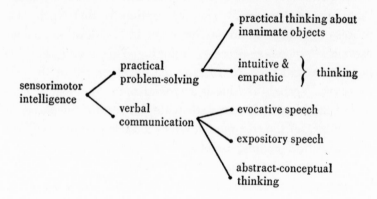

FIGURE XII-2

# CHAPTER XIII

## PRACTICAL THINKING AND VERBAL THINKING

### Practical Thinking

Practical thinking may be about inanimate objects, or it may be about people, about interpersonal relations.

#### PRACTICAL THINKING ABOUT INANIMATE OBJECTS

*Sensorimotor Intelligence.* Practical thinking about inanimate objects begins with what Piaget calls "sensorimotor intelligence." According to Piaget (1936), the acquisition of such sensorimotor intelligence culminates around the infant's eighteenth month in an ability to grasp spatial relationships in the range of his immediate perception and to manipulate objects purposefully and inventively within that range.

*"Signs and Symbols."* A decisive step occurs when the infant acquires the capacity to "evoke absent objects" in memory or imagination. Thereafter, the very young child becomes capable of recognizing objects actually perceived as "in-

dexes," or "signals," of objects not yet present to his senses. "For the hunter," Piaget (1947, p. 124) says, "tracks in the snow are an index of game, and for the infant the visible end of an almost completely hidden object is an index of its presence."

Piaget (1945) distinguishes such "indexes" or "signals" from "symbols," which the child, in symbolic play, can use to represent objects or persons who are either not present to the child's perception or at least not subject to the child's control. As an example, Piaget (1947) cites "a child, playing at eating," by whom "a pebble representing a sweet is consciously recognized as that which symbolizes, and the sweet as that which is symbolized." Such "symbols" enable the child to give to his fantasies a kind of imaginative external reality (French, 1952, Ch. XLIX). By using real objects to represent the persons or objects in his fantasies, he makes his fantasied objects seem more real.

It seems probable to the authors that what we have called the "substitution of analogous problems" in the dream thoughts dates, in part, from this period in the child's intellectual development.

*Understanding of Space, Time, Causality. Mechanical Sense.* From this point on, the child's intellectual development becomes closely intertwined with the development of his capacity to use language. Piaget (1937), in particular, has made extensive studies of the development of the child's concepts of space, time, and causality. His studies show that the child begins to make practical use of such concepts in the first half of his second year, at a time when speech could have contributed little if anything to his acquiring them.

One important variety of practical intelligence concerning inanimate objects is "mechanical sense." In some individuals, mechanical sense is developed in high degree, but is not accompanied by much capacity on the part of the same individual to explain in words what he is doing. This fact would seem to prove that such persons have acquired their mechanical sense and mechanical skills without much help from words.

From our patients, we rarely hear dreams that are really struggling with mechanical problems. Our patient's cement dream (Hour 15) is only an apparent exception, since in this dream he was not really preoccupied with mixing cement, but, rather, with a problem in interpersonal adaptation for which this mechanical problem had been substituted. In our clinical experience, it is at least rare to find a dream that has helped the dreamer discover anything about a mechanical problem that he did not know before. Yet, Kekule's famous dream that registered his discovery of the benzene ring (Chemistry Society, 1958) seems to prove that such a thing is possible. In our clinical experience (with adults), some dreams also seem to reflect discoveries (correct or incorrect) that the patient made as a child in the course of his investigations concerning the anatomical and physiological relations between the sexes. These, for the child, are often conceived as mechanical problems.

### PRACTICAL UNDERSTANDING OF PEOPLE

*Intuitive Understanding and Empathic Understanding.* The beginnings of practical understanding of other people's behavior probably occur very early. By watching his mother, even the infant learns, step by step, to anticipate what she will do next and, in particular, how she will respond to his own acts. He soon learns to be guided in his own behavior by what he expects his mother's reactions to be. Sometimes, he is even able to manipulate the mother by provoking responses that he (consciously or unconsciously) desires. It is not long before the young child is able to read, not only the mother's conscious intentions, but also impulses and emotional attitudes which she may not have intended to betray. Step by step, such signs become for the child the language of the mother's unconscious. This kind of practical intelligence we shall call, in accordance with common usage, "intuitive understanding." Step by step, the child acquires such intuitive understanding, not only of the mother, but of other persons in his environment as well.

Later, when the child begins to acquire an understanding of speech, his capacity for intuitive understanding also continues to expand. Long before the child has learned to talk, he is sensitive to the tones of the mother's voice. While he is slowly learning the factual or intellectual meaning of words, a speaker's intonation, her manner of speaking, and accompanying gestures continue to be just so many more signs, revealing—wittingly or unwittingly—the speaker's emotional attitudes. Also, many words have an emotional, rather than an intellectual, meaning (e.g., "good boy," "naughty"). Thus, while the child is slowly piecing together an understanding of expository language, he is also continuing to pick up an intuitive understanding of the evocative language of his parents and others.

We have been describing a first step in the development of intuitive understanding. After a time, this first step is supplemented by another one, by the development of "empathic understanding." By "empathic understanding," we mean understanding another person's feelings and behavior by identifying * with him, by imagining ourselves in his situation and motivated to act as he does. In order to perform this imaginative act of identification, we must make use of the same cues from the other person's behavior that made possible our more direct "intuitive understanding." When we understand another person's behavior empathically, we supplement our observation of the other person with knowledge of how we might behave under similar circumstances. In this way, we are often able to refine our intuitive understanding.

Thus, empathic understanding, like the more elementary "direct intuitive understanding," is essentially nonverbal. It is communicated most subtly and accurately without words, by intonations, gestures, and emotional language, rather than by the expository meaning of words. Indeed, as we know, it is often possible to understand empathically that what another person is really feeling is very different from what he says he

---

\* In the psychoanalytic literature, there are many subtle variations and attempts to make precise distinctions in the use of the concepts "empathy" and "identification."

In the case of empathy, Edoardo Weiss (1960, Ch. XXXI), in particular, has distinguished carefully between "empathy," "sympathy," "pity," and "compassion." These distinctions are important and valuable, but they go beyond what is necessary for our present discussion. Our present purpose is to try to understand in the simplest possible terms the underlying mechanism which makes it possible for one person to sense (correctly or incorrectly) what another person is feeling. This we call "empathic understanding." "Empathy," "sympathy," "pity," and "compassion," as defined by Weiss, involve differing ways of reacting to such "empathic understanding."

The concept of "identification" is sometimes restricted to a more-or-less permanent taking over of the attitudes and emotional orientations of another person in the process of character formation. What we have in mind in the present discussion is something more elementary and usually more transient than this. We are interested just now in the "act of identification" that makes possible "empathic understanding." This act we have tried to define precisely as "imagining ourselves in the other person's situation and motivated to act as he does." To distinguish this concept from other uses of the word "identification," we call it an "imaginative act of identification."

feels. This is, of course, the kind of understanding on which our psychoanalytic interpretive art is based.

*Learning to Imitate—a First Step toward Empathic Understanding.* The essential problem in trying to understand the development of empathy is to trace how the child comes to attribute to other people feelings similar to his own. This process is easiest to trace in the infant's learning to imitate the physical movements of others. In learning to imitate, two steps seem to be involved. First, the infant spends a great deal of time looking at his own hands and feet and other parts of his body while he moves them. In this way, he acquires a close association between what it looks like and what it feels like (kinesthetically) to make a certain movement (of hand or fingers, for example). It would probably be more accurate to speak of a fusion or condensation of what it looks like and what it feels like into a single (nonverbal) concept of a certain movement. Once such a concept has been acquired, the infant is ready for a next step. Another person's hand and arm, for example, look like the infant's own. Consequently, it is easy for the infant next to identify his own arm and hand with the arm and hand of another person. (Such identification may be so complete, indeed, that the child does not discriminate between another person's hand and his own. See Page 142, *infra.*) Once this identification has been achieved, the infant becomes capable of imitating with his own hand and arm an act which he sees another person perform with the same organs.

Piaget (1945) has studied this process in great detail through the first year and a half of the infant's life. Imitation "does not depend on an instinctive or hereditary technique," he says. "The child learns to imitate." He traces six stages in this learning process, corresponding to the six stages which he has described in the development of sensorimotor intelligence. The first acts that the infant imitates are those *that he can already perform spontaneously*. Such acts he imitates sporadically as early as his second month. At seven or eight months (Stage 3), he becomes capable of imitating such acts systematically, but *only when the act performed is visible to him*. Not until his ninth or tenth month (Stage 4) does he learn to imitate movements (such as opening and closing his mouth, for example) which he has already performed spontaneously but which he cannot see himself make.

For the purpose of our inquiry, this feat of imitating acts which the infant cannot see himself make is of particular interest because it is what we have called "an imaginative act of identification" with another person. Actually, this feat is somewhat difficult to learn. The infant must at first grope about in order to find the act that corresponds to the one that he is trying to imitate. For example, one of Piaget's children, at the age of eight and a half months, responded to her mother's opening and closing her mouth by biting her own lips. It was not until two months later that she learned to respond by opening and closing her own mouth. Piaget cites many such examples. Similar gropings occur (during Stage 5) while the child is learning to imitate new movements, i.e., movements which the child, herself, has never made before. For example, when his daughter was fourteen months old, Piaget struck his abdomen. The little girl responded by hitting first the table and then her own knees. It was only two months later that she responded immediately by hitting her own stomach.

These examples show plainly that the essential step in learning to imitate is learning to identify parts of the child's own body with corresponding parts of another person's body. In fact, numerous observations on children of one and a half to two years of age seem to indicate that the child often does not distinguish clearly between parts of his own body and the corresponding parts of another person's body. A child will sometimes try to feed another child of the same age or younger, for example. At this age, careful observers (Freud & Burlingham, 1943) insist, this is not usually an act of generosity on the child's part. It is based, rather, on identification with the other child (i.e., identification of the other child's mouth with his own).

It now seems reasonable to assume that continuation of the same kind of learning process is what later makes it possible for a child to identify his subjective feelings with those of another person. Thus, we can reconstruct a picture of the cognitive process that culminates in a child's becoming able to "imagine himself in the same situation as another person and motivated to act as the other person is doing."

*Development of Empathic Understanding—a Hypothesis.* We do not yet know what motivates this cognitive process. How does the child develop a *desire* to understand another person empathically? From this point of view, few, if any, studies have been reported on the development of empathy.* We shall, accordingly, try to fill in this gap by a hypothesis based on clinical observations.

In Chapter VIII, we found evidence of what we called "sympathic resonance." In his ninety-eighth hour, our patient told of having achieved, for a short time, a sense of oneness with

* In the psychological literature, interest in empathic understanding is just beginning. S. J. Beck (1963) hopes that analysis of Rorschach data will give us a new approach to the study of empathy or, better, "sympathy," in its original Greek sense of "feeling with" another person.

his wife. After telling her of his "acute sense of appreciating" her, he had embraced her. Feeling her increased heartbeat, he then "knew that she was feeling it, too." We decided to call this sense of emotional reunion "sympathic resonance." In the patient's ninety-eighth hour, such sympathic resonance was achieved and given expression in a number of ways— first, by evocative speech: he told his wife of his feelings and evoked similar feelings in her. Then his sympathic resonance found expression in an embrace—"two hearts beating as one" —and then (he says "naturally") in sexual union. Finally, at the end of the hour, he described it as "like falling in love all over again." In Hour 98, the patient's desire for sympathic resonance was one side of a conflict. The whole hour was "polarized" between his longing for sympathic resonance and his fear of losing it, his fear of estrangement.

One of the patient's presenting symptoms was neuroderma-titis. From psychoanalytic studies of patients suffering from bronchial asthma, neurodermatitis, or both,\* we have found that *conflicts* † *centering on* a need for *sympathic resonance* are characteristic of the emotional background of both these diseases. Starting with these tentative observations, we suggest a hypothesis something like the following: Before birth and for periods of varying length for some time afterward, there exists between mother and infant a relationship which

---

\* See French and Alexander (1941). In these studies, the term "sympathic resonance" was not used, but it was implied in the importance which was attached to "fear of estrangement."

† In order to avoid possible misunderstanding, we call attention to the words underlined in this sentence. What is particularly characteristic of patients with asthma and neurodermatitis is, we believe, not a capacity for sympathic res-onance, but rather a *conflict* between desires for sympathic resonance and fears of estrangement. A capacity for sympathic resonance is, of course, much more widely distributed in the general population, but the conflicts of asthmatics and neurodermatitis patients help to isolate this phenomenon for observation.

Benedek (1949) calls "symbiosis." It is best illustrated by the normal relationship, as analyzed by Benedek, Spitz, and other observers, between the mother and the nursing infant. According to these authors, this relationship is by no means a one-sided one. It is an exceedingly sensitive interaction between mother and infant which is highly satisfying to both. In order to anticipate its relationship to later developments, we shall call it "primary resonance."

Of course, such primary resonance cannot be continuous, even in earliest infancy. When the mother leaves him, the baby follows her with his eyes, listens to her in the next room, and later creeps or toddles after her, longing to continue his primary resonance with her. During periods of primary resonance, the infant possesses little, if any, individuality of his own. He is part of a "mother–child unit." As the child's own individuality begins to develop, it necessarily interferes with his primary resonance with the mother. Especially in his second and third years of life, the child struggles to assert his own individuality, by saying "no" to every suggestion, for example.

Still, from time to time, he is eager to regain his sense of resonance with the mother, later with the father and other adults if possible, and still later with other children. By subtle signs, he may give evidence of desires to have his mother participate in his delight in interesting sights. Or he may demand that she or his father participate in his active play, join him in "ridin' a horse," for example. What is often depreciated by adults as "merely a desire for attention" is often a longing to have the adults who watch him participate emotionally in the activities that he enjoys so much. Primary resonance, when regained temporarily after it has been lost, we call "sympathic resonance."

Often, desires for sympathic resonance may take the form of cravings for physical contact. Much of the delight of being cuddled, for example, probably comes from the sense of being, once again, "one with" the mother. This is probably the reason for the close association, in our patients, between neurodermatitis and frustrated longings for sympathic resonance.

In asthmatic patients, the longing for sympathic resonance takes other forms. An impulse to cry in these patients is usually in response to fear of estrangement. Fear of estrangement is fear of loss of sympathic resonance. If crying is suppressed, asthmatic wheezing results. Talking is another way of gaining or regaining sympathic resonance with a mother figure. This is particularly clear when the patient confesses impulses which he fears might offend the mother. If the mother will accept his confession, sympathic resonance is restored. If fear that the mother will reject his confession is too great, the confession is suppressed, and asthmatic wheezing again results. In adult life, probably the most complete sympathic resonance of which two people are capable is in the normal act of coitus.*

*Empathic Understanding and Empathic Grasp of Interpersonal Situations.* Sympathic resonance is not yet "empathic understanding." In order to account for a capacity for empathic understanding, there is still another step to explain. We must postulate a split in the ego † of the person who under-

---

* It is of interest that, in our patient's ninety-eighth hour, talking, bodily contact (physical embrace), and sexual intercourse were all utilized as means of achieving or giving expression to sympathic resonance.

† This "split in the ego" is something that we recognize introspectively whenever we reflect consciously on the phenomenon of empathy. It is probably implicit in everyone's concept of both empathic understanding and introspective

stands. With one part of his ego, he remains in sympathic resonance with the person who is understood. The other part of his ego, remaining detached, "understands" by observing the part of his own ego that is in sympathic resonance with the observed person.

Empathic understanding is not always limited to understanding one other person. It is also possible, at least to some degree, to understand two other persons at the same time. While watching a movie in which there are two actors, for example, one may identify predominantly with one of the characters. Usually there is also some degree of empathic understanding of the other character. If so, the observer has succeeded in achieving "empathic grasp" of an interpersonal situation.

---

insight. In the following discussion, we are trying to make this implicit concept explicit.

Such analyses of the concepts of empathy and introspection have, of course, been made before. One of the earliest and most significant was the thesis of the philosopher George Herbert Mead (1934) that the concept of "the self" has a social origin, arising when a human being first begins to be conscious of his own behavior and to see himself as others see him. In the psychoanalytic literature, Sterba attributed the corrective influence of the analyst in psychoanalytic therapy to his making possible a "dissociation" in the patient's ego. By interpreting the transference situation, Sterba (1934) points out, the analyst tries to help the patient dissociate an observing part of his ego which can then focus on understanding the other part of his ego that is directly involved in the patient's emotional responses in the transference. Fliess (1942) later attempted a similar analysis of the analyst's empathic understanding of the patient's transference responses. The analyst first identifies with the patient, he says, then "projects the [patient's] striving, after he has tasted it, back onto the patient." In a more recent article, Christine Olden (1953) characterizes empathy as "an interchange of the emotional experience of feeling as the object does and an intellectual process of observing, judging, understanding."

Finally, Paul Federn (1952) and Edoardo Weiss (1950, 1960) have developed much further than we have the study of interactions between various "ego states" in empathic understanding and introspective insight, as well as in many pathological conditions.

We have postulated that empathic understanding of one other person involves a functional splitting of the ego into two parts. Following this hypothesis, we would have to postulate a three-way splitting of the ego to account for empathic grasp of an interpersonal situation involving two persons. For example, a child may see two persons struggling with each other or in some kind of sexual embrace. With the detached, observing part of his ego, he sees what they are doing to each other. His "understanding" of the scene, however, may go much further than just looking. He also participates in the scene with his imagination, as though he were one or both actors. We say that he identifies with one or both of the actors. To explain the thought processes involved in such acts of identification, we assume that, in the observer's imagination, a part of his ego gets into sympathic resonance with one of the actors. If there is double identification, two parts of the observer's ego get into sympathic resonance, one with each of the actors. Then the detached, observing part of the ego projects these feelings of sympathic resonance back into the observed scene and experiences them as the feelings of the two observed persons, respectively.

Empathic grasp of an interpersonal situation is sometimes possible, though much more difficult, when the observer himself is also one of the actors. In such a case, also, a three-way split of the ego is necessary. Let us suppose, for example, that the observer, O, is trying to understand objectively his own emotional interaction with another person, A. Then, to achieve objectivity, the observer's ego must be functionally split into an observing part, an emotionally reacting part, and a third part which is in sympathic resonance with A. The observing part of O's ego must then achieve an adequate degree of detachment from the emotionally reacting part of his own ego, as well as from that part of his ego which is in sympathic resonance with A.

*Practical Utilization of Empathic Understanding.* Empathic understanding is only occasionally an end in itself. Occasionally, empathic understanding of another person or of a personal relationship is an important source of aesthetic pleasure, as in the enjoyment of a play or of a novel, for example. More frequently, empathic understanding is utilized as a guide in efforts to achieve other purposes. In psychoanalytic therapy, it is essential as a guide for our therapeutic efforts. It is equally important as a guide for a wise parent or for a statesman and, generally, for anyone who is responsible for the welfare of another person or of a group, large or small.

An ability to understand the motivations of other people can also be used for more utilitarian purposes. For example, a salesman is usually more successful if he understands the needs of his prospective customers and how they are likely to react to his sales approach. In other situations, a man may use his empathic understanding of other people to manipulate or exploit them. On the other hand, a sensitive appreciation of the feelings of others plays an important role in seduction, in courtship, in love, or in the tactful handling of social situations.

*Empathic Understanding and Introspective Insight.* According to the hypothesis just outlined, empathic understanding of another person involves three steps. First, in the observer's imagination, the observer's ego must get into sympathic resonance with the observed person. This is an act of imaginative identification. Second, there follows an act of introspection. The observer's ego splits into an observing and an observed part, with the observed part remaining in sympathic resonance with the observed person. In the third step, the observing part of the observer's ego, remaining detached, projects these feelings of sympathic resonance back into his picture of the observed person, experiencing them as the feelings of the observed person.

From this analysis, we learn that there is a close structural similarity between empathic understanding of another person and introspective insight into one's own feelings. Both involve a split in the ego. Introspection is much the simpler process. In introspective insight, only one step is involved: the ego is functionally split into an observing part and an emotionally reacting part that is observed. In empathic understanding, the act of introspection is only one of three steps. It has been preceded by an act of imaginative identification and followed by an act of projection. In empathic understanding, what is introspectively observed is not the ego's own immediate emotional response, but its sympathic resonance with another person. After it has been introspectively recognized, this response, based on sympathic resonance, has been projected back into the observer's picture of the other person.

Empathic understanding of another person and introspective insight into one's own feelings also differ quantitatively. In introspective insight, the feelings that one recognizes in oneself may be rather intense. In empathic understanding, on the other hand, identification with the other person should be only a token identification, just intense enough to permit the observing part of the ego to sense the quality of the other person's feelings. If identification is too intense, it impairs the necessary degree of detachment of the observing part of the ego. The observing part of the ego becomes too much of a participant, to the impairment of its role as observer. As a result, the objectivity of the observer's understanding suffers.

*The Role Structure of Empathic Thinking.* In dreams, we can often recognize patterns of introspective insight with particular clarity. Even more frequently, we encounter pathological patterns intermediate between introspective insight and empathic understanding of other persons. A few examples will suffice to illustrate possible variations on the basic pattern common to introspective insight and empathic understanding.

A dreamer will sometimes say: "I was in this dream in two roles. In one role, I was only an observer. I was also in the dream as another person who was doing so and so."

Another variation on a pattern of introspective insight is a dreamer who dreams of a certain actual person, X, but also subjectively feels this person, X, to be himself. If translated into words, this insight would be, "My feelings are like those of X."

In still another case, the dreamer's own feelings would again be projected into X, but this time X would not be recognized as the observer himself. In this case, the feelings would be attributed rather to the real person, X (perhaps incorrectly). Thus, this time the result would be a distortion of reality, what in waking life we would call a pathological projection.

All three of these patterns, as well as the pattern of empathic understanding of other persons, are variations on the same pattern of ego organization. The feature common to all these variations is the understanding of personal relations in terms of a role structure. A role structure is like the plot of a play, the roles of which can be taken interchangeably by various actors. From the age of three or four on, many children spend a great deal of time in role-giving and role-taking play.

Such play probably contributes greatly to the progressive expansion of their capacity to think in terms of role structure. Thinking in terms of role structure is what we call "empathic thinking." In empathic thinking, role structures, undergoing change and being substituted one for another, become the units of more complexly organized fantasy or thinking.

*Difficulties in Studying Empathic Thinking.*   We tend to underestimate the importance of empathic thinking in everyday life. According to our definition, any thought processes which involve attempts to understand other people by identifying with them should be recognized as empathic thinking. Any thinking which tries to understand or to fantasy interpersonal situations in terms of role structure is empathic thinking.

Empathic thinking is practical thinking, interested primarily in influencing interpersonal situations, rather than in being communicated to others. It has no necessary connection with language. When it does use speech, it prefers evocative speech, calculated to influence the behavior of others directly by arousing desired feelings in them. It uses expository (propositional) speech only secondarily, if at all. When one thinks empathically, he senses that explanations are futile unless the hearer is emotionally predisposed to listen to them.

It is easy to understand why empathic thinking is often taken for granted instead of being made a subject of serious study. Empathic thinking is unobtrusive and evanescent. If we succeed in understanding another person well enough for our practical purposes, we need not retain in memory how we arrived at our correct conclusions. We seem to have "understood" by a kind of mystical "intuition." For this very reason, scientists sometimes dismiss empathic thinking as not being thinking at all.

We should, of course, abandon the notion that "intuition" and empathic understanding are something mysterious. On the contrary, a person's conscious fantasies or errors and slips in his thinking or in his overt behavior often give us clues for the reconstruction of the steps in his empathic thinking. The utilization of such clues is, of course, the basis of our art of psychoanalytic interpretation, as well as of the methods proposed in these studies for refining and checking our interpretive art.

*Role-giving Play, Empathic Fantasy, and Empathic Thinking.* The role-giving and role-taking play of children is often particularly transparent for the purpose of reconstructing the steps in empathic thinking. In the symbolic play of very young children, inanimate objects are substituted freely in the roles of persons or animals. In genuine role-giving play, roles are given to imaginary or real persons whose imagined motives and feelings are lived out empathically with more or less intensity. We may call this kind of play "empathic fantasy." In its purest form, empathic fantasy is dominated by a wish-fulfilling tendency. It seeks to modify real interpersonal situations in the direction of fulfillment of the wishes of one or more of the participants.

In other play of this kind, the real difficulties in the way of wish-fulfillment are given more or less recognition. With increasing recognition of real difficulties, empathic fantasy is increasingly transformed into efforts to find solutions for interpersonal problems. When thus transformed, empathic fantasy increasingly approximates "empathic thinking."

*The Structure of Empathic Thinking.* The interpretive method that we have outlined in the preceding pages has been especially designed to reconstruct the continually changing and developing cognitive structures of empathic thinking. As we have pointed out, the functional units in practical thinking are problems. Wishes are the dynamic stimuli that activate problems. Wish-fulfilling fantasies are attempts—often only fleeting attempts—to solve problems.

The problems which become focal for empathic fantasy and empathic thinking arise out of interpersonal situations. An interpersonal situation that has been (more or less) understood empathically gives rise to a wish to change it. This wish finds temporary fulfillment in a wish-fulfilling fantasy. Then the difficulties in the way of wish-fulfillment demand attention, and empathic thinking becomes a search for possible solutions to the resulting problem.

Thus, both empathic fantasy and empathic thinking involve substitutions, often a series or hierarchy of substitutions of interpersonal situations, one for another. Our thesis is that these substitutions are always motivated, always in the direction of wish-fulfillment. In empathic fantasy, a desired interpersonal situation will be substituted for a painful or less desirable one. In the defensive substitutions of the dream work, a less disturbing problem is substituted for a more disturbing one.

*Interchange of Roles in a Role Structure.* Interchange of roles in a role structure is one of the most frequent patterns of substitution in empathic thinking. This kind of substitution plays an important part in character formation. The structure of the personality, as analyzed by Freud (1923) is based on this kind of interchange of roles. Both the superego and important parts of the ego, at least, are built up by identification with the parents and others. The ego or superego has taken over a role formerly played by the parent. Then, in dreams, the superego or parts of the ego or of the id * may be projected back into the external world and perceived again as persons. The superego may become a policeman or some other person in authority. Some part of the id may be recognized as a criminal.

An example of interchange of roles in the defensive structure of a dream is our patient's use of the puppy analogy in the gold-plate dream. In the thoughts underlying this dream, the patient has given an inverted picture of his own feelings toward the analyst by describing how "the Colonel" followed him around like a puppy. Such reversal of roles in an interpersonal situation should not be regarded as a distortion, but rather as a normal wish-fulfilling mechanism in empathic fantasy. In this case, the patient's intense longing for sympathic resonance with the analyst embarrasses him and even threatens him with fear of being rejected. By reversing roles, he has relieved himself temporarily of his embarrassment and fear.

*The Use of Analogy in Empathic Thinking.* Another kind of substitution in empathic thinking is more radical. The whole pattern of a problem in interpersonal adaptation may be replaced by an analogous problem. Empathic thinking uses analogy freely, both in its attempts to grasp its problems cognitively and in its search for solutions to its problems. For example, in the cement dream, the notion of "hiring" the analyst to help with the patient's family problem was suggested by his having "hired someone" to do his tuckpointing for him. In the dinosaur dream, a trip in an automobile into unknown territory has been substituted as a venture analogous

* Edoardo Weiss (1950, 1960) would say, "egotized parts of the id."

to committing himself to undertaking the analysis (whose dangers are even more mysterious). Often, the analogies utilized by the dream work do much to enhance for us the vividness of our understanding of a dreamer's conflict. For example, in the beautiful-mansion dream, the mother-in-law's criticisms together with the patient's description of the first year of his marriage give us a much more vivid picture than we could otherwise have, both of the critical attitude that the patient expects from the analyst and of the distress that he himself will experience if he allows his conflict about his family to be exposed in his treatment.

Such dependence on analogy for delineating problems and arriving at solutions is an important consequence of the fact that empathic thinking is practical thinking, focused on concrete, practical problems. Practical thinking lacks the capacity for formal generalization which is made possible in conceptual thinking by words. Reasoning by analogy is a rudimentary substitute for the generalization that might have been made possible by words. In practical thinking, such reasoning by analogy may give an exceedingly vivid understanding of the essential nature of a problem to be solved.

### Verbal Thinking

Verbal thinking is thinking in words and sentences. We often regard thinking and talking as identical. Talking to oneself is "thinking out loud," or thinking may take the form of talking to oneself silently.

This notion that thinking and talking are identical is an illusion. Words and sentences have meaning. Somewhere in the background of all verbal thinking is a nonverbal meaning. At the most elementary level, concrete particular things or events, which are perceived or intuitively understood, are described or explained in words. This is descriptive or expository speech.

Language has two main contributions to make to thinking. (1) It puts thoughts in a form that can be communicated to others. (2) It makes abstract, conceptual thinking possible. These two contributions of language to thinking are closely related. To make clear their relations, we shall consider three stages in the development of verbal thinking.

### INTELLECTUAL MASTERY BY MEANS OF SPEECH

Very early in the child's learning of words, naming an object serves the purpose of intellectual mastery. A young child can often be observed naming objects that he is playing with and talking (to himself) about what he is doing, even when he does not know that anyone is watching or listening to him.

Even in naming objects, the very young child is making a first step toward concept formation. One of the first concepts that he acquires is that of the constancy of objects. An object has many appearances, depending on its position, from what distance and from what direction it is seen, whether it is at rest or moving, and so forth. Very early, the child begins to learn that it is the same object even though its appearance keeps changing. He begins to discover for himself a world of real objects that have a continuity of existence beneath their changing appearances. The first beginnings of this process occur before the child has learned to use words. Then, giving a name to an object greatly facilitates recognizing the object as the same the next time it is seen. Even more, it facilitates the process of distinguishing one object from another by giving the two objects different names.

Later, sentences can be used to register an understanding of relationships or even to master what might otherwise have been a disturbing experience. For example, a two and one-half-year-old boy had just been excluded from his father's consultation room with the explanation, "Daddy is busy." After this, he kept repeating, "Daddy is busy, Joe." (He had recognized that his father was busy with a patient, whom the little boy called "Joe." "Joe" was the grocery boy, whose name had become a class name for all other males except "Daddy.") By focusing his interest on repeating his father's explanation, the little boy was protecting himself from what might have otherwise been experienced as rejection by his "Daddy."

### COMMUNICATION BY MEANS OF SPEECH

Communication is the most obvious function of language. For purposes of communication, perceptions, insights, fantasies, and the like are formulated in words or sentences. That which is designated (named) by a word or described or formulated by a sentence is its "meaning."

In evaluating descriptive language, it is important to distinguish what is being communicated. For example, a father had pointed out a woodpecker to his little boy. He had explained that the bird had received its name because it pecks at the tree. A little later, the boy called out, "See, Daddy, there is another tree-knocker." In this case what had been communicated to the little boy was the (nonverbal) meaning of the word "woodpecker." In another case, if the little boy had repeated exactly the word, "woodpecker," it would be clear that what had been communicated was the word. (In this latter case, whether the meaning of the word had also been conveyed to him would not yet be clear.) Similarly, if a mechanical operation is described and the hearer is then able to perform the operation, this proves that the meaning of the instructions has been understood. Whether the hearer has been able to remember the exact words of the instructions may be unimportant. In such a case, the thinking that has been communicated is practical, mechanical thinking. Words have been used only as a device to communicate the speaker's mechanical thinking.

In descriptive language, for purposes of communication, the meaning of a sentence has usually been subjected to analysis and resynthesis. Consider the sentence, "John is running." Let us compare this sentence to a moving picture of the scene described. In the moving picture, a single act is shown. It would be impossible to find a single word to describe this act to someone else. So, in the sentence, making use of the concept of object constancy, the single act has been analyzed into an object and its appearance. Then the two words have been put together as the subject and predicate of a sentence. The two words have been fitted, each into its place, into the syntactical structure of a sentence.

It is of interest now to note that, in the picture, there is nothing to correspond to either of the two words of the sentence alone. There is no John who is not running, no one running except John. The two words in this sentence have each abstracted one feature of the observed scene. There are also features in the picture that have been left unmentioned in the sentence—how John is dressed, for example.

Even more important is the fact that the syntactical structure of the sentence has no point-to-point relationship with the event being described. The structure of the visually perceived event has been changed by formulating or translating it into a sentence. This is the most characteristic feature of verbal thinking; it has been given a syntactical structure of its own that is not derived wholly from what is being described or explained. This syntactical structure is based in large part on a system of conceptual analysis prescribed by the language being spoken.*

On the other hand, the syntactical structure of descriptive speech does come closer to reproducing the role structure of empathic understanding. Consider the sentence, "John loves Mary." In this sentence, no one of the three words alone corresponds to anything in our empathic understanding of the relationship between John and Mary. There is no John who does not love, no Mary who is not loved, no loving except that uniting John and Mary. Still, there is a correspondence be-

---

* This dependence of the logical structure of thinking on the syntactical structure of the language spoken has been beautifully demonstrated by Benjamin Lee Whorf (1941) by comparisons of similar thoughts as expressed in English and in American Indian languages (Shawnee or Nootka), respectively. To illustrate Whorf's thesis, we quote one of his examples:

" 'I push his head back' and 'I drop it in water and it floats,' " he writes, "though very dissimilar sentences in English, are similar in Shawnee." "I push his head back" is, in Shawnee, "ni-kwaskwi-tepe-n-a." "I drop it in water and it floats" is "ni-kwask-ho-to." In these two sentences, the common root, "ni-kwask," means "a condition of force and reaction, pressure back, recoil." "Tepe-n-a" identifies this action and reaction as one between head and hand. "Ho-to" refers the action and reaction to the surface of water interacting with something inanimate.

"The point of view of linguistic relativity changes Mr. Everyman's dictum," Whorf concludes. "Instead of saying, 'Sentences are unlike because they tell about unlike facts,' he now reasons: 'Facts are unlike to speakers whose language background provides for unlike formulation of them.' "

Another way of stating Whorf's concept might be: "The differing syntactical structures of two languages will make a speaker sensitive to one kind of relationships in one case, to another set of relationships in the other case, in describing the same events." Thus, in the example just given, a person who speaks Shawnee is sensitive to recognize "a condition of force and reaction, pressure back, recoil." One who speaks only English does not notice this state of dynamic interaction. The speaker of English, therefore, describes the two acts in words that pay no attention to their essential similarity.

tween the syntactical structure of this sentence and our empathic understanding of its meaning. The word "loves" might be compared to a (very short) one-act play. There are two roles in the dramatis personae. In this particular performance, these roles have been assigned to John and Mary. The syntactical structure of the sentence, when analyzed in this way, does correspond rather accurately to the role structure of the relationship between John and Mary.

It is important, further, to recognize that communication by means of speech usually involves not syntactical thinking alone, but, rather, an integration of verbal and empathic thinking. We have already discussed (in Chapter VIII) the close relation between empathic thinking and evocative speech. Even in descriptive or expository speech, moreover, what is to be communicated must first be adapted to the hearer's understanding. In other words, the speaker must identify in his imagination with the listener in order to make sure that what he is saying is intelligible. In composing what he has to say, the speaker must be guided by empathic understanding of the hearer. The need for this kind of empathic understanding becomes obvious when it is lacking. For example, when a little boy tries to tell a story that he has seen in a movie, he tells the incidents in the story in whatever order they may occur to him. He does not realize that, in order for the hearer to understand each incident, he must usually have some idea of what has happened before.

### ABSTRACT, CONCEPTUAL THINKING

The detachment of thinking from direct perception and its dependence on the syntactical structure of the language become much greater in abstract, conceptual thinking. In abstract, conceptual thinking, the meanings of words are defined, not by reference to the immediate data of perception, but in terms of other verbal concepts. In this way, the concepts of abstract, conceptual thinking are two or more steps removed from the immediate data of perception. For example, kinetic energy is defined as equal to one-half the product of the mass of a moving object multiplied by the square of its velocity. In other words, kinetic energy cannot be directly measured, but is defined in terms of two verbal concepts, mass and velocity, which can be directly measured. Mass is measured (roughly) by the weight of the object, and velocity, by measuring the distance traversed in a unit of time. Thus, the concept of kinetic energy is two steps removed from data of direct observation. By thus building up conceptual systems that are two or more steps removed from the data of immediate perception, abstract, conceptual thinking is able to arrive at broad generalizations whose validity could not be recognized by direct observation.

Psychologists, other scientists, and philosophers rightly regard this as a momentous step in the development of thinking. It is the step that made possible, first, such practical disciplines as arithmetic; later, many differing philosophies; and, finally, the widely ramifying conceptual structure of modern science. In the study of human relationships, we have attempted to do something similar, though much less successfully. Our empathic understanding of one another's behavior is often not good enough to serve as a trustworthy guide for our relations to other people. So we keep trying to devise abstract concepts, ethical and legal, to standardize behavior. It is much easier to predict what we or another person should do according to accepted ethical rules (not to steal, for example) than it would be to guess what we or he would do if there were no rules.

On the other hand, the very fact that the acquisition of a capacity for abstract thinking has been such a momentous step in the development of civilization is probably the main reason for a widespread tendency to undervalue the thinking of which dreams, neurotic symptoms, psychotic delusions, poetry, and religious inspiration are some of the end products. Our analysis of verbal thinking now begins to give us an inkling as to why, at first, the thought processes involved in dreaming seem so illogical. The logic that we miss in the dream work is the syntactical logic of speech—the *syntactical logic* that is essential for the framing and testing of propositions and reasoning from them. Speech was designed primarily for communication. When we dream, we are not particularly interested in communicating our thoughts to others or in reasoning from propositions.* Therefore, we can dispense with syntactical logic. What is present in the dream work, on the other hand, is a practical, empathic understanding of interpersonal relations. This kind of understanding does not need syntactical logic.

* When a person seems to be dreaming about abstract propositions, there is usually a highly personal concrete problem close by, in the background.

# CHAPTER
# XIV

## THE DREAM WORK FROM
## A NEW POINT OF VIEW

### Three Parts of the Dream Work

We have proposed the thesis that the really significant thought
processes in the dream work involve practical (usually empathic) thinking, rather than verbal thinking. When reconstructed carefully, we said, the impression grows on us that
the thought processes underlying dreaming have a much
greater similarity to the thought processes underlying rational
waking behavior than they often seem to have.

We contrasted this impression with Freud's description of
the "primary process." We concluded that the difference between Freud's concept and our own must be a result of differences between Freud's way and our way of studying the dream
work. We tried to sketch these differences. In particular, we
called attention to the fact that Freud reconstructs the dream
work by tracing chains of association, whereas we believe that
all concrete practical thinking is in terms of total *Gestalten*, in
terms of "practical grasp" of concrete problems to be solved.
Still, we are puzzled to explain why tracing chains of associa-

tion yields a different picture of the dreamer's thought processes than does our method. The answer that we suspect is that these two methods are focused on different parts of the dream work.

### EVIDENCE FOR FREUD'S CONCEPT OF THE DREAMER'S THOUGHT PROCESSES

Let us now re-examine the evidence on which Freud based his concept of the dreamer's thought processes. Freud's first and basic discovery was the wish-fulfilling function of dreams (1900, Chs. II-III). Then, in order to account for the distortion in dreams, he introduced a distinction between the latent dream thoughts and the manifest dream (1900, Ch. IV). The process by which the latent dream thoughts are converted into the manifest dream is the dream work. Later (1900, Ch. VI), Freud devoted himself with great thoroughness to reconstruction of the dream work by tracing the chains of association that lead from the latent dream thoughts to the manifest dream.

From the beginning, Freud insisted over and over that dreams are not nonsense. This was Freud's basic discovery— dreams have sense and meaning, similar to and continuous with the wishes and thoughts of everyday life. In particular, the latent dream thoughts make logical sense. Only the chains of association that lead from the latent dream thoughts to the manifest dream seem to give evidence of displacement of energy without regard for reality or logical relations.

Freud's explanation of these facts was the one with which we are familiar—that the dream work successively involves two kinds of thought process. The latent dream thoughts, with which the dream work started, are the products of logical and reality-oriented thought processes, which Freud called the secondary process. In the next phase of the dream work, however, these logical and sensible thoughts had been subjected to another kind of thought process. This was the primary process, which seemed to involve "free and massive displacement of energy from one psychic element to another, guided only by the pleasure principle, along any available associative pathway, without regard for reality or logic." Freud thought of these two ways of thinking as the characteristic features of different systems of the mind. Thinking in the systems Cs and Pcs (conscious and preconscious) was secondary-process thinking, whereas primary-process thinking was characteristic of the system Ucs (the unconscious). In Freud's analysis of the dream work, the latent dream thoughts were preconscious, secondary-process thoughts. In the course of the dream work, these preconscious thoughts had been "drawn down into the unconscious" and elaborated according to the primary process.

### TWO APPROACHES TO INTERPRETATION

Instead of this classical explanation, the authors suggest an alternative explanation of the same facts. Our starting point is the distinction between empathic thinking and verbal thinking that we discussed in Chapter XIII.

When we carefully study Freud's many samples of dream analysis, we find that he has two ways of listening to the dreamer's free associations. Part of the time, he is listening to catch the meaning that is hidden behind the dreamer's words. He is "listening with the third ear," as Theodor Reik calls it. In Freud's own words, which we have already quoted, he is using his own unconscious as a receptive organ to resonate to the patient's unconscious. At other moments, Freud is interested in the words themselves, rather than in their meaning. He is trying to analyze how the dreamer's words and verbally expressed thoughts are linked together. His aim is to trace the chains of associations that lead from the latent dream thoughts to the manifest dream.

What interests us now is that, when he listens for the meaning of the dreamer's words, Freud finds that the dreamer's thoughts make sense. He discovers the latent dream thoughts, which make sense, and, underlying these latent dream thoughts, he discovers the wish-fulfilling function of the dream. On the other hand, when he listens primarily to the dreamer's words, he finds that the chains of associations that lead from the latent dream thoughts to the manifest dream do not make sense.

The authors now suggest that Freud's two ways of listening to the dreamer's associations correspond to the two kinds of thinking that we have postulated. "Listening with the third ear" is empathic listening. When the interpreting analyst succeeds in listening empathically, what he hears is the dreamer's empathic fantasy and empathic thinking, which make good sense. On the other hand, when the interpreting analyst concentrates his interest on studying how the dreamer's words are linked together in chains of associations, what he then finds is disintegration products of the dreamer's verbal thinking. *The dreamer's chains of associations,* we believe, *are not the dreamer's actual thought processes.* They are, rather, disintegration products, which have become a mask behind which the really significant empathic thought processes are hidden.

The latent dream thoughts are the link between the dreamer's empathic thinking and his verbal thinking. They are expressed in words, but, like all verbal thoughts, they have a nonverbal meaning. They are the product of the dreamer's empathic fantasy and empathic thinking, concerned with the dreamer's wishes and emotions. Then this empathic thinking has been translated into words. In the dream work, the resulting verbally expressed thoughts have undergone disintegration, involving *destruction of their syntactical structure*. The result is what seems to be a free displacement of energy without regard for reality or syntactical logic.

### A COMPOSITE PICTURE

We shall now try to build up a composite picture showing how these two parts of the dream work fit into each other. Figure XIV-1 is a much oversimplified diagram of our concept of the part of the dream work that can best be understood empathically. We shall call this Part A of the dream work. It is the part of the dream work in which empathic fantasy and empathic thinking are predominant.

In this diagram, we have divided Part A of the dream work into two parts, centering on the dreamer's focal conflict. Part $A^1$ is the historical background of the dream, represented in the diagram by lines leading upward and converging on the dreamer's focal conflict. In Part $A^2$ of the diagram, we have represented the empathic thought processes in which the dreamer is trying to find a solution for his focal conflict. These problem-solving efforts are represented in the diagram by lines leading upward from the dreamer's focal conflict to the various parts of the manifest dream.

In Chapter XV, we shall discuss Part $A^1$, the relation of a dream to its historical background. We shall discuss this part of the dream work only briefly.* A more complete discussion

* For a more extended discussion of the historical background of dreams, see French (1953).

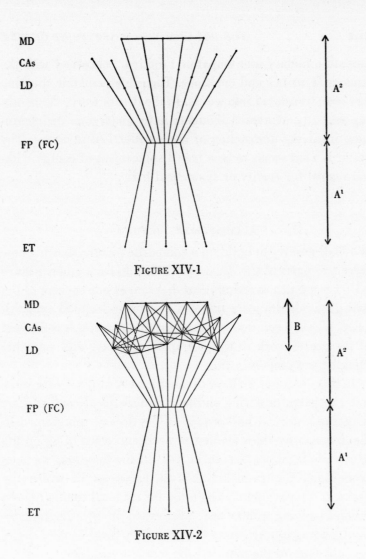

FIGURE XIV-1

FIGURE XIV-2

MD = manifest dream
LD = latent dream thoughts
CAs = conscious associations
FP = focal problem
FC = focal conflict

ET = early traumatic conflicts
A¹ = historical background
A² = problem-solving
B = (transverse) secondary chains of association

would require study of many more dreams of one patient than we have yet attempted in these essays.

In our discussion thus far, we have been principally interested in Part $A^2$. On its way upward, this part of the dream work has activated emotionally charged fantasies and memories, each of which was a different attempt at solution of the dreamer's focal conflict. These fantasies and memories are the really significant steps in the dreamer's search for a solution to his problem. (In the dream of the beautiful mansion, for example, such significant fantasies and memories are: the dreamer's unhappy memories of the first year of his marriage in his mother-in-law's home, his memory of rescuing the lady next door when she had locked herself out, his fantasy of suddenly achieving harmony in his family as a result of his treatment, and the like.) In reconstructing this part of the dream work, we trace these significant memories and fantasies upward into the manifest dream. (For example, in the manifest dream, the mother-in-law's criticisms of the patient as a husband become her criticisms of the neighbor's lawn. His fantasy of suddenly achieving harmony in his family becomes the sudden transformation of the neighbor's house into a beautiful mansion, and so on.) In this way, we trace the dreamer's actual problem-solving efforts in the dream thoughts.

We shall now turn to that part of the dream work that is concerned with the fate of the dreamer's preconscious verbal thinking. We shall call this Part B of the dream work. In Figure XIV-2, we have tried to make a composite diagram of how Parts $A^2$ and B fit together in the dream work. When we trace chains of associations, we find chains that cut transversely across the vertical lines of Part $A^2$. These are verbal chains of association that have established secondary connections between the nonverbal memory and fantasy images which are the significant steps in the empathic problem-solving thinking of Part $A^2$. These secondary transverse chains of association constitute Part B of the dream work.

They are these transverse secondary chains of Part B that give an impression of free displacement of energy without regard for reality or logic.* What is the functional significance of these secondary associative connections? This question requires further study. In many dreams, at least, careful study reveals the fact that the displacement of energy from one psychic element to another is not automatic and mechanical, but deliberately playful. The authors have the impression that such secondary associative chains are produced most prolifically by dreamers adept in verbal thinking and fond of playing with words. In *The Interpretation of Dreams* (1900), Freud has devoted a special section to absurd dreams. Many of his examples show that absurdity in the manifest dream or in the dream thoughts is willful, intended as ridicule of some person or of some train of thought in accordance with the

---

* It may be of interest also to distinguish between a Part $B^1$ and a Part $B^2$ in the dream work. In the dreams that our patients tell us, it is of interest to distinguish between the manifest dream and the dream text. Before the manifest dream can be reported, it must be translated into words. This involves translation of the visual or other imagery of the manifest dream into descriptive language.

We may now distinguish between a Part $B^1$ of the dream work, which contributes directly to the manifest dream, and another part, $B^2$, which we discover by study of the descriptive language of the dream text and of the associated trains of thought.

Description of the manifest dream is only the most superficial meaning of the dream text. The dream text and the associated verbal dream thoughts also find ways of alluding to all levels of the empathic thinking that has shaped the manifest dream. Language is incomparably rich in possible associative links between words and between verbal thoughts. Consequently, the dream text and the associated dream thoughts furnish an enormously fertile field for the kind of play with words and ideas that constitutes what we call Part B of the dream work.

dreamer's wish. We shall return to this Part B of the dream work after a short theoretical discussion.

### Varying Degrees of Commitment in Practical Thinking

In Chapter X, we described an operational procedure by which we try to estimate the degree of a dreamer's commitment to a conflict. Making use of this concept, we can improve our understanding of both Part $A^2$ and Part B of the dream work by a preliminary consideration of fluctuations in a person's degree of commitment to his practical problem. Efforts to find a solution for a practical problem may be playful or serious or may involve intense preoccupation with an excessive and insoluble conflict. We shall next discuss these three degrees of commitment to a practical problem.

#### PLAYFUL FANTASY AND EARNEST PURPOSE

In its purest form, daydreaming is playful. It is dominated by a wish-fulfilling tendency and does not take seriously difficulties in the way of wish-fulfillment. Yet play often becomes earnest. Children may take their play very seriously, and stubbornly resist any attempt to interrupt it. Fantasy is often contrasted with reality-adjusted behavior. Yet fantasy plays an important part in all but the most routine forms of rational behavior. Perception of external reality is only one pole of the thought processes underlying rational behavior. The other pole is fantasy. The contribution of fantasy is of course greatest in the more imaginative and creative forms of rational behavior.

Daydreaming grades into making plans. When we begin to take our daydreams seriously, they become tentative plans.

Rational, purposive behavior involves first an exploratory phase and then an executive phase. In the executive phase, one already has a plan. He thinks that he knows how to solve his problem and is trying to carry out his plan. Suppose that a person does not yet have a satisfactory plan for achieving his purpose or that he does not even have a definite purpose. Perhaps he has only a dim sense of a problem to be solved. In such a case, the executive phase of problem-solving must be preceded by an exploratory phase.

### REGULATION OF COMMITMENT. DANGER OF BECOMING INVOLVED IN EXCESSIVE CONFLICT

While a person is only exploring his problem, it is desirable that he not let himself become too involved in it. At first, he should only play tentatively at planning. Suppose he lets himself be committed to one plan too soon. Suppose then that his plan turns out badly. His efforts to carry it out end in failure or in other disturbing consequences. In such a case, he will be frustrated.* His reactions to frustration will seriously interfere with his search for a better plan.

In order to forestall frustration, it is better not to let oneself become committed to any plan until one is sure of it. One tries out one plan after another. At an earlier stage of exploration, one may play with the task of understanding the problem. One may puzzle first over one part of the problem, then over another part, until he finally arrives at an understanding of the whole.

Unfortunately, it is not always possible to regulate judiciously the degree of one's commitment. Sometimes a person may become prematurely committed to an excessively disturb-

---

* This follows from the fact that commitment to a purpose is, by our definition, irreversible involvement in it.

ing problem. There are three possible kinds of reaction to commitment to an excessively intense conflict:

A person may continue to struggle desperately in some disorganized way to understand his insoluble problem and find a practical solution to it. His frustration will, of course, continue and will result in panic or in an acute confusional state.

As defenses against being overwhelmed by the full intensity of his disturbing problem, he may try to protect himself from full commitment to this problem by substituting analogous but easier problems. In this way, he may or may not succeed in forestalling the development of overt neurotic or psychotic symptoms.

A third possible kind of reaction is to try desperately to abandon commitment to the insoluble problem. One tries to make play of his conflict and of serious attempts to find a solution for it. A commitment cannot, of course (by our definition), be abandoned. The result will be a kind of humor with an undercurrent of frustration and bitterness. One of the purest examples of this kind of "flight of ideas" is a manic psychosis.

### The Nature of Dreaming

#### DIFFERENCES BETWEEN DREAMING AND RATIONAL WAKING BEHAVIOR

By paying close attention to fluctuations in the nature and degree of a dreamer's commitment to his focal problem, it is possible to get a much better picture of the part played by the integrative function of the dreamer's ego in dreaming.

We shall turn back first to the part of the dream work, $A^2$, that is most concerned with practical problem-solving. (See Figure XIV-1.) Just now, we are interested in the differences

between the thought processes in this part of the dream work
and the empathic thinking underlying rational behavior. These
differences can be reduced to two. (1) The dreamer is sleeping and wishes to continue sleeping, and (2) most dreams are
struggling with problems that are too disturbing for the
dreamer to solve. We shall discuss these two differences in
turn.

*The Influence of Sleep.* During sleep, the dreamer has
withdrawn his interest as far as possible from disturbing
stimuli in the real world. He concentrates his attention on
wishing, on dreaming that his wishes are fulfilled. This is
Freud's fundamental formulation—that dreams aim to preserve sleep by representing wishes as fulfilled.

In order to understand the relation between wish-fulfilling
dreams and the empathic thinking underlying rational behavior, we must recall that wish-fulfilling fantasy is not something different from rational behavior. It is one pole, a very
important part of the thought processes underlying rational
behavior. Even dreams are not able to ignore disturbing reality
entirely. Careful analysis of the chronological order of emergence of dream episodes in the manifest dream suggests that
this ability of the dreamer to ignore disturbing reality depends
on the depth of sleep.* Increasingly, as the depth of sleep
diminishes, the dreamer must take account of the fact that his

---

* See French (1952, Sec. VI). The hypothesis is that the state of sleep
"absorbs" or "neutralizes" painful pressures in proportion to its depth. Recently, Rechtschaffen *et al.* (1962) (see also Foulkes, 1962) have reported that
dreams reported from the deepest stage of sleep (Stage 4 in the electroencephalo-
graphic record) resemble ordinary waking thoughts much more than they do the
dreams reported from a lighter stage of sleep (Stage 1 of the electroencephalo-
graphic record). Rechtschaffen's report corresponds to our hypothesis insofar as
our hypothesis, too, postulates that in deep sleep the dreamer's thinking is much
less distorted by excessive affective pressures.

wish-fulfilling fantasies are only unfulfilled wishes. Increasingly, he must struggle with the problems that arise out of his unfulfilled wishes and their possible consequences.

Nevertheless, the emphasis in dreams is on wishing. When the pressure of an unsolved problem or of the need to find a solution for his problem becomes too great, the dreamer must awaken from his sleep.

*Influence of excessive conflict.* In Chapter V, we suggested a somewhat new concept of the function of defenses. Ordinarily, one speaks of a defense against a disturbing drive or impulse. When our purpose is to study the dream work, we get a much more intelligible picture by studying the dreamer's defenses against reactivation of his conflict (French, 1958, Ch. 8, esp. p. 31, n. 2). The best defense that the ego has to protect itself against a disturbing conflict is to delay or prevent the conflict's being activated. If a conflict has already been activated, the ego must try to postpone or forestall becoming further involved in or committed to it. In either case, such delay of further commitment can be achieved only by diverting the dreamer's interest.

We also distinguish between a "prophylactic defense," which diverts a person from a potentially disturbing conflict at a time when it is only slightly activated, and a less successful defense, in which defensive substitution occurs only after there has been considerable commitment to a disturbing conflict.

We shall now make use of these concepts in an attempt to compare and explain the ways in which dreams and waking life, respectively, deal with problems that are too disturbing. In waking life, so long as he remains rational, a person does not let himself become committed to a problem that is too disturbing. If such a problem arises, he quickly turns back to some problem in the real world that is soluble, to some goal in the real world that is achievable. When he sleeps, he does not have this recourse. He has withdrawn his interest from the real world. In other words, in waking life one is able to utilize a soluble problem in external reality as a prophylactic defense. If this prophylactic defense fails, an individual's conflict will be activated, and he will become emotionally disturbed or develop neurotic symptoms. In sleep, it is no longer possible to employ the prophylactic defense of turning away to a soluble problem in the real world.*

The dreamer has another recourse. In deep sleep, he can wish his disturbing problems away. For the moment, at least, he can replace his disturbing problems with wish-fulfilling illusions. This increased capacity for wish-fulfilling illusion has a paradoxical, seductive effect. Just because deep sleep dulls his pain, it allows him for the moment to let himself be preoccupied with what would otherwise be an excessively disturbing problem. When the depth of sleep diminishes, he may discover that he has let himself become too deeply involved in a problem that is too disturbing for him to solve.

This seductive influence of deep sleep explains the relationship between a dream and its precipitating stimulus. The precipitating stimulus of a dream was usually some event of the preceding day that threatened to stir up an excessively disturbing conflict. While he was awake, the dreamer did not allow himself to become preoccupied with this disturbing conflict. He withdrew cathexis from it and busied himself instead with activities oriented toward soluble problems in external reality. Not until he has withdrawn in sleep does this diverting influ-

* Except just at the moment of waking. French (1952, Ch. XLII) has described a mechanism which he called "pseudo-awakening."

ence of activities in the real world cease. Then, after a time, the dreamer begins to let the disturbing conflict emerge. This conflict is masked at first by wish-fulfilling illusions, and its pressure is absorbed by deep sleep. Then, as the depth of sleep diminishes, the disturbing pressures of the conflict emerge progressively until the dreamer is forced to awake and realize that he has only been dreaming. In the meantime, he has tried to turn back to the reality-oriented activities of everyday life. Still he does not awake immediately. For a time he continues to dream.

### COGNITIVE GRASP IN DREAMS

Our next task is to study how the thought processes in dreaming are influenced by this seductive activation of disturbing conflicts and by the progressively diminishing depth of sleep which follows. We just stated that the dreamer often finds himself too deeply involved in a problem that is too disturbing for him to solve. Actually, he often finds himself committed to a problem that he is not even able to grasp cognitively. He seems to have become committed to trying to answer a practical (i.e., nonverbal) question without even knowing what the question is.

At first, this statement sounds paradoxical. How can a dreamer try to solve a problem that he cannot grasp? Fortunately, there is an answer to this paradox. There are various possible ways of achieving cognitive grasp of a problem. Even though the dreamer may not have an adequate detailed understanding, there seems to be always in the background a kind of schematic delineation of his problem as a whole. The interpreting analyst is not the only one who must employ a jigsaw-puzzle technique. The dreamer, too, has often worked at his problem as though it were a jigsaw puzzle. He is able to deal with essential phases of his problem only one at a time. Yet he does repeatedly become aware (preconsciously) of the blank spaces that are yet to be filled in.

For example, in the beautiful-mansion dream, the patient never seemed to lose track of his underlying reluctance to expose his distress about his family to the analyst. Yet this problem never did become manifest. In the manifest dream, he dealt with this problem successively in several ways. In many cases, the dreamer's attempts to solve his jigsaw puzzle have one defect. When he turns to the task of piecing together another part of his puzzle, he often loses track of the part that he has already begun to solve. He seldom succeeds without help in assembling his partial solutions into an adequate understanding of the whole.*

### CREATIVE, IMAGINATIVE, EXPLORATORY THINKING

We begin to get a new insight into the nature of dreaming. Most dreams are groping to understand problems that cannot yet be adequately grasped. This is true both of dreams and of many daydreams. Then there are the problems with which poets, poetic philosophers, and religious seers play—universal human problems; problems whose ultimate solutions must be lived, not only dreamed about; dreams which it may take many centuries to realize, even imperfectly.

### UNSUCCESSFUL REGULATION OF COMMITMENT IN DREAMS

We have already discussed the complications that ensue when one becomes prematurely committed to an excessively disturb-

* The only exceptions are the simple wish-fulfilling dreams of children and occasional "resolution dreams"; but resolution dreams, too, *start* with a problem that the dreamer cannot yet master.

ing conflict. In waking life, the result is neurotic (or psychotic) behavior. In dreams, premature commitment may result in the dreamer's awakening with anxiety. In other cases, the dreamer's too-late attempts to ward off further commitment to a disturbing problem may result in a dream that seems confused and relatively incomprehensible.

We earlier discussed three possible reactions to commitment to an excessively disturbing conflict. The second and the third of these correspond, respectively, to Part $A^2$ and Part B of the dream work.

The dreamer is usually able to protect himself from full commitment to his disturbing conflict by turning away to analogous or related, but less disturbing, problems. For example, in the dinosaur dream, the dreamer focused not on the disturbing problem itself *but on the question of whether to permit further commitment* to his disturbing conflicts to occur. In the cement dream and in the beautiful-mansion dream, he substituted an inanimate house for his family as the object of his conflict. In the beautiful-mansion dream, as already described, he also dealt with various aspects of his problem, one at a time, as in a jigsaw puzzle.

In Part B of the dream work, on the other hand, the dreamer's seemingly free displacements of energy from one psychic element to another can be best understood as attempts of the dreamer to escape from frustration by making play of his conflict. The excessive intensity of the dreamer's conflict would result in any case in diminution of his cognitive span and in the consequent destruction of the syntactical structure of his verbal thinking. The dreamer's ego tries to make this disintegration process harmless by making play of it. Still, one cannot really get rid of frustration in this way. The trend of bitterness underlying the dreamer's ridicule is evidence of the fact that one cannot get rid of a commitment merely by repudiating it.

Such a trend of frustration underlying ridicule is well illustrated by our patient's gold-plate dream (100). In the thoughts underlying this dream, the dreamer is energetically repudiating the idea of being in love with the analyst. He must repudiate love because he bitterly anticipates that revealing his love would be followed, not by loving response, but by rejection. His frustration finds expression in ridiculing the notion that brothers love each other. "Are you related?" he asks Jack Benny's brother. Everybody laughs. Soon afterward in the dream text, he finds it ridiculous that Jack Benny, who has millions, does not help his brother.

If we now turn back to our report of this patient's twelfth hour, we realize that at that time the patient's bitterness about disharmony between brothers was much more intense.

"The whole damn thing is rotten to the core," he blurted out, after relating many instances of hostility between his brothers and in their families. "I don't like all these people from my past," he said. He spoke very harshly, swearing at them—"unpleasant memories of a bunch of related people—a vicious circle. . . . I want it different for my children."

Now, comparing this outburst to his dream in Hour 100, we recognize that, in the dream, he has been able to mitigate his bitterness considerably by humor. Thus, in Part B of the dream work, we get the impression that the dreamer's ego has deliberately chosen to abandon serious thinking and to merely play with words and ideas. This is an example of what Kris (1936, 1950) calls "regression in the service of the ego."

The purpose of such playful repudiation of reality and logic becomes clearer when we take account of its relation to the dreamer's practical thinking. Under the seductive influence of sleep, the dreamer has approached or momentarily achieved (nonverbal) cognitive grasp of his emotional conflict. As the depth of sleep diminishes, his dawning insight proves excessively disturbing. Then he may turn away to analogous but less disturbing problems. If he fails in this, he may next try to repudiate serious thought altogether and to play with the fragments of his previous thinking. If he has turned away soon enough, his play may be really playful. If he has become too intensely committed to his conflict, his frustration will find expression in more or less bitter ridicule of the frustrating situation.

# XV

## COMPARISON OF FREUD'S AND THE AUTHORS' CONCEPTS OF DREAM WORK

An important innovation in the authors' approach to dream interpretation is the way of studying the dreamer's defenses that we have just been expounding. By focusing our interest on the ego's problem of protecting itself against premature commitment to disturbing conflicts, we have brought the dreamer's defenses into much simpler and more intelligible relationship to the problem-solving function of the dreamer's ego.

The primary and essential difference between our concepts and Freud's, however, is our more explicit recognition of a distinction between verbal and empathic thinking. This has led us to a somewhat new terminology whose relation to Freud's terminology needs further clarification. Our most important distinction is between parts A and B of the dream work. Part A is that part of the dream work in which empathic fantasy or empathic thinking (more or less adequate) is dominant. In Part B, we find disintegration products of verbal thinking.

The clearest correspondence between our system and Freud's is between Part B in our system and those latent dream thoughts in the system Pcs which, according to Freud, have been "drawn into the system Ucs" and elaborated according to the primary process. We are not so sure about where our Part A fits, because we are not clear how Freud would classify a number of kinds of empathic fantasy or empathic thinking. For example, how should simple (i.e., undistorted) wish-fulfilling empathic fantasy be classified? Is such fantasy to be regarded as primary-process or secondary-process thinking? And how about the jigsaw-puzzle technique of the beautiful-mansion dream?

### SUGGESTED BREAKDOWN OF THE PRIMARY-PROCESS CONCEPT

In general, Freud has tended to include in the primary-process concept not only the disintegration products of verbal thinking, but all thinking that does not have a syntactical structure. Our chief objection to this expanded primary-process concept is that classing together empathic thinking and the disintegration products of verbal thinking involves gross undervaluation of empathic thinking. Empathic thinking is never irrational. Even those patterns of empathic thinking that are least adequate for solving practical problems have sense and meaning, once we learn how to read them.

A further objection to the expanded primary-process concept is that it satisfies us too easily. When we talk of primary-process thinking, we usually mean little more than strange and unaccountable thinking. By using this term, we remove the stimulus for us to study carefully the many kinds of thought processes that cannot be understood in terms of verbal logic. To clarify our understanding of the dream work, it is helpful to break down the primary-process concept into a number of more precisely defined categories of thinking.

First, we should distinguish between relatively inadequate forms of empathic thinking and the disintegration products of verbal thinking. The disintegration products of verbal thinking do not need further discussion at this point. They do deserve further study.

Of the imperfect forms of empathic thinking, the least inadequate are those that have been successful in postponing activation of and commitment to disturbing problems. Empathic fantasy is the simplest of these, as in playful daydreams and in simple wish-fulfilling dreams. Other dreams succeed in diminishing the dreamer's conflict by substituting an analogous or related, but less disturbing, problem. The thinking in such dreams may be characterized as "empathic thinking with diminished involvement." The dinosaur and cement dreams are good examples. Of these, the cement dream is of particular interest because, behind the mask of a protective symbolism, it succeeded in finding a solution to the dreamer's practical problem of the moment. Dreams that succeed in achieving momentary resolution of the dreamer's focal problem are, in fact, usually the products of "empathic thinking with diminished involvement."

Still other dreams employ a jigsaw-puzzle technique of empathic thinking because the dreamer is unable to span all aspects of his problem at one time. We shall call this kind of thinking "empathic groping." * Our best example is the

---

* We have borrowed the term "groping" from Piaget (1936), who uses it to characterize his fifth stage in the development of sensorimotor intelligence.

beautiful-mansion dream. Still other regressive patterns of empathic thinking involve condensation and splitting of roles in a role structure. These patterns we shall call "condensed empathic thinking."

In Freud's discussion of the dream work, we can distinguish at least two kinds of condensation. Many of Freud's examples involve condensation of words in the dreamer's chains of association. Such condensations, in our system, belong to Part B of the dream work. Another kind of condensation plays a really central part in the empathic fantasy of Part A of the dream work. What we have in mind are condensations of different roles in a single role structure. In Chapter XVII, we shall analyze one example to illustrate the central significance of this kind of condensation in this dreamer's attempt to find a solution to his practical problem.*

Until now, we have concerned ourselves chiefly with the substitutions in the empathic thinking in Part A of the dream work. Our thesis is that every such substitution is intelligibly motivated, that the substitutions in empathic fantasy are always in the direction of wish-fulfillment. The same principle, we believe, also applies to the condensations in Part A of the dream work. In empathic fantasy, condensations, too, are intelligibly motivated. In many cases, such condensations serve an important purpose in the integrative function of the ego.† They make it possible for the dreamer's ego to achieve

---

* See French (1953, Chs. XXXI, XXXIV), in which two similar examples are analyzed.

† The historical background of the dinosaur dream (to be discussed in Chapter XVII) is only one of many possible patterns which involve condensation and splitting of roles in a role structure. This particular pattern of shrinkage of the span of an interpersonal field is one that seems to be particularly characteristic of patients subject to bronchial asthma or neurodermatitis. (The two dreams analyzed by French [1953] were from a case of bronchial asthma.) In other dreams, as one of Freud's (1900, pp. 147–151) examples shows, the con-

a shrinkage of integrative span and thus to adapt its integrative capacity to a conflict that would otherwise be excessive.

---

densation pattern may correspond to the mechanism of hysterical identification. Indeed, it is probable that careful study would show that each neurosis has its own characteristic patterns of condensation and splitting of roles in a role structure.

CHAPTER

# XVI

## THE CAMBIUM LAYER
## OF THE MIND

In our discussion of the dream work in this chapter, our primary emphasis has been on Part $A^2$. One reason for this emphasis is that, until recently, this area has been relatively neglected in psychoanalytic and psychological literature.* An-

* There are, however, a number of notable exceptions. The "autosymbolic" phenomenon, which occurs during the hypnagogic state between waking and sleeping, was early described by Herbert Silberer (1909). This phenomenon should undoubtedly be assigned to what we call Part $A^2$ of the dream work. There were also early studies of daydreaming by Varendonck (1921), which have more recently been discussed by David Rapaport (1951). We have already mentioned Ernst Kris's "On Unconscious Mental Processes" (1950), with special reference to his concept of "regression in the service of the ego." Outstanding are the extended experimental studies of Charles Fisher (1954, 1956, 1957; Fisher & Paul, 1959), following and extending Otto Poetzl's (1917) earlier experiments on the role of subthreshold perception in the dream work. In studies which are broadly based on neurophysiological as well as psychoanalytic and other data, Lawrence S. Kubie (1953a, 1953b, 1958) has also been greatly impressed with the importance of what he calls "preconscious" thought processes. He has called attention to the enormous number of perceptions, many of them subthreshold perceptions, that are spanned by preconscious thought processes, and he is impressed by the tremendous speed and efficiency of these thought processes in problem-solving. He also attributes artistic creativity to this kind of thinking. In view of the latter fact,

other is that we, as well as others, are beginning to realize the great importance of this part of the dream work for our understanding of the integrative function of the ego.

Just under the bark of a tree, is a layer of cells which botanists call the cambium layer. This cambium layer is the actively growing area in the tree trunk. Above, it lays down ever-new and replaceable layers of protective bark. Below, the cambium layer keeps building up new rings of wood.

Somewhat similar to the cambium layer of a tree trunk is the focal-problem level of the mind. This is the level where active growth, problem-solving, and learning all take place, probably the only level that is directly accessible to therapeutic influence. Above, this living, growing level of the mind keeps generating new attempts at solution for problems that arise. Below, it solidifies into the more stable structures of a healthy ego or into the rigid patterns of a neurotic ego.

Such is the picture that begins to emerge when we resolutely try to abandon stereotypes in our psychoanalytic interpretations and to keep our intuitive imagination always alert and sensitive to what is focal in a patient's thinking.

---

it is clear that the empathic thinking that we call Part A[2] of the dream work would be included by him in his concept of the preconscious system. Calvin S. Hall (1947, 1953) has emphasized that, in the dream, the ego attempts to solve a current conflict. Walter Bonime's recent book (1962) also deals, almost exclusively, with what we call Part A[2] of the dream work. Finally, Edward S. Tauber and Maurice R. Green (1962) have surveyed from many angles the work that has been done in this field.

# CHAPTER

# XVII

## FRAGMENTS OF
## A HISTORICAL ANALYSIS

From a re-examination of the first dream analyzed by Freud in the light of other events known about Freud's life, Erik H. Erikson (1954) * has reconstructed a series of "crises" in the dreamer's past—crises which have presumably been of central importance in the dreamer's ego development. This reconstruction corresponds to what we have called the "historical background" of a dream. French (1953) has also utilized analysis of latent dream thoughts to reconstruct nuclear problems from the dreamer's past. Our basic assumptions are that the dreamer's focal conflict is a derivative of one or more nuclear conflicts from his past and that the successive steps in the dreamer's attempts to find a solution to his focal conflict are based on a hierarchy of successive attempts in the dreamer's past to find solutions to these nuclear conflicts. This

* Erikson's method of dream analysis has since been elaborated by Richard M. Jones (1962). The features in which Erikson's and Jones's methods differ from ours are not important for our present purposes.

hierarchy of problems and attempts at problem solution is what we call the "historical background" of a dream.

A good technique for making such a reconstruction is to compare the focal conflicts of a number of the patient's most significant dreams and to study how these dreams fit into what we can learn directly from his conscious memories and from his emotional responses in the course of treatment.

The four dreams that we have studied in these essays are a rather small sample on which to base such a historical reconstruction. Nevertheless, they will suffice to illustrate our method. One great advantage of historical reconstructions is that they can be repeatedly checked, revised, and expanded as long as the patient continues to bring new material or, indeed, as long as there continues to be material in the patient's record that has not yet been adequately exploited for interpretive purposes.

## A CONFLICT CENTERING ON MOTHER'S PREGNANCY
### WITH YOUNGER BROTHER

For the purpose of historical reconstruction, we often get valuable hints from dream symbolism.* We shall start with the dinosaur dream of Hour 5. Two sets of symbols in this dream seem promising.

In the universal symbolism, a cave is often a symbol of the mother's body. The "huge animal" in the dream might be the father standing guard over the mother, but we do not yet find anything further to confirm such an interpretation. Another set of symbols suggests another possibility. We count the number

* Symbol interpretation is a method that is easy to misuse. We should remember that a symbol gives us only a hint for a working hypothesis. This working hypothesis should be elaborated and then checked against other evidence.

of people riding in the car. They are five—the patient, the business associate and his wife, and another couple. The dinosaur makes six. The patient was the fifth of six children.* At the time of dreaming, the patient's wife was pregnant.

The fact that the patient's wife is pregnant suggests a probable precipitating stimulus for a dream about a cave. The fact that the dinosaur is a prehistoric animal suggests that the wife's pregnancy has begun to reactivate a historical conflict concerning the mother's pregnancy. Since there was only one sibling younger than the patient, the pregnancy involved must have been the one with his youngest brother.

We get an unexpected suggestive confirmation of this hypothesis when we discover that the number of people in the car with the patient corresponds to the number of his older siblings. In the dream, the five older siblings are investigating the dinosaur in possession of the cave, which, according to our hypothesis, corresponds to the mother's pregnancy with the youngest brother. All this implies, not phallic competition with the father, but envy of the unborn child inside the mother's body.

### ELABORATION OF THIS WORKING HYPOTHESIS

The chief difficulty with this interpretation is the huge size of the animal. We shall skip this difficulty for the present and return to it later. We next inquire how this historical interpretation fits our earlier interpretation of this dream.

The focal conflict in the dinosaur dream was fear of be-

---

* In a surprisingly large number of cases, the number of persons in a dream and the relations between them reflect the number of and the relations between the siblings in the dreamer's family or the number of persons in some other equally significant constellation from the dreamer's early life.

ginning analysis, fear of free association and of the conflicts that might be reactivated by free association. Just what conflicts the patient feared we were not able to guess at the time —except that the "huge animal" of which he was afraid was a prehistoric animal. Our study of the dream symbolism now suggests that the patient is thinking of the investigation of his unconscious which he is planning to make, in his analysis, as though it were a reliving of his and his older siblings' investigations of the mother's pregnancy with his youngest brother in his early childhood.

This hypothesis receives some confirmation later in the hour when the patient identifies the analyst with his next-older brother. Other associations to the dream also seem to identify the analyst with the business associate, who is one of the four other persons in the car with the patient. In other words, according to our interpretation of the symbolism also, the analyst seems to be an older brother figure.

In our earlier discussion, we concluded that the dinosaur represented hostile impulses dating back to this patient's childhood. The dream symbolism now suggests that these were hostile impulses against the younger brother inside the mother's body. We reconstruct this early conflict somewhat as follows: Seeing another baby inside the mother reawakened a desire for this most intimate kind of union with her. On the other hand, the unborn baby threatened to come between the child and his mother. Hostile impulses toward the unborn baby threatened the child still further with estrangement from the mother.

We now have, first, a question and, then, a probable explanation for another detail of the manifest dream. We have identified the four other persons in the car as the patient's four older siblings. We have not yet discovered what these four older siblings have to do with the problem that the dreamer is trying to solve. His conflict is one of rivalrous hostility toward his unborn brother. What have his older siblings to do with this problem?

The answer is suggested by the symbol of five persons in one car. The car, too, is a symbol of the mother's body. In the dream, the five siblings are sharing this maternal symbol. This is a possible solution to the patient's sibling-rivalry conflict. If the siblings are willing to share the mother, then there need be no hostility among them. The symbol of the car with five people in it suggests that, for the moment at least, the patient has achieved this kind of solution with his four older siblings. Threatened with estrangement from the mother on account of her pregnancy with still another child, the five older siblings have found consolation by clinging to one another and sharing a maternal symbol.

Nevertheless, the patient's hostility to the mother's pregnancy cannot be wished away, even with the help of a symbolic consolation of solidarity with the older siblings. We have already concluded that the dinosaur is itself a symbol of the patient's awakening hostility toward his mother's pregnancy.

### THE MEANING OF A CONDENSATION

We seem to be faced with a discrepancy. The dream symbolism has suggested that the dinosaur represents the patient's unborn brother. Now we are returning to our earlier interpretation that the dinosaur represents the patient or at least that part of the patient which is hostile. If our interpretive reasoning so far has been correct, we are forced to the conclusion that there has been a condensation. The dinosaur represents both the patient who is hostile * and the baby who is the object of his hostility.

In our approach to interpretation, the basic assumption is that every step in the dream work is intelligibly motivated. So far, we have applied this principle to the substitutions in the dream work. Now we propose the thesis that the condensations in the dream work also make sense.

In the context of our interpretation, it is not difficult to recognize the significance of the condensation that we have just found. In this particular case, by condensation, the patient has achieved, in fantasy, a kind of fusion of identity with his brother. The dinosaur is in possession of the cave which represents his mother. By fusing with his brother, the patient, too, comes into possession of the mother. In this way, this condensation achieves reunion with the mother even more vividly than the intrauterine sharing fantasy did.

To make this possible it has been necessary only to reverse the direction of his hostility—away from the cave and the unborn brother and toward the five persons in the car who are intruding on their intimate union. Instead of attacking the brother, he has fused with him and made common cause with him in resenting the intrusion.

---

* Why is it not enough to say simply that the patient has projected his hostility toward his brother, we might ask—as though to say, "My brother hates me," instead of, "I want to get rid of him." In this way, he would get rid of guilt owing to hostility toward his brother. One objection to this interpretation is that it would imply that the patient's reactive motive was guilt. Actually, there is no evidence of this. On the contrary, the patient's intrauterine sharing fantasy plainly indicates that his reactive motive was fear of estrangement or of separation from the mother—to be answered by a fantasy of sharing her with his rivals. There is no evidence that this fear of estrangement from the mother has been internalized, that it is being reacted to as fear of estrangement from his own conscience (i.e., as guilt).

### COGNITIVE STRUCTURE OF THIS DREAM

According to this interpretation, we now notice, the patient's ego has been split into two parts. The result is a role structure which might be compared to a gang war. The five persons in the car (five older siblings) are investigating the mother's pregnancy, with hostile intent. The dinosaur, representing both the patient and his younger brother, stands ready to resist. The patient's ego has been split into two parts, one in each gang. He is one of the five, but also participates in the dinosaur's reaction, of possession of the mother and of resistance to intrusion.

We can now complete our picture of the cognitive structure of this dream by studying how the gang war in the role structure of the dreamer's infantile conflict has been transformed at the next higher (more superficial) level—at the level of his focal conflict over becoming committed to his psychoanalytic treatment. At this next higher level, the investigation of the mother's pregnancy in the infantile conflict has become the investigation of the patient's unconscious required by his analytic treatment. One of his brothers has become the analyst. The cave and the dinosaur have become part of his unconscious. And now a new split in his ego has developed, replacing the earlier one. The patient's conscious ego is in the driver's seat, bent on continuing his journey into the unconscious, but his fear and resistance have been attributed to the other four persons in the car.

### CHECKING THIS RECONSTRUCTION

Historical interpretations are difficult to check from the evidence of one dream and its associations alone. In this case, our interpretation has succeeded in bringing into intelligible relationship a number of facts that seem otherwise unrelated. Yet, there are still a number of unexplained details in the dream text and in the dreamer's associations. In particular: (1) We have not yet accounted for the huge size of the prehistoric animal. (2) The four people in the car with the dreamer are referred to as two couples, not just as four people. Actually, the patient has three older brothers and one older sister, not two and two. (3) We have not found any specific meaning for "driving on the rocks." (4) In the associations, we have not accounted for the emergence of a memory about the dreamer's brother in which "pissing" and "fire" played such a prominent role. We have not yet any further insight on the third and fourth of these points.

The huge size of the animal may refer to the intensity of the patient's hostility at the time of the mother's pregnancy. This explanation seems probable, but it is still not entirely satisfying. In any case, there still does not seem to be much evidence suggesting that the dinosaur is the father.

The reference to two couples instead of just four people suggests the following thoughts: The historical background of a dream usually consists of not just one memory, but of a constellation of memories. For example, an early traumatic conflict may have been relived many times in the dreamer's later life. Then the structure of the dream may reflect the whole hierarchy of original and derivative conflict situations.

In the dream that we are now studying, the patient's envy of his younger brother's relationship to his mother was a triangular conflict. Perhaps this patient has a pattern of living out this early conflict in other triangular situations, i.e., in relation to other couples. In our earlier discussion, we called attention to the patient's reticence about telling his wife of his analysis. We suspected then that he feared becoming involved in a triangular conflict with his wife and the analyst.

### EVIDENCE FROM LATER DREAMS

The evidence for checking a historical interpretation is not all in when we have studied the dream under consideration and the dreamer's associations in the same hour. Our ultimate check is to inquire whether evidence of the conflict that we have postulated also emerges in other dreams. If a conflict in the past has been important enough to influence a patient's behavior once, it will do so many times.

### RECONSTRUCTION BASED ON HOUSE SYMBOLISM

In our discussion of the house symbolism in the cement dream (Hour 15) and in the fantasy of fixing up a house (Hour 12), we have already arrived at a historical reconstruction that closely parallels the one suggested by the dinosaur dream. To account for the patient's intense need to hold his family together, we postulated that the patient's brothers and sister had intruded between him and his longing for harmony with his mother and that hostility toward his brothers threatened to estrange him still further from his mother. Then, to regain harmony with his mother, his only hope was to include the brothers and sister in the harmonious circle and become one happy family. This reconstruction is identical with the one that seems to be necessary in order to account for the five persons in one car in the dinosaur dream.

## LATER "SYMPATHIC RESONANCE" WITH
## WIFE AND ANALYST

In our conceptual analysis of this patient's ninety-eighth hour, we concluded that, for a short time, the patient had achieved sympathic resonance with his wife. He ended the hour with a feeling "like falling in love all over again." During this hour, this patient's longing for sympathic resonance was in conflict with fear of estrangement.

We now recognize a close parallel between this feeling of sympathic resonance and the sense of intimate union with the mother implied by the intrauterine symbolism of the dinosaur dream. In the intrauterine state, the unborn baby has almost no identity. He is a part of the mother. In his fantasy of being inside the mother, the child is longing for a state in which he is intimately fused with the mother.

In our discussion of Hour 98, we recognized that the patient and his wife were not the only ones involved in the patient's feeling of being in love at the end of Hour 98. Preconsciously, the analyst was also included in the patient's feeling of sympathic resonance. In fact, it was his repressed fantasy of sympathic resonance with the analyst to which the patient reacted most intensely in the next two days (hours 99 and 100). Thus, at the end of Hour 98, there was sympathic resonance involving the patient, his wife, and the analyst—three persons. When we think of the intrauterine state as one of primary resonance (and a fantasy of the intrauterine state as one of sympathic resonance), this feeling of being in love with both his wife and the analyst becomes closely parallel to the dream imagery of the dinosaur in the cave. In the image of the dinosaur, the patient and his younger brother have been condensed into one person. There could be no more complete symbolization of sympathic resonance. Moreover, the dinosaur that represents their union is in possession of the cave that represents the mother.*

In Hour 98, the patient's longing for sympathic resonance with his wife was at first in conflict with fear of rejection by her (fear that he might stick his neck out and find that she, like Bertha, "did not care much for him"). This fear of rejection corresponds to the fear of estrangement from the mother in the background of the dinosaur dream.

Thus, in both Hour 98 and the dinosaur dream, there is longing for sympathic resonance, fear of estrangement, and a solution of the conflict by sympathic resonance including three persons.

### THE POSSIBILITIES OF HISTORICAL ANALYSIS

So far, we have checked our historical interpretation of the dinosaur dream against only four later hours (12, 15, 16, 98) of this patient's psychoanalysis. If we were continuing our discussion of this case further, we should want to make many more such checks.

In the meantime, we have made an unexpected discovery. It is not only the content of the dinosaur dream that has historical implications. The mechanism of condensation that led to the symbol of the dinosaur has also played an essential part

---

* We are skipping a discrepancy at this point. In the manifest dream, the dreamer is represented as fused, not with the mother, but with the unborn brother. The mother herself has been replaced by a deanimated symbol, the cave. At this point, we shall not take time to spell out the explanation for this apparent discrepancy. We shall only suggest the answer. The dreamer's longing for sympathic resonance with the mother in the intrauterine state is in conflict with fear of estrangement from her. The dream work has protected him from activating this disturbing fear of estrangement by substituting a deanimated symbol for the mother.

in the search of the dreamer for a solution to his practical problem. By means of this condensation, the dreamer has obliterated his awareness of being in conflict with his unborn brother and has made possible an illusion of being one with the brother in his possession of the mother.

The way that this condensation mechanism fits into the cognitive structure of this dream also fits beautifully our theory of the genesis of empathic understanding. We have suggested that empathic understanding is made possible by a split in the ego of the person who understands. With one part of his ego, he remains in sympathic resonance with the person who is understood. The other part of his ego, remaining detached, understands by observing the part of the ego that is in sympathic resonance with the observed person. In the mechanism of condensation that we have just reconstructed, we see a reversal of this development from sympathic resonance to empathic understanding. In this condensation, the split in the ego that made possible empathic understanding has been obliterated, restoring the original sympathic resonance.

Our reconstruction of the condensation mechanism in this dream is only one example of the light that can be thrown on early stages in the development of the ego by careful analysis of the cognitive structure of a dream. Furthermore, even this fragment of a historical analysis, incomplete as it is, does give us a glimpse of the precision with which we can reconstruct significant problems from a patient's early past. The unsolved problems of a patient's past have left accurate traces—like fossils in a rock. All that is necessary is that we learn to read these traces by carefully reasoned analysis of recurring constellations of fantasies in the cognitive structures of his dreams.

# *PART 4*

———

# SUMMARY

# CHAPTER XVIII

## SUMMARY

### DIRECT, INTUITIVE APPROACH TO INTERPRETATION

Psychoanalytic interpretation is an intuitive art. We usually make no claim for it as a rigorous scientific procedure. Direct, intuitive interpretation is like understanding a foreign language. We cannot really understand another language by translating it word for word into a language with which we are already familiar. We must first catch the spirit of the strange language so that we can understand it directly. Freud conceived of understanding the language of the unconscious as a kind of resonance between the unconscious of the interpreter and the unconscious of the patient. We call this resonance "empathic understanding."

We often think of empathy as something mystical. We forget that empathic understanding, too, must be based on evidence. Often, we do not like to have our empathy questioned. Empathic understanding is based on total impressions. When we make an interpretation by the direct, intuitive method, we usually do not stop to think how we arrived at it. Often, we do not know on what evidence we based our interpretation.

For this reason, direct, intuitive interpretations are difficult to check.

## OUR OBJECTIVELY CRITICAL APPROACH
## TO INTERPRETATION

The method of interpretation that we propose adds one feature to the direct, intuitive approach to interpretation. We try to systematically check the evidence on which our empathic understanding is based. We often do this against some resistance. We do not like to give up the sense of mystical understanding that our empathy gives us. This resistance is often strongest in those who are most gifted intuitively.

Our empathic understanding may be erroneous. Often, it is distorted by some emotional bias of the interpreting analyst. Such a bias may be impossible to correct. Only if the interpreting analyst can discover his bias can he correct it.

Another source of error in our direct, intuitive interpretations is simpler. We may not have examined the evidence carefully enough. Fortunately, not all errors are due to emotional bias. Even when little or no bias is present, our direct, intuitive impressions may not have evaluated the evidence correctly. The remedy that we propose is to spell out conscientiously the evidence and the reasoning on which our interpretations are based. Often, our initial intuitive impression was based on only part of the evidence. In such a case, we check whether the rest of the evidence supports our interpretation. Our initial intuitive interpretation may even be in conflict with some part of the evidence. If so, we should revise our initial interpretation or even look for a better one to replace it.

Our objectively critical approach to interpretation involves two steps. Both of these steps are intuitive. Our method differs from the direct, intuitive method chiefly in the fact that we use intuition alternately in two ways—first imaginatively, then critically. We first use our intuition imaginatively, just as we do in the direct, intuitive method, searching for promising hypotheses. Then we use our intuition as a basis for critical appraisal of the products of our intuitive imagination.

Often, in a dream and its associations, the facts are so abundant and so complex that it is impossible to grasp them all at once. In our objectively critical method, we try to renounce the illusion that we can take account of all the evidence in a single glance. We must often build up our interpretations by successive small steps, alternating with somewhat more comprehensive critical surveys. We begin by selecting just those bits of evidence that we are surest that our intuition can grasp. Step by step, we then take account of other parts of the evidence, until we can build up a trustworthy understanding of the whole.

From time to time, we interrupt our building operations to subject our picture to critical intuitive appraisal. Sometimes, our critical appraisal suddenly opens up a new perspective, making understandable many facts that we had not yet used in building our hypotheses. Such an opening up of new perspective is our best confirmation of the work that we have done so far. On the other hand, we must keep ourselves alert to gaps and discrepancies in the evidence. When we find discrepancies, we must be ready to revise our intuitive picture.

### COGNITIVE STRUCTURE

Every dream has many meanings. This fact can be used to buttress our resistance to checking our interpretations. Even if some of the evidence seems to point in another direction, we can still maintain that we have only found another one of the dream's overdetermined meanings. In opposition to this resistance, we propose the working assumption that the various meanings of a dream fit together intelligibly. Each dream must also fit intelligibly into the dreamer's real-life situation at the moment of dreaming. These two working hypotheses prevent us from being content with a mere list of possible overdetermined meanings of a dream. They are our most rigorous check, indeed, our only adequate check, on our interpretations. We try to make our standards very strict. When we really succeed in interpreting sensitively and correctly, the parts fit like the most beautifully constructed jigsaw puzzle, and each new bit of evidence makes the fit more perfect.

We use the term "cognitive structure" to designate the way in which the meanings of a dream fit together and the way that they fit into the context of the dreamer's situation in real life. We think of the cognitive structure of a dream as a constellation of related problems. In this constellation, there is usually one problem on which deeper problems converge and from which more superficial problems radiate. This was the dreamer's focal problem at the moment of dreaming. Every focal conflict is a reaction to some event or emotional situation of the preceding day which served as a "precipitating stimulus." As a check on our whole reconstruction, it is most important to find the dreamer's focal conflict and the precipitating stimulus which activated it. In Chapter VII, we have described at some length how we try to reconstruct the cognitive structure of a dream.

### THE DREAMER'S ACTUAL THOUGHT PROCESSES

What we are trying to reconstruct is the actual thought processes of the dreamer while he was dreaming. Thinking is a living, dynamic process, but it does have a continuing structure (*Gestalt*) which is also continually, often rapidly, undergoing change (e.g., growth, learning, problem-solving, and regressive changes). What we call cognitive structure is probably best conceived, at least roughly, as a cross-section of this living process at a particular moment or moments in the process of dreaming.

### PROBLEM-SOLVING IN THE DREAM WORK

Our reconstructions of the thought processes of the dreamer differ in one important way from the usual psychoanalytic approach to interpretation. The practical, empathic thinking that underlies dreams becomes much more intelligible when we recognize that the functional units in this living process are problems, not wishes or fantasies. Wishes are the dynamic stimuli that activate problems. Wish-fulfilling fantasies are attempts, often fleeting attempts, to solve problems. Both wishes and wish-fulfilling fantasies are only parts or phases of a more comprehensive problem-solving effort.

This is our third methodological assumption, namely, that every dream is struggling, more or less successfully, to solve a problem. The problems with which dreams struggle are always practical problems and usually problems of inter-personal adaptation. Our working assumption is, further, that the dream work can be resolved into a series or hierarchy of substitutions of one problem for another. Most important is our assumption that each of these substitutions was intelligibly motivated. Condensations in the dream work, too, we assume, were intelligibly motivated.

### EMPATHIC UNDERSTANDING AND CONCEPTUAL ANALYSIS

Up to this point, we have been discussing only the first phase of our interpretive approach, the phase of "empathic understanding." Empathic understanding can be vivid and precise. It can be communicated to others by gestures, by tone of voice, or by the evocative language of an artist, but it cannot be explained or analyzed without being translated into another language, the expository language of the scientist.

We call this process of translating our empathic understanding into an expository language "conceptual analysis." In order to translate it into expository language, we have to analyze our empathic understanding. When used evocatively, words activate total impressions. In the art of conceptual analysis, we use words analytically. We break down fantasies or even feelings into parts or aspects. We use different words to designate separately each aspect that we have recognized. For example, in Chapter VIII, we analyzed our patient's feeling of "being in love" with his wife into two components, one of sympathic resonance with her and one of mutual honor bestowed by each on the other. In Chapter IX, by studying fluctuations in the quantitative relations of these two components during three analytic sessions, we were able to follow intelligently the patient's successive ways of dealing with his underlying conflict.

### RELATION OF INTERPRETATION TO THEORY

We compared this procedure of analysis and resynthesis to a chemical procedure—first evaporating the water from milk (in order to diminish its bulk), then reconstituting the original milk by mixing the dried powder with water. We used this analogy to illustrate the misuse of theory as a frequent source of error in psychoanalytic interpretation. When our purpose is to reconstitute the milk with which we started, we must take care not to mix in extraneous substances. In the interpretive method that we propose, we try to avoid the contaminating influence of preconceived theories on our interpretations. We advocate an *operational approach* to both interpretation and theory. We try to let our interpretations *shape themselves* out of the colorful words and vivid analogies which the patient himself uses. Instead of letting our theories influence our interpretations, we hope, rather, to use our interpretive procedure as an ever-renewed check on our theories. If bits of theory are legitimately applicable, we argue, we should be able to rediscover them in the material that we are studying. Insofar as our theories are valid, each case should confirm them anew.

These principles are applicable to both phases of our interpretive procedure. In the phase of empathic understanding, we try to forget our theories. We concentrate attention, rather, on resonating empathically with what the patient is feeling and thinking. In the phase of conceptual analysis, in order to let our interpretations "shape themselves," we employ, as our method of analysis, an adaptation of John Stuart Mill's "joint method of agreement and difference." We take note of parallel responses in a dreamer's behavior—responses that have at least one significant feature in common. We then note the differences between these parallel responses. By thus comparing parallel responses, we can analyze each into two or more factors as follows:

$$\text{Response (1)} = AB$$
$$\text{Response (2)} = AC$$
$$\text{Response (n)} = An$$

We have illustrated this procedure at some length in Chapter VIII.*

---

\* French (1952) has also described this procedure of "analysis by comparison" at some length.

### APPLICATIONS OF INTERPRETATION TO THEORY

In our operational procedure, theories should ideally be built by generalizing from well-checked interpretations. Interpreting the behavior of many patients one at a time is an essential first step in building theories of more general validity. Building theories has not been our primary purpose in these essays. Still, our interpretive reconstructions of four dreams (as a small sample of many dreams interpreted by the authors) do have some theoretical implications.

In Chapter XVII, we sketched briefly how, by comparing the cognitive structures of different dreams of the same patient, we can reconstruct with considerable precision significant problems from the patient's past. This kind of reconstruction is an elaboration and extension of the phase of empathic understanding in our operational procedure. Of particular interest are the inferences that can be drawn from our thesis that both the substitutions and the condensations in the dream work are intelligibly motivated.

In the preceding chapters, we also sketched a few of the many possibilities of conceptual analysis. By this method, we were able to define operationally and precisely a number of important concepts—the notions of involvement in and commitment to a conflict, of prophylactic and less successful defenses, of sympathic resonance and estrangement, and of empathic understanding. Starting with these few concepts, we sketched a picture of the nature of empathic fantasy and empathic thinking and of some of the forms that empathic thinking takes when confronted with excessive conflict.

Turning to study of the dream work, we tried to break down Freud's concept of the primary process into a number of more precise categories. In particular, we stressed the difference between disintegration products of verbal thinking and a number of more or less regressive forms of empathic thinking. Making use of these distinctions and of the concepts of involvement in and commitment to a conflict, we focused our interest on the ego's problem of protecting itself against premature commitment to excessive conflicts. In this way, we can bring the dreamer's defenses into simpler and more intelligible relationship to the integrative function of the ego.

This kind of study of the dreamer's defenses gives us access to study of what we call the cambium level of the mind (corresponding, though only roughly, to Freud's system preconscious). This level of the dreamer's focal problem—the level where active growth, problem-solving, and learning take place—is probably the only level directly accessible to therapeutic influence.

In conclusion, our procedure, with its step-by-step checking of evidence and its insistence on an operational method, makes possible a sureness, precision, and depth of theoretical formulation that would not otherwise be possible.

# REFERENCES

ALEXANDER, FRANZ. Remarks about the relation of inferiority feelings to guilt feelings. *Int. J. Psychoanal.*, 1938, **19**, 41–49.

BECK, SAMUEL J. Rorschach's *Erlebnistypus:* An empiric datum. *Rorschachiana*, 1963, **8**, No. 45.

BENEDEK, THERESE. The psychosomatic implications of the primary unit: Mother–child. *Amer. J. Orthopsychiat.*, 1949, **19**, 642–654.

BOISEN, ANTON. *The exploration of the inner world.* New York: Willett, Clark & Co., 1936.

BONIME, WALTER. *The clinical use of dreams.* New York: Basic Books, 1962.

CHEMISTRY SOCIETY. *Theoretical organic chemistry Kekule symposium.* London: 1958.

DEUTSCH, HELENE. *Psychoanalysis of the neuroses.* London: Hogarth, 1932.

ERIKSON, ERIK H. The dream specimen of psychoanalysis. *J. Amer. psychoanal. Ass.*, 1954, **2**, 5–56.

FEDERN, PAUL. *Ego psychology and the psychoses.* New York: Basic Books, 1952.

FISHER, CHARLES. Dreams and perception: The role of preconscious and primary modes of perception in dream formation. *J. Amer. psychoanal. Ass.*, 1954, **2**, 389–445.

FISHER, CHARLES. Dreams, images, and perception: A study of unconscious–preconscious relationships. *J. Amer. psychoanal. Ass.*, 1956, **4**, 5–48.

FISHER, CHARLES. A study of the preliminary stages of the construction of dreams and images. *J. Amer. psychoanal. Ass.*, 1957, **5**, 5–60.

FISHER, CHARLES, & PAUL, I. H. The effect of subliminal visual stimulation on images and dreams: A validation study. *J. Amer. psychoanal. Ass.*, 1959, **7**, 35–83.

FLIESS, ROBERT. The metapsychology of the analyst. *Psychoanal. Quart.*, 1942, **11**, 211–227.

FOULKES, W. DAVID. Dream reports from different stages of sleep. *J. abnorm. soc. psychol.*, 1962, **65**, 14–25.

FRENCH, THOMAS M. Clinical approach to the dynamics of behavior. In J. McV. HUNT (Ed.), *Personality and the behavior disorders*, Vol. I. New York: Ronald Press, 1944. Pp. 255–268.

FRENCH, THOMAS M. *The integration of behavior. Vol I. Basic postulates.* Chicago: University of Chicago Press, 1952.

FRENCH, THOMAS M. *The integration of behavior. Vol. II. The integrative process in dreams.* Chicago: University of Chicago Press, 1953.

FRENCH, THOMAS M. *The integration of behavior. Vol. III. The reintegrative process in a psychoanalytic treatment.* Chicago: University of Chicago Press, 1958.

FRENCH, THOMAS M., ALEXANDER, FRANZ, et al. *Psychogenic factors in bronchial asthma.* Washington, D.C.: National Research Council, 1941.

FREUD, ANNA, & BURLINGHAM, DOROTHY T. *Infants without families.* London: Allen & Unwin, 1943.

FREUD, SIGMUND. *The interpretation of dreams. Standard Edition.* Vols. IV-V. 1953 *et seq.* [1900].

FREUD, SIGMUND. Recommendations to physicians practicing psychoanalysis. *Standard Edition.* Vol. XII. 1953 *et seq.* [1912]. Pp. 109–120.

FREUD, SIGMUND. On narcissism: An introduction. *Standard Edition.* Vol. XIV. 1953 *et seq.* [1914]. Pp. 67–104.

FREUD, SIGMUND. Instincts and their vicissitudes. *Standard Edition.* Vol. XIV. 1953 *et seq.* [1915]. Pp. 109–140.

FREUD, SIGMUND. The ego and the id. *Standard Edition.* Vol. XIX. 1953 *et seq.* [1923]. Pp. 12–59.

FREUD, SIGMUND. Inhibitions, symptoms, and anxiety. *Standard Edition.* Vol. XX. 1953 *et seq.* [1926]. Pp. 75–175.

FROMM, ERIKA, & FRENCH, THOMAS M. Formation and evaluation of hypotheses in dream interpretation. *J. Psychol.,* 1962, **54,** 271–283.

FROMM-REICHMANN, FRIEDA. A preliminary note on the emotional significance of stereotypes in schizophrenics. In Dexter M. Bullard (Ed.), *Psychoanalysis and psychotherapy: Selected papers.* Chicago: University of Chicago Press, 1959 [1942].

HALL, CALVIN S. Diagnosing personality by the analysis of dreams. *J. abnorm. soc. psychol.,* 1947, **42,** 68–79.

HALL, CALVIN S. *The meaning of dreams.* New York: Harper, 1953.

JONES, RICHARD M. *Ego synthesis in dreams.* New York: Schenkman, 1962.

KASANIN, JACOB S. & FRENCH, THOMAS M. A psychodynamic study of the recovery of two schizophrenic cases. *Psychoanal. Quart.,* 1941, **10,** 1–22.

KRIS, ERNST. Psychology of caricature. *Int. J. Psychoanal.,* 1936, **17,** 285–303.

KRIS, ERNST. On preconscious mental processes. *Psychoanal. Quart.*, 1950, **19**, 540–560.

KUBIE, LAWRENCE S. Problems and techniques of psychoanalytic validation and progress. In Eugene Pumpian-Mindlin (Ed.), *Psychoanalysis as science.* Stanford, Calif.: Stanford University Press, 1952. Pp. 46–124.

KUBIE, LAWRENCE S. The distortion of the symbolic process in neurosis and psychosis. *J. Amer. Psychoanal. Ass.*, 1953, **1**, 59–86. (a)

KUBIE, LAWRENCE S. Psychoanalysis as a basic science. In Franz Alexander and Helen Ross (Eds.), *Twenty years of psychoanalysis.* New York: Norton, 1953. (b)

KUBIE, LAWRENCE S. Some implications for psychoanalysis of modern concepts of the organization of the brain. *Psychoanal. Quart.*, 1953, **22**, 21–68. (c)

KUBIE, LAWRENCE S. *Neurotic distortion of the creative process.* Lawrence, Kans.: University of Kansas Press, 1958.

LANGER, SUSAN K. *Philosophy in a new key: A study in the symbolism of reason, rite, and art.* Cambridge, Mass.: Harvard University Press, 1942.

LANGER, SUSAN K. *Problems of art.* New York: Charles Scribner's Sons, 1957.

MEAD, GEORGE H. *Mind, self and society.* Chicago: University of Chicago Press, 1934.

MILL, JOHN STUART. *A system of logic—ratiocinative and inductive.* New York: Longmans, 1958 [1843].

OLDEN, CHRISTINE. On adult empathy with children. In Ruth S. Eissler, Anna Freud, Heinz Hartmann, & Marianne Kris (Eds.). *The psychoanalytic study of the child.* Vol. VIII. New York: International Universities Press, 1953. Pp. 111–121.

PIAGET, JEAN. *The origins of intelligence in children.* New York: International Universities Press, 1952 [1936].

PIAGET, JEAN. *The construction of reality in the child.* London: Routledge, 1955 [1937].

PIAGET, JEAN. *Play, dreams and imitation in childhood.* New York: Norton, 1951 [1945].

PIAGET, JEAN. *The psychology of intelligence.* London: Routledge & Paul, 1950 [1947].

PIERS, GERHART, & SINGER, MILTON B. *Shame and guilt: A psychoanalytic and cultural study.* Springfield, Ill.: Charles C Thomas, 1953.

POETZL, OTTO. Experimentell erregte Traumbilder in ihren Beziehungen zum indirekten Sehen. *Z. f. Neurol. u. Psychiat.,* 1917, **37,** 278–349.

RAPAPORT, DAVID. *Organization and pathology of thought.* New York: Columbia University Press, 1951.

RECHTSCHAFFEN, ALLAN, WHEATON, JOY, & VERDONE, PAUL. Reports of mental activity during sleep. *J. Canadian Psychiat. Ass.,* 1963, **8,** 409–414.

REIK, THEODOR. *Surprise and the psychoanalyst.* New York: Dutton, 1937.

STERBA, RICHARD. The fate of the ego in analytic therapy. *Int. J. Psychoanal.,* 1934, **15,** 117–126.

TAUBER, EDWARD S., & GREEN, MAURICE R. *Prelogical experience.* New York: Basic Books, 1962.

TOYNBEE, ARNOLD. *A study of history* (Abridged ed.). New York: Oxford University Press, 1946 [1934].

VARENDONCK, JULIAN. *The psychology of day-dreams.* New York: Macmillan, 1921.

WEISS, EDOARDO. *Principles of psychodynamics.* New York: Grune & Stratton, 1950.

WEISS, EDOARDO. *The structure and dynamics of the human mind.* New York: Grune & Stratton, 1960.

WHORF, BENJAMIN L. Languages and logic. In *Language, thought and reality: Selected writings.* New York: M.I.T./Wiley, 1956 [1941].

ZEIGARNIK, BLUMA. Uber das Behalten von erledigten und unerledigten Handlungen. *Psychol. Forsch.,* 1927, **9,** 1–5.

# INDEX

went quickly and without any trouble. . . . Now he's starting at the bottom, at the toes of my left foot . . . he's just sucking my foot up into him . . . he's going up the left side just like a vacuum cleaner, all the way up and turning in the shoulder and my arm and he's finished . . . and he's starting at the shoulder and going to the head . . . ah . . . now he's just sucking me in like a rag. I'm all gone already. Just sucking me in like . . . not even biting, just wooshing me in. . . . Now he's starting at the feet, he's taking both feet at the same time . . . he's chomping up and his mouth is wide and he is taking everything up past the knees, the hips up to the chest . . . going in like a salami into a meat grinder, up all the way to my chest, my hands are at my side and going . . . he's gnawing away at my face . . . [m,m] . . . ah . . . all the way up . . . yes, I'm all gone again . . . he's starting at the top and he's going at it really fast and furious . . . [m] . . . oh, yes, he's snapping away at me like at a carrot . . . he's just chomping away now, down to the hips . . . that was fast, he took everything, he took me at three gulps just about . . . I can't even tell what kind of dog it is any more . . . oh . . . I see some sort of a dog. He's looking at me, sort of smiling . . . ah . . . just keeps looking at me . . . doesn't want to . . . maybe it isn't a dog . . . it's a bird. . . . That looks like one of those silly birds that dip their beaks into a glass of water and stand up again. It works by evaporation and condensation, it's sort of two tubes . . . I see this dickie bird or something like that going up and down . . it's sort of a crazy children's toy . . . yes, that's what it is, going up and down. . . . There comes the bulldog this time, sort of sneaking up at me . . . yeah, he's taking his time about nibbling away at me . . . he's taking his sweet time. Doesn't seem to want to take it . . . he's just going at it very slowly. Now he's going up a bit faster . . . my left leg up to my thigh . . . feels very relaxed to sort of have him eat me up . . . he's taking my arm and hand together at one crack now . . . up across, head and all, shoulder, arm . . . more like a vacuum cleaner really . . . I'm nearly all eaten up . . . yeah, there goes the last of my toes . . . very calm now . . . sort of tan color. . . . I seem to see a chicken leg . . . nothing really to see . . . I get the impression of this Roman haircut again, this forehead and some hair . . . I think that chap is wearing one of these skullcaps, yarmulke I think is the word for it. . . . Ahh, I think I see a big polar bear. He's yawning, I don't know . . . I'll see if he feels like . . . ah, he is taking a nibble at me . . . yeah, he's chomping away . . . he's taking his time, he's up to the knees. This is a big boy . . . he's taking everything at once . . . he's taking me in . . . yes, he swallowed me just about whole . . . yes, I'm inside . . . it seems to be like inside a tube, there's still a little bit of light . . . I'm sort of slithering down, sort of dark . . . there's pressure from the sides on me . . . I don't know, it seems . . . I've the impression of feathers for some reason . . . for some reason or other. . . . Yes, now I see what looks like a falcon sitting on a perch . . . looking . . . though it could be a horned owl . . . I don't know . . . I don't think so . . . yes, now it is an owl looking at me . . . he did eat me up, just sucked me, started at the right leg. I was very tiny and he just . . . as if I were a worm. Somehow it did not bother me too much . . . He's eating me again. . . . Now I see those ribs of beef again . . . like I saw in one of the earlier trips, except I don't think they are ribs of beef . . . its my own chest . . . I don't know, something looks like a big cat eating through them . . . ripping them, chomping through them . . . looks like a black panther . . . yes, he's eating me up again, except this time he's biting, and not swallowing me as a whole like the others . . . the left shoulder, my head, my right shoulder, right arm, there's only my left are hanging there . . . by nothing, he took it in one snap . . . now he's going down on the right side . . . going down . . . yes, a black panther . . . he's slowing down considerably . . . he's sort of chomping away . . . going down my right foot . . . down to my ankle, there goes my foot . . . Now I see a goose . . . now I got gobbled up like a worm again. Whew! I'm just seeing some concentric circles . . . I don't know, I'm seeing some abstract shapes that don't mean anything . . . looks perhaps like a door handle, European style. . . . Now I see a little frog . . . I guess I'm a fly and he's just taking a snap at me . . . I felt about three times like that, like a fly . . . sort of light violet color, a little bit of shimmering. . . . I get the impression of being under water. . . . Now I can't see anything . . . that looks like a duck, or something . . . he's chasing after me . . . I'm a little bug skittering along, and I'm trying to get away, and he's chasing me . . . ah, there I go, he snapped me up . . . ah, I don't know, I got mad all of a sudden, I said I'm not a bug, I turned around and I took the duck, and I just swung him around and flung him away . . . I got very aggressive or independent . . . I felt I didn't want to get eaten up any more . . . I see sort of a texture, like sharkskin, or something like that . . . I seem to have a different sort of shape it isn't really me . . . I don't know . . . I'm sort of a shapeless blob . . . a tiny miniature thing, a bug or something. . . . Now there is a robin . . . he's pecking at me . . . yeah, I feel his beak going into me . . . ah, that's funny, I took the robin by the beak and sort of threw him over my shoulder, in a sort of judo hold, or I just flipped him over me . . . I don't want to get pecked to death . . . I can see the bird sort of lying there, he's much bigger than me, but I just sort of threw him over me and he crashed down on his back. . . . Now I'm walking away from him . . . I seem to be walking on a beach or something . . . it's sort of mud colored. . . . Ahh, I seem to see a snake . . . hmm . . . the snake had wide-open jaws and I just walked up and put my foot up and my other hand on the other jaw, and reached in, and turned the snake inside out. . . . That's a good trick. . . . Now I feel very calm. . . . [Can you describe the visual field?] . . . Sort of stripes, wavy stripes, and sort of monochromatic colors in shades of light gray . . ." (termination).

## SYNCHRONIZED THEMATIC MULTIPLICATION

A specific brain-designed maneuver of thematic repetition involving visual elaborations (e.g., stages III-VI; see Table 33, p. 188) consists of a synchronized repetition of the same thematic elements (see Case 73, p. 168; Case 122). Depending on the prevailing level of differentiation of visual elaborations, synchronized thematic multiplication may assume static picture-like characteristics of symbolic nature (see Case 124), or may involve highly differentiated cinerama-type dynamics with multiplication of self-involvement (see Case 122, Case 123). Such phases of synchronized thematic multiplication are preceded by thematic repetitions of the same elements which follow a pattern of serial repetition as a part of the sequential type of thematic programming (see p. 273 ff.). From pattern analyses of processes of neutralization which precede and follow such phases of synchronized thematic multiplication, it was assumed that this brain-designed maneuver is a self-facilitating time-saving device which accelerates the brain-desired progression of neutralization, and as such may be considered as a convenient substitute for slower processes of sequential monothematic patterns of repetition.

*Case 122:* A 37-year-old housewife (hysterical personality, posttraumatic anxiety reaction, moderate depressive reaction, ecclesiogenic syndrome). In the following passages, during the neutralization of masochistic and accident-related material, the brain changes from a pattern of sequential repetition to a facilitating and apparently more efficient pattern of synchronized thematic multiplication.

"Yes, I'm up against the wall . . . and I see the truck coming . . . I see it and I'm scared . . . and it crashes into me . . . it crushes me against the wall . . . and it stays there . . . and I start over again . . . I see it advancing, I know that it's going to hit me, it crushes me against the wall . . . I start over again . . . *there are ten trucks . . . there are ten of me . . . and it's a row of trucks advancing . . . and me, there are ten like me . . . and I'm crushed, all at the same time . . . it starts over again . . . and the trucks crush me . . . it's like an advancing army . . . and they crash into me* . . . and they crush me, I know that it would come someday, but I didn't think that it was necessary . . . I return to the wall, on my own, it's as if it was to punish myself . . . it's worse if I'm alone, and if there's only one truck because . . . in other words, if there's a row of me, we can support each other, but if I'm all alone in front of a truck, it's worse . . . it crashes into me, but it didn't crush me. . . ."

*Case 123:* A 38-year-old housewife (hysterical personality, anxiety reaction, multiple psychophysiologic reactions). A phase of synchronized thematic multiplication occurs as brain-disturbing material related to the general topic of death and inadequate identifications with a number of deceased persons undergo thematic neutralization.

"It is on the theme of funerals, it is the salon, the little coffin. I saw another coffin, white coffin, the *B* child died of cancer at the age of five . . . I was what? eight . . . nine . . . so I am in both of those as a child . . . I don't know, it could be in Quebec, at the funeral home . . . and I see my father in his coffin . . . and I see my grandmother. But I did not see her . . . I don't think I saw my grandmother laid out . . . grandfather, so *I am in all of those coffins* . . . D.C.'s son . . . I am also in that coffin . . . different stages of my life . . . *about ten simultaneous funerals* . . . they could be in different places . . . they could be all in one place . . . I am in each one of these coffins . . . can hear the earth . . . most of the time, it is like dry hard earth falling on the coffin. . . ."

*Case 124:* A 30-year-old social worker (anxiety reaction, moderate depression, multiple phobic and psychophysiologic reactions, ecclesiogenic syndrome). In this patient, AA 6 shows a pattern of visual elaborations which are still restricted to stages III and IV (see Table 33, p. 188), and frequent functional regression to more elementary elaborations of stages II and I. During this and previous autogenic abreactions the dynamics of neutralization emphasized elaborations of thematically distorted thematic repetitions, heavily disguised elements of a sexual and ecclesiogenic nature. Interjected phases of synchronized thematic multiplication (see example below) occurred repeatedly.

"The shape of a sailboat . . . noise in my stomach . . . my hands feel numb, my arms also . . . [sigh] . . . toes, very clear presentation with toenails . . . *thousands of toes,* those which are very close to me are bigger in size and they get smaller and smaller as the row of toes goes into the endless distance . . . [sigh] . . . a gable . . . something like a road . . . a big circle which is getting smaller . . . in the center it is purplish blue. . . ."

Very similar to the phenomena of synchronized thematic multiplication of visual elaborations are phases of generalized motor or sensory discharges which, from a physiologic point of view, may be considered as a synchronized release of a quantitative multiplication of the same thematic elements (see Case 92, p. 228; Case 121, p. 278).

## ROTATIONAL MULTITHEMATIC REPETITION

The observation that processes of serial monothematic repetition lead progressively toward greater degrees of thematic flexibility with facilitated engagement in other brain-selected areas of disturbing material led to the tentative conclusion that more flexible patterns of multithematic rotational repetition are a brain-preferred form of neutralization. Such patterns may be temporarily restricted to repetitions of a relatively limited number of topics as, for example, alternating thematic antitheses (see p. 308) or rotational repetitions of autosexual, heterosexual, homosexual and transsexual dynamics (see Fig. 6, p. 60; Fig. 15, p. 285). However, in many instances patterns of rotational repetition involve functionally interrelated material composed of a larger number of thematic elements. When such multithematic patterns are adopted, the brain-desired goal of progressive neutralization is brought about by periodically occurring thematic shifts from one pressure area (see p. 270 ff.) to the next, until a certain number of brain-desired topics are covered; and another round of rotational neutralization follows. As

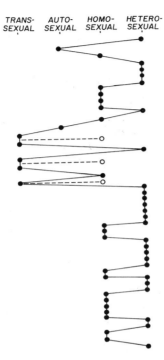

FIG. 15. Pattern of multithematic rotational repetition of autosexual, heterosexual, homosexual and transsexual elaborations (24-year-old male student, personality disorder, sexual deviation, anxiety reaction, obsessive-compulsive manifestations, multiple phobic and psychophysiologic reactions, ecclesiogenic syndrome, hypothyroidism).

different although interrelated thematic areas undergo repeated processes of neutralization, progressively oriented (see Table 11, p. 57) modifications of content, dynamics and the patient's reactivity can be noted. Certain initially important elements and dynamics lose their importance and finally disappear from the rotational program. As the brain directed processes of multithematic neutralization keep advancing, the appearance of new thematic elements and previously unobserved dynamics characterize progressive developments of brain-programmed self-normalization. After a brain-directed number of multithematic repetitions have taken place, the self-regulatory brain mechanisms invariably indicate by relevant elaborations that their program of neutralization has ended for the time (see p. 78 ff., p. 329 ff., Case 16, p. 66 ff., Case 50, p. 125 ff.; Case 125, p. 286 ff.).

*Case 125:* A 26-year-old student of theology (personality disorder, sexual deviation, anxiety reaction, multiple phobic and psychophysiologic reactions, ecclesiogenic syndrome). The following autogenic abreaction is a good example of progressively advancing multithematic processes of neutralization which conveys various characteristics of rotational patterns of thematic repetition.

"I see a snake in my room . . . it's a boa, and the boa is very big . . . and he takes up most of the floor, and he comes up to me and stings me . . . and now I'm dead . . . and now I'm in a grave . . . and now I'm being taken to the cemetery . . . and now I'm going into a very deep pit . . . and the devil takes me by the neck and slits my throat . . . and now he stops . . . he then puts my nose in some crap and throws me head first into it . . . and I get stabbed in the head and in the ribs with a pitchfork . . . and now there's a whole gang of devils, and they scratch me with their nails, they pull my skin off and put me in a soup caldron of boiling water . . . and I'm at the bottom . . . and now I'm put into a furnace, and I'm burning . . . and I'm still burning . . . and then they take me out and I see the devil before me, and he wants to slit my throat, and he punches me, and he tears off my penis and my testicles . . . and he pulls out my teeth, my eyes, and my hair . . . and he puts a red-hot iron into my mouth and my eyes . . . he puts some red juice into my body . . . and then he begins to eat . . . and he eats the skin . . . and he takes out the intestines, the stomach and the rest . . . and he squashes the testicles . . . he tears off my penis again . . . and he twists my legs, and he crushes me onto the floor . . . and another gang arrives, and they pull me about in all sorts of ways . . . and they throw me into a snake bath . . . and there are many stinging and biting me . . . and they're still stinging me . . . and one eats my head, and others my legs . . . and others sting my body . . . and a crocodile nibbles at me with his teeth . . . and he bites my face . . . and the boa opens his mouth and eats me up . . . and I go down through him, and I come out by the anus . . . and some snakes are stinging me . . . and the crocodile eats me . . . and the snakes surround me from all directions and sting me again . . . and there I crash my head against the wall . . . and my head cracks open and blood flows . . . and big claws are scratching me . . . I'm put into a flaming fire . . . and there, I'm burned . . . and I hear the screams of the people suffering around me . . . a devil chokes me and another crushes my testicles, and another tears off my penis . . . and one pulls my eyes out and twists my hands and feet . . . and one tears off my skin . . . and he throws me up into the air . . . there are pitchforks . . . and a knife passes through my stomach and cuts my head off and splits me in two. . . . I'm back with the boa again, and a snake stings and bites me, and another stings me . . . and I see my bedroom . . . and there's still a big boa there . . . and I'm in my bed . . . and he moves around the bed . . . and he passes in between my legs and stings me again . . . and I fall onto the floor . . . and the devil enters, and he is looking for me . . . and the snakes follow us . . . and we go down the stairs and we enter into a tunnel . . . and there's a slope there, and we go down into the cavity . . . and there are bats all around, and one flies right in my face . . . and there are birds, and they pull my eyes out and my head and bite my stomach with their beaks . . . and I'm walking on snakes . . . and the devil leads me into another tunnel, and there are all sorts of mouths eating my skin . . . and a snake bites me . . . and he eats my penis . . . and my testicles . . . the snake climbs up and eats my head . . . and my head is in the snake and my body on the outside, and two other snakes take my legs and bite me all over and twist around me in all sort of ways . . . and spiders climb up on my body . . . and on my face . . . and I'm walking, and I squash some underfoot . . . and there are others sucking at me and stinging my legs, and they're sucking up the blood . . . and there are little adders and octopuses taking me by the body and stinging me all over . . . and they're stinging me . . . and they eat my head . . . and I feel its stomach on mine . . . and the tentacles . . . all around me . . . I'm in a sort of bath . . . full of octopuses taking me in all sort of ways, and snakes as well . . . and the crocodiles all around me . . . and spiders also . . . and as soon as I rise, the crocodiles bite me and spiders sting me . . . and there are spiders crawling all over my body . . . and the devil comes and takes me and puts me into the flaming fire . . . and it's full of devils . . . screaming in all sorts of ways, and now I see them . . . and a steamhammer falls and crashes me in a continuous motion . . . and they throw me back into the bath full of snakes and octopuses . . . and the same game begins again . . . I'm in the corridor and there are snakes all over, and my heels are being bitten, and I'm stung, and I fall . . . and snakes sting my eyes . . . and the shoulders and the buttocks and the legs . . . and again the devil is there before me . . . and there's a sort of dragon, and he doesn't scare me as much . . . it's the torturing that especially scares me . . . and I feel the heat, and it's black . . . and the doors are black . . . and the doors are closed hermetically . . . and I'm still in the fire . . . and I'm in the snake bath . . . and there are octopuses also grabbing me in every which way. . . . I see myself in my bedroom again . . . and there are snakes on my dresser and in the drawers and behind the bookshelves and on the ceiling . . . and in my bed and on the sheet . . . and the floor is crowded with snakes . . . and I leave them be, and the snakes leave and go down the corridor and down the stairs into hell . . . there are still a few left in my bed, but they aren't dangerous . . . and I take one and play with it . . . it tires me . . . and I see a big boa approaching me, he stings me and opens his mouth, and he takes me up in his mouth, and we walk together, and we go down the stairs, and we walk into the tunnel . . . and we go down into hell again . . . and there are big boas down there with large iron 'lancets' . . . and they sting me in every which way, and they put some kind of juice into my body, and I catch on fire . . . and they burn me . . . and my hair burns as well . . . and the snakes eat me up each in turn . . . and I go into a snake and stay there . . . it regurgitates me, and I go into another, and again into another, and again into another, and again into another . . . and I take away all their lancets . . . and there are little blocks of dirt, and I'm playing around with their mouths . . . and they go away quietly . . . and once again, I find some little snakes and octopuses . . . they have a sort of hole underneath with which they take my head and squeeze it, and they kill me, and it's all quite sickening . . . and each octopus does the same thing . . . now I see my room . . . and there are snakes in it . . . and I'm lying down on my bed amidst the snakes . . . and they sting me . . . and they fall onto the floor . . . and now a sort of snake comes and gets me, and it's an immense boa . . .who leads me down the corridor . . . and we go down to hell . . . and it's an immense animal . . . and in hell . . . there's another big animal which opens his mouth . . . and I go into it . . . right to the end, and I go down inside the snake right through to his head . . . and he has an immense lancet . . . and this animal has huge eyes . . . I tear his eyes out . . . they are big ball bearings . . . and I also tear out the lancet . . . and I sit on the snake's head . . . and with my foot I put him on the ground, and I walk on him . . . and I make a sort of rug with this . . . and I return to my room . . . and there's still a boa in there moving about, and he licks my face with his tongue, he stings me with his lancet . . . but a juice is flowing out from his lancet, flowing into my insides . . . and I go on sleeping . . . and the snake is on the edge of the bed, sleeping as well . . . and I go around my room to see if there are any more snakes . . . yes, there's one underneath my dresser . . . and he stings me in the buttocks . . . and lies down beside me in bed . . . and I see some more bats on the ceiling, and they stay caught in my hair . . . and they're biting my head . . . and my legs . . . and they open their mouths . . . and I see another lancet, and it stings me. . . . And I see the devil walking alongside me in the corridor . . . we're leaving the college . . . then he pushes me into a car, and the car drives and crushes me . . . and the funeral takes place at the college . . . and there is singing . . . now they set me down on the ground . . . and I go down into the grave . . . now I'm on a slide . . . it's a sort of shaft . . . very deep, and below there are two snakes biting my legs . . . and a boa is eating my penis and my testicles . . . and I'm in my room with some boas . . . and they're coiled tightly around me . . . and I'm struggling with them . . . and they're everywhere, and one is biting me all over, and I'm struggling . . . and a grate open up . . . and I fall into a huge space . . . full of crap and full of snakes and fire and human heads, and I see some octopuses . . . and I'm in the crap, and I'm eating crap, and my eyes and nostrils are full of this crap . . . and worms are going into my ears . . . and now I get out . . . and then it starts all over again . . . my mouth and my body are full of crap . . . and I get out again . . . and I stay there . . . and there again, I go back into it and I swallow some more crap . . . and there are snakes as well, and they're coming out from my behind . . . and I get out of there again . . . and the snakes have stopped coming out . . . and I go back into it again, and I eat crap, and I eat some snakes . . . and the snakes enter by the mouth and come out from my behind . . . and I get out again, and I stay there . . . and this time I walk in it, and with each step, they sting me with forks, and I go into it once more, and I again swallow some, and I'm still walking in it, and I'm drowning in it . . . and there are still some snakes entering my mouth . . . and coming out from my behind . . . and I go outside . . . and there's a snake there . . . and I walk with the snake . . . and he stings me all over . . . and I take the elevator . . . and

I arrive at my floor . . . and I go into another room . . . and I'm still looking for some snakes . . . there are no more snakes . . . and from my bed I look around . . . there's still one . . . and he climbs up and stings me in the neck . . . and I look at the snake . . . and I tear out his lancet . . . and he bites my hand . . . and I see a sort of crocodile which eats my head . . . and the crocodile is on my bed . . . and I'm lying down on my bed . . . and I see the crocodile, and the crocodile leaves the room, and I follow the crocodile with my eyes until he gets to the other side . . . and I see another crocodile with large teeth, and I go into the crocodile . . . and I come back out . . . and I look at the crocodile's eyes . . . and I open up the crocodile . . . and I send him to hell . . . and I see myself once more in my bedroom . . . there's another crocodile there . . . and I open the window, and I get into the crocodile, and I'm inside it now . . . and I come out of it and the crocodile pursues me, and he bites my heel . . . and I go down into hell . . . and there are still many crocodiles . . . and I go into an open mouth . . . and I come out . . . and they grab me lengthwise and crush me . . . and they eat me up . . . and they still have their mouths wide open . . . and they go on eating me . . . and I'm on the outside, and I'm walking toward the elevator . . . and the crocodiles come . . . and I walk on their heads . . . I look into their eyes . . . and they've calmed down . . . and I take the elevator . . . and I'm in my room . . . and there's still another snake . . . twisting about me . . . he stings me and bites me . . . it's a big boa . . . and with his lancet, he pierces through my body . . . and he takes me in his mouth, and we're in the corridor, and we go down into hell . . . and there are more boas down there eating me, and I'm inside them . . . I come out . . . and they eat me up once more . . . and I come out . . . and now, I see my room, and I'm lying down on my bed . . . and there's nothing . . . but I still have the feeling there's something else . . . and I go around my room . . . to see if there are still more snakes. . . . And I see none . . . a slightly colored background . . . it's bluish . . . the background is bluish . . ." (termination).

## CHANGES ASSOCIATED WITH THEMATIC REPETITION

Quite contrary to many patients' impression that thematic repetitions seem to be a waste of time and do not contribute anything new to their treatment process, clinically oriented observations and detailed pattern analyses indicated that therapeutically significant changes take place as thematic repetitions are allowed to proceed. Of general therapeutic interest are, for example, some of the following changes:

1. A trend of progressively decreasing brain-antagonizing thematic resistance. This may be indicated by:
   (a) A shift from initially hesitant, inhibited, restricted, slow (or un-
       usually fast) abortive or otherwise incomplete elaborations, and
       engagement to progressively more facilitated, more differenti-

ated, more dynamic, more spontaneous, more appropriate, more efficient thematic elaborations and engagement.

(b) A progressively decreasing need for supportive interventions as, for example, non-specific encouragements (e.g., "It's going very well, please continue") or thematically adapted support designed to overcome brain-antagonizing forms of resistance (e.g., *thematic evasion, abortive engagement, repetition resistance;* see Part I, Vol. VI; see also Case 16, p. 66 ff.; Case 121, p. 278 ff.).

(c) A change from initially more dissociated, more impersonal, more indirect forms of self-involvement (see Table 44, p. 296) to less dissociated, more involved, direct forms of active self-participation (e.g., initially: "I would hit my mother"; later: "I am hitting my mother").

2. Various manifestations reflecting a progressive development toward improvement and normalization as, for example:

(a) A progressive decrease of negatively accentuated emotional and psychophysiologic reactivity (e.g., anxiety, disgust, nausea, dizziness, pain, motor discharges) which were originally or during a transitory initial phase associated with the topic of thematic repetition.

(b) A slow but progressive increase of more neutral and more positively oriented thematic elements and emotional and psychophysiologic reactions (e.g., enjoying attacking mother, feeling that one is getting something out of it, feeling relaxed, experiencing flowing warmth and comfort).

(c) A progressively increasing thematic flexibility with interjected or progressive shifts toward closely related themes.

(d) Positively oriented developments during advanced phases of thematic neutralization (e.g., terminal phase of the abreactive period).

3. A trend of progressively increasing manifestations of reintegrative dynamics as, for example, indicated by:

(a) Progressive changes from less differentiated to more detailed and complex elaborations with augmentation of reality features (see Case 16, p. 66 ff.).

(b) Progressive decrease of brain-disturbing thematic dynamics (e.g., homosexual, transsexual, dependence, inadequate passivity, inadequate identifications), and gradual increase of brain-desired elements and dynamics (e.g., heterosexual, independence, adequate initiative, disappearance of inadequate identifications).

4. Various improvements in areas of case-specific complaints and disorders during (a) the interim period and (b) over longer periods of treatment (e.g., disappearance of abdominal complaints, of episodes of paroxysmal tachycardia, of headaches, of interest in homosexual activities, of negatively colored religious orientations, of difficulties at work, increase of inner harmony, creativity and productive efficiency; see Table 11, p. 57).

# 22. Thematic Modification

In many instances processes of autogenic neutralization are composed partly or completely of brain-directed elaborations which in one or another respect are not in accordance with reality. From the endless variety of thematic modifications which may involve a large variety of psychodynamically and psychophysiologically brain-directed elaborations at different levels of functional integration, it may be concluded that the brain either cannot or does not want to proceed otherwise. The reasons why, at certain times, such and such thematic modifications (e.g., symbolic) are preferred and why such a combination of different forms of modifications are selected require further investigation.

So far it has been found helpful to distinguish three major categories of psychodynamically and psychophysiologically oriented thematic modifications: (a) thematic disintegration, (b) thematic dissociation, and (c) thematic distortions. All three categories of thematic modification help to disguise and reduce the disturbing potency of relevant thematic material and thus contribute to a facilitation of the self-regulatory processes of thematic neutralization.

## THEMATIC DISINTEGRATION

The brain-directed functional dissection of complex brain-disturbing material into its constituent parts is called *thematic disintegration*. It is assumed that processes of thematic disintegration are manifestations of adaptional exigencies which facilitate a successful engagement in brain-desired neutralization of complex disturbing material (e.g., accidents, traumatic sexual experiences, traumatic medical procedures) by proceeding in a piecemeal fashion. In other words, it appears that brain mechanisms find it undesirable to engage in neutralization of, for example, a "complete picture" all at once, and prefer to break it down into thematic components like a jigsaw puzzle. Then each piece is submitted to thematically adapted processes of neutralization until the entire material is sufficiently neutralized and the brain can present large sections, or the "entire picture," without eliciting undesirable reactions. This brain-designed procedure of thematic disintegration appears to entail a number of functional advantages which facilitate, economize and help to advance the dynamics of thematic neutralization. For example, by engaging in piecemeal neutralization, the original disturbing potency inherent in the "complex picture" is significantly reduced and

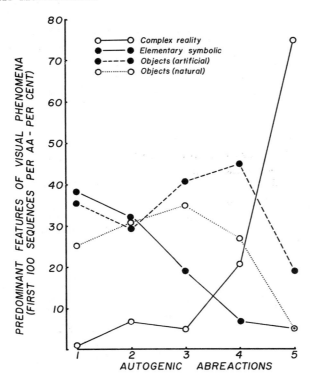

FIG. 16. Progressive increase of reality features in visual elaborations during the first five autogenic abreactions (24-year-old male student, anxiety reaction).

each "piece" can be released and repeated without eliciting undesirable degrees of disturbing reactions and without approaching the systems level of tolerance too closely or causing changes to its own system (e.g., by damaging intensities of unloading). Thematic disintegration also seems to facilitate the release and neutralization of very specific and particularly disturbing thematic elements, without eliciting undue excitation or activation of the functionally associated but yet undesired parts of the same or closely related material. Furthermore, it is hypothesized that the fractioned release of thematic material passes more easily through the existing barriers of resistance and is generally less prone to evoke the patient's apprehension and thus result in mobilization of additional forms of brain-antagonizing resistance. In other words, thematic disintegration and processes of piecemeal neutralization make it easier for the patient to maintain a brain-desired attitude of passive acceptance. Other thematically camouflaging effects which are assumed to facilitate the brain's self-curative work appear to result from patterns of neutralization which are characterized by alternating brief phases of elaborations which emphasize a simultaneous repetition of a variety of "functional fragments" which are released in seemingly random combinations. As such patterns permit efficient simultaneous neutralization of many small, thematically disintegrated pieces, faster progress in brain-desired directions is possible. In the course of advancing piecemeal neutralization, progressively more differentiated and complex pieces appear, and larger reality-related sections become discernible. Finally, like a completed jigsaw puzzle, the entire theme (e.g., car crash) evolves in an undistorted manner. In other words, as autogenic neutralization progresses in piecemeal fashion, there is progressively less need for thematic disintegration and a development toward higher levels of integration (and realism) while progressive functional readjustment can be observed (see Case 126).

*Case 126:* A 29-year-old housewife who was hit by a car while crossing a street (cerebral concussion, multiple contusions and hematomas; see also Case 12, p. 54; Case 79, p. 181; Case 102, p. 242; Case 146, p. 328). The unusually long and difficult neutralization of this accident followed a characteristic pattern of thematic modification with thematic disintegration and alternating phases of piecemeal neutralization. Several examples of passages from different autogenic abreactions reflect the progressively oriented patterns of advancing neutralization.

*From AA 5:* ". . . the car again, but rather blurred . . . now it's all gray . . . I see the sky . . . I see the sky as if I was lying on the pavement of the street . . . the clouds . . . now gradually it is getting gray . . . starts turning . . . turning . . . and now it's gradually becoming brighter . . . it is very bright now . . . and glittering . . . again all gray and turning . . . this sort of hollow empty cavity. . . ."

*From AA 6:* "Now the car again . . . I see the upper part only . . . the hood and the windshield . . . the windshield wiper, shiny and glittering . . . my stomach aches, my left arm hurts quite a bit . . . now I see the lower part . . . the chrome . . . it is very dark under the chrome . . . and I see a shoe, an overshoe, must be my own . . . now the car is in the middle of the road in the snow . . . the street corner . . . and the other corner . . . I feel like turning again . . . I am afraid I am going to fall . . . I have the impression as if I am turning in front of the car . . . it is as if I do a somersault in the air in front of the car . . . the car comes close . . . I only see the car . . . it is dark . . . there are no lights on the car . . . I see the car from a front view, but I don't know where I am . . . I see it from the front . . . and now I am half sitting on the car . . . oh, everything is hurting . . . I have the feeling as

if I am going to drop forward . . . I am lying in front of the car . . . get up . . .
again up on the car . . . down . . . and the car is standing . . . my abdomen
is hurting. . . ."

## THEMATIC DISSOCIATION

When during autogenic neutralization the release or elaboration of
thematic material is characterized by a loss, decrease or weakening of
what may be considered as its normal or original functional context of
thematically related emotional and psychophysiologic reactivity (e.g.,
engaging in neutralization of aggression without experiencing a proportional feeling of aggression; having the impression that the brain-
directed elaborations have nothing to do with oneself), then the term
*thematic dissociation* may be applied. Self-regulatory phenomena of
thematic dissociation are encountered as a consistent feature of various
processes of neutralization at different levels of thematic disintegration
and in association with all kinds of modalities of thematic discharges
or elaborations.

It is assumed that phenomena of thematic dissociation play in combination with other brain-designed dynamics of thematic modification
(e.g., thematic disintegration, thematic distortion) a decisive role in
facilitating advances of thematic neutralization in a brain-desired direction. Furthermore it is hypothesized that the psychophysiologic changes
which are associated with the autogenic state (see Vols. I-VI) and the
patient's attitude of passive acceptance provide particularly favorable
functional conditions for the brain-directed activities which bring about
and which maintain desirable levels of thematic dissociation. Varying
degrees of thematic dissociation are encountered in a great number of thematically related combinations. These range from an apparently absent or
extenuated functional association, response or reactivity with attitudes
of seemingly complete indifference of non-involvement to significantly
less attenuated, reality-related levels of thematic dissociation with variable forms of self-involvement (see Table 44, p. 296).

The level and frequency of thematic dissociations are adapted to the
nature and the disturbing potency of the material selected for neutralization. During initial periods of neutralization of complex and thematically very disturbing material, phenomena of thematic dissociation
are encountered more frequently than during more advanced phases
of thematic neutralization.

Apart from the particular nature of brain-directed elaborations, phenomena of thematic dissociation are also conveyed by the manner in
which the patient formulates his description (i.e., impersonal, sub-

TABLE 44. *Forms and Degrees of Self-Involvement during Autogenic Abreactions Associated with Visual Elaborations*

A. *Direct active self-participation* (e.g., "Now I am opening the window," "I take the knife and stab him," "I am driving down the road")

B. *Passive observation:* being present at the scene, as a bystander who is reacting to, but not directly participating in, the happenings

C. *Indirect self-participation:* watching and describing another self doing something

D. *Passive indirect self-participation:* watching and describing another self who observes yet another self doing something

E. *Passive involvement:* not being actually present on the scene, but rather reacting as one watching a cinerama which concerns him

F. *Indifferent non-involvement:* reacting and describing as one who is watching a film in a disinterested indifferent manner.

junctive: e.g., "One could . . ."; "I could . . .") during the abreactive period, certain statements he makes during the postabreactive discussion, the nature of his commentary and his reactivity during thematically related technical discussions during the preparatory mobilization phase (see Case 127).

*Case 127:* A 35-year-old engineer (moderate depressive reaction). After a 45-minute period, largely focussing on relatively minor incidents of an army camp episode (e.g., being drunk, embarrassing situations at a dance, etc.), the brain gradually shifted to the field of aggression (i.e., games, tossing firecrackers into rooms, water fights). Then followed a long period (51 min.) of aggressive engagement (beating, punching, kicking, killing someone) with many repetitions.

After the autogenic abreaction, the patient wondered why he actually had not experienced any aggressive feelings during this part of the abreactive period (although his voice got quite loud and sharp at times). He remarked also that he might have bottled up some aggression, but nothing of the nature which (according to him) would justify such actions. He wondered whether these aggressive dynamics were "artificial" and had actually very little or nothing to do with him. Further manifestations of thematic dissociation and related forms of resistance were conveyed by the nature of the patient's commentary. While three type-written pages were devoted to comments about the military training episodes, there was no comment on the major part of the abreactive period dealing with violent and vicious aggression. When we attempted to discuss this matter by asking him why he had made no comments on the aggressive material, he misunderstood the therapist's question on four occasions, thus avoiding again any thematically related discussion. Finally, after repeating the same question again, he stated: "No, there is no comment, I did not know what to think of it, I had no ideas."

Dynamics of thematic dissociation and related forms of indirect thematic involvement which may also consist of, for example, description of what others are doing, a certain film shown, a dream depicted or content of stories told by others, are usually characteristic features of thematically-related preparatory phases which tend to be followed by more direct forms of involvement and self-participation. Various patterns of alternating levels of thematic dissociation and different forms of self-involvement (see Table 44) can be more readily observed and studied when processes of thematic neutralization are associated with intermediate and advanced stages of visual elaborations (i.e., stages IV-VII; see Table 33, p. 188).

Depending on the nature of elaborations in the visual field, different degrees of thematic dissociation can be distinguished. During elementary (i.e., I-III) and intermediate (i.e., IV and V) stages, patients frequently wonder if it is at all possible that "these things" have anything to do with them. During filmstrip and film-like elaborations (i.e., stage VI) many patients tend to feel like a describing spectator, who

TABLE 45.   *Dominant Patterns of Various Forms of Self-Involvement during the First and the Second Autogenic Abreaction of Psychosomatic and Neurotic Patients*

| Phases of Autogenic Abreaction | Forms of Self-Involvement (see Table 44, p. 296) (%) | | | | | |
|---|---|---|---|---|---|---|
| | A | B | C | D | E | F |
| *Initial Section of AA* | | | | | | |
| AA 1 (N = 100) | 46.0 | 15.0 | — | — | 5.0 | 2.0 |
| AA 2 (N = 96) | 61.4 | 3.1 | — | — | 8.3 | 5.2 |
| *Central Section of AA* | | | | | | |
| AA 1 (N = 100) | 56.0 | 9.0 | — | 1.0 | 6.0 | 1.0 |
| AA 2 (N = 96) | 68.7 | 2.1 | — | — | 8.3 | 2.1 |
| *Terminal Section of AA* | | | | | | |
| AA 1 (N = 100) | 52.0 | 7.0 | — | — | 6.0 | 2.0 |
| AA 2 (N = 96) | 63.5 | 6.2 | — | — | 9.4 | — |

accepts more readily that the "happenings on the screen" have something to do with him or are actually depicting certain aspects of himself. More direct forms of self-involvement are usually associated with
cinerama-type patterns (i.e., stage VII). However, even when self-participation does occur, it is easy to distinguish different forms and dynamics
of thematic dissociation (see Table 44, p. 296; Fig. 17a and b).

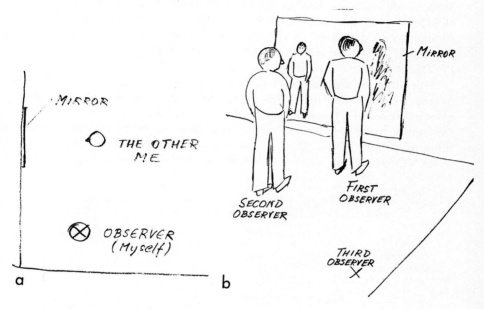

FIG. 17. Examples of indirect selfparticipation.
(a) *Indirect self-participation.* "I stand about ten feet from a mirror, as
    *observer,* right near the wall that the mirror is mounted . . . and I
    vaguely see the image that the other one is seeing, some intangible
    unwelcome image . . . there is a wolfish image. . . ."
(b) *Passive indirect self-participation.* I look at the mirror again . . . the
    face is blackish-brownish . . . and I pretended it was a mask and pulled
    it off . . . and now there is some kind of pink image . . . and the
    *second observer* behind me sees that the *first observer* is myself and the
    second observer is standing slightly behind to one side, and the first and
    the second observer look at the mirror, and the observers see in the
    mirror just the second observer in a distance, not the first observer
    (myself). The *third* observer is watching this, so as the first observer
    (myself) goes away, the second observer disappears, and the third ob-
    server is able to see the second observer in the mirror. . . ."

## Thematic Distortion

The brain-selected release or elaboration of specific elements of more complex brain-disturbing material in combination with other camouflaging elements or elaborations which thematically appear to be of different origin and nature than those which were originally or which are normally integral parts of the particular disturbing material under neutralization is called *thematic distortion* (e.g., during cinerama-type neutralization, a big ferocious bird starts clawing and pecking at precisely the bodily area where the patient sustained lacerations during a motor scooter accident; see also Case 103, p. 243; Case 128). Countless variations of such brain-directed presentations of potent brain-disturbing elements in a disguising, out-of-context manner are a consistent feature of various types of autogenic abreactions. Since our understanding of the exact reasons for these brain-directed phenomena awaits further exploration, it is hypothesized that thematic distortions are a specific category of thematic modifications which, similar to processes of thematic disintegration and dynamics of thematic dissociation, are designed to facilitate thematic neutralization by circumventing existing barriers of resistance and reducing or eliminating the possibility of undesirable arousal of reactive forms of brain-antagonizing resistance (e.g., thematic evasion, abortive engagement, intentional resistance; see Part I, Vol. VI).

From pattern analyses of thematic distortions, which also include elaborations of transferential and paratransferential nature, it was learned that those elements which constitute the distorting camouflaging "wrapping" are not just randomly selected substitutes for certain original or normal thematic components. In most instances these thematically distorting elaborations appear to be composed of disintegrated thematic elements belonging to functionally related areas of disturbing material. This led to the tentative conclusion that the elaboration of thematic distortions also serves as an economizing time-saving device for purposes of preparatory piecemeal neutralization of material which has a different position in the program-related order of thematic priorities. In this connection it appears justified to consider many types of thematic distortions as efficiency-enhancing multithematic products.

*Case 128:* A 24-year-old office girl (anxiety reaction, moderate depression) who at the age of 13 lost control of her bicycle while racing downhill. She suffered multiple contusions and multiple superficial lacerations on both hands and particularly the left arm. While discussing this accident she remarked: "For three or four years after the bike accident I was self-conscious about all the scars. I felt marked and used to put on dresses with long sleeves. I had a terrible complex about it." During several autogenic abreactions, phases of thematic modification (i.e., distortion) containing specific elements of the bike accident and injuries which involved both arms and hands occurred. Since no other events of thematically related nature could be remembered, these brain elaborations were viewed as thematic distortions related to material accumulated in connection with her bicycle accident.

*From AA 16:* "I walk away from the village *down the road* and there is a *huge mountain . . . I keep walking down the road,* and I see a boy coming toward me *on a bicycle* and I hit the boy off the bicycle and take it and ride away . . . and *as I am riding along the road I hit a rock and I fall from the bicycle and I hit my head on the ground . . . I see everything go black when my head hits the ground and when I try to get up I feel very dizzy* so I go over to a little brook and wash my face. . . ."

*From AA 17:* "I see a bear running toward me and I try to run away from him by climbing one of the trees, but the tree is not high enough and the bear pulls me down and starts *ripping me apart* and *I can feel him biting my arms . . .* and I try kicking him, but the more I kick him, the more he bites me . . . finally *I feel myself go weak* and faint and the bear runs away . . . and I drag myself over to the stream to wash myself but *I feel very weak. . . ."*

*From AA 19:* "Then a lightning bolt hits the boardwalk and *the whole thing falls on me* and starts burning . . . but I can't seem to get out fast enough and I get caught in the fire . . . it feels very hot and I try to push all the logs away from me but *each time I touch the logs I burn my hands . . . I feel mostly that my arms are burning . . .* I keep touching the burning logs and then *I feel as if I had a lot of blisters on my hands . . .* and when I had pushed all the logs away from me I ran into the the ocean but *the salt in the water seems to make it worse and I feel my arms and my hands swell up . . .* so I come out of the ocean again and *I can hardly move my arms . . . .* I go into the house on the beach and the two men are still there and *they put some kind of a cream on my arms and it feels very cool and slowly I can feel the swelling go down . . .* one of the men is a policeman. . . ."

*From AA 20:* "I come to a small wooden house, it looks rather old and it is made of round logs . . . the inside of the house is all dirty and there is a table with benches on each side . . . there is a stove in one corner, and I make a fire and the room begins to feel a little bit warmer . . . I sit at the table but it is made of rough wood and *I get all kinds of splinters in my arms . . .* I try to take the splinters out and *my arms feel very sore . . .* then I go and wash them and it feels a little bit better. . . ."

The polythematic nature of many types of thematic distortions may, for example, manifest itself in variations of series of thematic analogies (see p. 302) and a continuity of modifications of antithematic elaborations (see p. 308). The degree and nature of thematic distortions may be regarded as an indicator for the power of brain-antagonizing forces of resistance which are (a) directly associated with the specific theme undergoing neutralization and (b) other inhibitory functions which may interfere through connections with other areas of thematically related material. In other words, in many instances there is evidence that interfering forces of resistance are not limited to the specifis theme in question, but are of heterogenous nature. This may be one of the reasons why, in certain cases, a high degree of thematic distortion is maintained throughout many periods of repetitions of thematic analogies and thematic antitheses. However, as neutralization continues there is a consistent although not linear trend characterized by a decrease of thematic distortion, a decrease of associated forces of resistance and increasing evidence of facilitation of integration-promoting processes aiming at functional readjustment. It is in this respect that a comparison of initially encountered degrees of multithematic distortions with the nature of thematic distortions encountered during later phases of neutralization has been found helpful in evaluating the therapeutic progress.

Thematic distortions as expressed through elaborations in the visual field permit more detailed studies of the dynamics involved. The mechanisms responsible for the elaboration of, for example, color, illumination, structure and dynamic features may or may not be distorted to a different extent. Progressive readjustment toward better agreement with reality may occur in synchronized fashion involving simultaneous changes in all participating variables of visual elaborations or may be restricted to one dimension (e.g., structure; see Case 129). While the reasons for such desynchronized changes of chromatic, dynamic or structural features of visual elaborations remain to be investigated, there exists a very flexible functional interdependence between the various mechanisms participating in the elaborations of visual phenomena. This observation led to the assumption that a highly differentiated coordinating mechanism, at a higher level of functional integration (hypothetical Reality Mechanism) determines the degree of reality relatedness of, for example, chromatic structural or dynamic elaborations at lower levels of functional integration with great precision and selectivity. It is in this respect that further investigation of the appearance, modification and disappearance of thematic distortions in the area of visual elaborations may provide information which may advance our understanding of certain abnormal and normal dynamics in other areas of mental function.

# 23. Thematic Analogies

Phasic processes of neutralization characterized by sequences of thematic elaborations which resemble each other thematically in one or more ways but which differ in other respects are called *thematic analogies* (see Fig. 18, p. 304).

Such thematic analogies may be of variable complexity and may, depending on the nature of their central theme, emphasize a repetition of psychodynamically or psychophysiologically oriented elements of brain-disturbing thematic (or antithematic) material.

This type of sophisticated thematic repetition tends to advance toward brain-desired functional readjustment by sticking to elaborations which are recognizable as closely interrelated versions of the central theme of neutralization, and by combining such repetitions of thematically central elements with complementary elaborations which appear to be essential for facilitating and promoting further progress along the main line of thematic neutralization (see Case 129).

*Case 129:* A 36-year-old priest (personality disorder, homosexuality, ecclesiogenic syndrome). In this case the brain-directed elaborations were initially very slow and largely restricted to intermediate stages of differentiation (see Table 33, p. 188) with a prominent lack of dynamic features. Of particular interest is the pattern of thematic analogies and the progressive trend from initial, largely symbolic elaborations to less disguised more direct confrontations which also include an increasing brain-directed emphasis on heterosexual features.

| **The patient's description as recorded during AA 5** | **The patient's commentary (homework)** |
|---|---|
| "I see a tree planted in a flower pot, there's dirt inside it. . . . | "This is probably a recollection of trees I planted at my cottage in early spring. The fact that this tree is planted in a flower pot could symbolize my actual frame of mind which is stifling and preventing me from giving my full capacity. [*Comment*\*: *avoidance of sexual interpretation*]. |
| For example, I see church columns holding up the roof . . . I see something like the summits of buildings or church steeples. . . . | These summits and steeples symbolize the high ideal that I've traced for myself and that I'm forever trying to attain. [*Avoidance of sexual interpretation*]. |

---

\* By therapist.

**The patient's description as recorded during AA 5**

**The patient's commentary (homework)**

I see a bridge seemingly passing overhead, this bridge is very high, it's held up by enormous structures. . . .

This bridge could symbolize a penis. These giant structures holding it up could symbolize the lack of security that I experience when I go up on a bridge or on an elevated highway.

I see a man in front of me, I especially notice his shirt and tie . . . I see another one here whose shirt is opened at the top. . . .

This man before me whose shirt and tie I particularly notice refers to my homosexual behavior. According to the shirt and tie a boy wears, I can judge him and know in advance what his sexual behavior is.

I see someone lying down on a hospital bed. . . .

It's the impression I kept of a person I visited recently in a hospital; she was in bed. [*First heterosexual confrontation*].

I see a very high steeple standing out against the sky; it gives the effect of a rather dark shape against a lighter-toned sky. . . .

I see an outdoor fountain in a circular shape; birds are drinking out of it. . . .

It's a recollection of the fountains I saw in Europe mostly; ones that I would have liked to see near my summer cottage.

I see mushrooms, there are many, they're quite large. . . .

These mushrooms symbolize penises and my desire to see many of them.

I see ocean waves coming up on the shore, washing up on the sand, then retreating. . . .

These waves are recollections of the ocean and waves in San Juan. [*Place where the patient had homosexual relations*].

I see woman's breasts forming two circles. . . .

As in previous trips, these breasts could symbolize the desire to really see a woman's breasts, to touch and caress them. [*Second heterosexual confrontation*].

Now there aren't too many shapes or designs . . . I see a hand, it clenches, I now see a fist. . . .

This clenched fist is probably referring to the punches I received from a person at whom I had made homosexual advances in a Turkish bath; this time I came back with two black eyes.

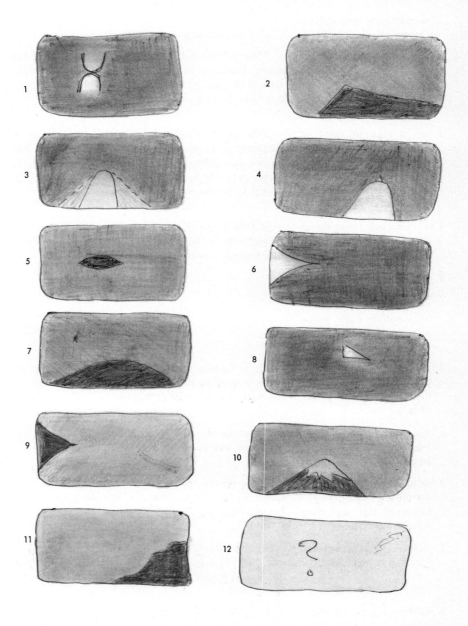

FIG. 18. Thematic analogies in visual elaborations during elementary stage III (AA 7, 30-year-old male patient, personality disorder, sexual deviation, posttraumatic anxiety reaction).

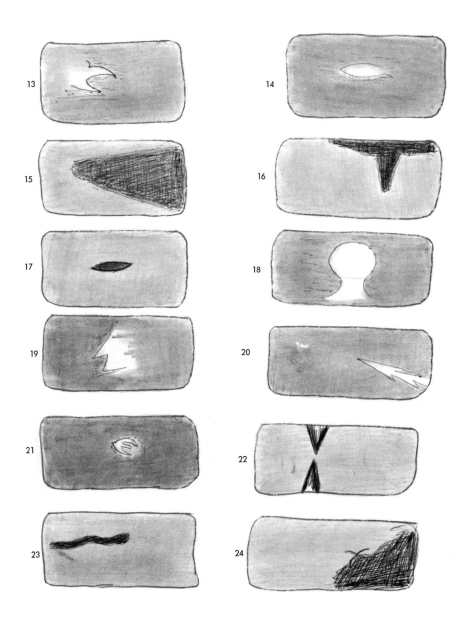

**The patient's description
as recorded during AA 5**

**The patient's commentary (homework)**

I see someone standing overhead looking down at me. . . .

I see the breasts of a woman who is advancing toward me; the nipples are very tiny, they form buttons. . . .

A repetition. [*Third heterosexual confrontation*].

I see a man's huge penis, it's in erection, its tip is rather like a mushroom, it's just above me, it's very big, the tip is shiny. . . .

There is certainly a link between the woman's nipple as described in detail in the preceding paragraph and the tip of the penis as described in this paragraph. [*Analogy between the tip of the nipple and that of the penis*].

I now see the penis entering the woman's body through the vagina. . . .

This description indicates my desire to see a penis entering a woman's vagina. This description also indicates my desire to have intercourse with a woman. [*Fourth heterosexual confrontation*].

I seem to see an immense candle placed upright. . . ."

It symbolizes a penis in erection."

Sequences of thematic analogies may be associated with variable degrees of thematic modifications (e.g., disintegration, dissociation, distortion) and thematically contrasting elements of antithematic nature (see Case 131 ff.; see p. 308 ff.). Depending on the prevailing pattern of neutralization, thematic analogies may be restricted to, for example, intellectual elaborations or to an emphasis on certain physiologically oriented modalities (e.g., falling, sliding down, sinking, turning, swinging, spinning, dizziness; sensory: olfactory, auditory, gustatory). When dynamics of thematic analogies are associated with visual elaborations, they may occur at different stages of structural, chromatic and dynamic differentiation (e.g., stages III-VII; see Table 33, p. 188), and may be of monothematic or multithematic nature. However, independent from the prevailing stages of visual elaborations (e.g., elementary, highly differentiated), thematic analogies tend to be increasingly associated with antithematic elements or alternating sequences of progressively more complex antithematic elaborations (see p. 308 ff.) as the brain-directed processes of thematic neutralization keep advancing toward functionally desirable levels of functional integration. When further advanced levels of neutralization are reached, the initial functional importance of thematic analogies and contrasting antithematic elaborations seems to decrease as higher degrees of thematic and dynamic flexibility result from progressive processes of neutralization.

*Case 130:* A 36-year-old male patient (personality disorder, sexual deviation, anxiety reaction, mild depression, ecclesiogenic syndrome). The following passages of AA 5 are characteristic of thematic analogies and the role of thematically related associative functions which seem to participate in linking different episodes from various phases of the patient's past.

"I see us (13-14 years old) fooling around with our penises, our pants are down, and we're on a sofa . . . and again on another occasion when their little maid was about our age . . . she was with a girl friend. . . . Michael and I were in the basement, we were talking about the penis . . . I was shy because of the girls, but Michael seemed to be much bolder, and finally the girls seemed to be daring us to show them our organ, which we did . . . it ended as such . . . the image remains fixed. . . . I now find myself on the back porch at home . . . I'm doing little odd jobs in the shed . . . my memory brings me back to when I was about seven or eight years old, wanting to cut some wire, I used an ax instead of getting a pair of pliers. The result was that of cutting the thumb that was holding the wire on the log, because when I went to chop with the ax, it missed and struck my thumb . . . I went into the house to wash my wound, I didn't feel any pain as I washed it under cold water; the tip of my thumb hanging, I went to show it to mother who somewhat panicked. . . . We left immediately for St. Mary's Hospital. . . . I see myself later on when my thumb had healed, the nail was gone . . . the surface of the tip was rough . . . I was told to be careful about infection because I often played in the sand with my toys. . . . Again I see the scene when the ax hit my thumb. . . and I drop everything and go inside the house . . . I don't seem to be suffering; and I recalled the dressings, that they put on at the hospital, that resembled a 'dolly' . . . I see myself on our street at the foot of the staircase . . . and I see myself in a doctor's office where there is talk that I would have to be circumcised . . . after some discussion, I chose to be hospitalized rather than having the operation done in the doctor's office. . . . Upon my return from the hospital, some friends who had just bought a cottage up north invited me to join them . . . it was a pal with whom I had often masturbated . . . we knew each other quite well, therefore he was well aware of my circumcision. . . . The problem of urinating in bed during the night somewhat bothered me, I was not going out because of this . . . I informed him as well as his parents . . . they agreed to have me come to the cottage with their children. We were 16 or 17 years old. . . . I mention all this because Andre wanted to see what a circumcision looked like . . . his brother as well, younger by two years . . . I see myself in the bedroom at the cottage showing them my bandages, and we commented on how big my finger was, and they somewhat laughed at me . . . I see their older brother's face who was a priest and. . . ."

# 24. Thematic Antitheses

A brain-directed change of thematic elaborations to other elaborations, the nature of which are the opposite of the preceding ones is called *antithematic shift*.

The contrasting element or combination which determines the opposite nature of the new sequence of neutralization is distinguished as *thematic antithesis*. Antithematic elaborations are encountered at various levels of thematic complexity. They may be limited to one particular thematic element (e.g., darkness to brightness; descending to ascending, swelling to shrinking), or they may consist of synchronized antithematic changes involving a certain number of psychodynamically or psychophysiologically oriented thematic elements. Accordingly, a technical distinction between monodimensional and multidimensional antithematic changes is indicated. Antithematic elaborations may be of very brief duration (e.g., Case 131) or they may take up larger portions of an abreactive period (e.g., Case 132, p. 310 ff.).

*Case 131:* A 38-year-old priest (personality disorder, sexual deviation, ecclesiogenic syndrome). The following passages (AA 14) reflect the dynamics of thematic antitheses (A, B) in still relatively restricted visual elaborations.

"Now it's a rather dark gray, uniform gray . . . I see a darker circle (A) . . . it's rather uniform . . . in the center there seeme to be a lighter circle (B) . . . it's uniform . . . I see what seems to be a circle surrounded by a much bigger circle (A) . . . I see the tip of a uncovered penis (B) . . . now there's no picture . . . there's absolutely nothing definite . . . I see (A) the end of a pipe, this image disappears . . . now I see (B) what seems to be a tent with an opened flap, it seems to be in darkness, it seems to be night (A) . . . now it's somber . . . now it's as if I was sleeping out in the open, and there seems to be sunshine (B), and I see the sky above me, which has absolutely no clouds, it seems quite clear and sunny (A) . . . now I see myself under an enormous mass which could be a stone or it's as if I was underneath a building (B) . . . it's uniform gray. . . ."

In many instances the antithematic elaborations appear to be associated with either distinctively positive connotations or distinctively negatively ones. Since the mainstream of processes of autogenic neutralization focusses on brain-disturbing material and consequently is prone to be negatively loaded (e.g., difficult, disagreeable, disgusting, unpleasant), it has become a technically not quite justified (see Case 132; ,Table 11, p. 57) practice to apply the term *antithematic shift*, particularly to changes from negatively loaded to positively oriented (e.g., agreeable, pleasant, relaxing, easy, recuperative) elaborations.

TABLE 46. *Examples of Thematic Antitheses*

| | | | |
|---|---|---|---|
| Above | Below | Frustrating | Satisfying |
| Afraid | Courageous | Hell | Heaven |
| Aggressive | Affectionate | Historic | Ultra-modern |
| Artificial | Natural | Homesexual | Heterosexual |
| Bad weather | Pleasant weather | Indoors | Outdoors |
| Black | White | Left | Right |
| Child | Adult | Masculine | Feminine |
| Close | Far away | Masochistic | Sadistic |
| Cold | Warm | Old | Young |
| Confined | Free | Passive | Active |
| Dark | Light | Round | Angular |
| Dead | Alive | Static | Dynamic |
| Depressive | Joyful | Stress | Recuperation |
| Descending | Ascending | Tension | Relaxation |
| Deserted | Crowded | Turbulent | Calm |
| Dirty | Clean | Vagina | Penis |
| Disagreeable | Pleasant | Weak | Strong |
| Dressed | Naked | Wet | Dry |
| Dwarfed | Gigantic | Winter | Summer |

Agreeable, relaxing and in a larger technical sense positively oriented antithematic (as far as its contrast with the bulk of the preceding material is concerned) phases tend to be purposefully interjected during processes of neutralization which are particularly disagreeable and demanding, and after a certain brain-desired progress has been achieved. Such temporarily agreeable, calming and relaxing antithematic phases appear to have a recuperative purpose which also seems to function as an encouraging stimulus to the patient to continue the largely disagreeable autogenic abreaction. Particularly pleasant antithematic phases are frequently followed by particularly disagreeable sequences of neutralization of very disturbing material. In such cases the preceding positively loaded antithematic elaborations appear to perform a preparatory task which seems to facilitate the subsequent presentation of a heavily negatively loaded topic.

The brain-programmed "strategic interjection" of such agreeable, calming and otherwise positively oriented antithematic elaborations during the central abreactive phase may sometimes lead to the erroneous conclusion that these phenomena are brain-directed indications that the terminal phase has been reached and the termination procedure can be applied. To avoid the error of inadequate premature technical termination, it is advisable to remain patient and to wait and see what is going to happen. If the brain wishes to continue with neutralization of disturbing material, it will indicate its course of action within less than two minutes. If the brain really wishes to terminate its work for the time, and brain-antagonizing resistance can be reasonably excluded, brain-directed elaborations as characteristic for *delayed termination* (see p. 84 ff.) will confirm the earlier impression that the autogenic abreaction can be terminated.

*Case 132:* A 50-year-old priest (anxiety reaction, multiple psychophysiologic reactions, ecclesiogenic syndrome). In the following passages of cinerama-type elaborations, thematic analogies and elements of thematic antitheses are used in a very loose pattern of flexible combinations as processes of neutralization (i.e., burning in hell) continue to proceed with thematic repetitions. Of further interest is a transitory, very positively oriented antithematic Bright Light Phase with unusual dynamic features.

"Now I'm falling into flames . . . I'm falling into the fire . . . it's not too hot . . . it's not as much the flames as . . . it's as if the air was, was red . . . the air was white . . . it's as if it was the air . . . and I go down into this sort of luminous air . . . I'm going down . . . my body has started burning . . . nice . . . I have nice brown skin . . . I go down into that . . . now I spread my arms out again, and I'm soaring in this sort of incandescent air . . . it's not unpleasant, it's not too hot . . . I turn over on my back, I'm getting my back tanned . . . I turn over on my stomach, I'm getting my stomach tanned . . . I'm soaring about in there . . . of course it'll be hotter down there . . . so I kick and plunge downward . . . I plunge down another few hundred feet . . . because of the rubbing as I go down, my head is in flames . . . but I don't feel anything . . . my head is in flames . . . so I soar some more . . . now I'm closer . . . and now I feel that . . . I'm no longer brownish, I turn deep brown. I turn black from the fire there . . . and now I plunge down into it . . . it's liquid fire . . . and I plunge in with a splash, a splash that becomes one of sparks, of flames, in this liquid fire . . . and I'm swimming in the liquid fire . . . I'm submerged in the liquid fire . . . I can swim in this . . . I can swim like I could in water . . . like we swim in a swimming pool, like I swim in a swimming pool . . . now I'm doing some deep-sea diving in this liquid fire . . . it's very clear . . . my body is entirely black . . . I'm still very much alive in this . . . I can swim with agility . . . I'm swimming with agility, I see . . . it's as if I was making a projection, I was seeing my body entirely black, very limber in this, this liquid flame . . . my body is fooling around in there, taking all sort of postures . . . I dive into the bottom, I come back up, I float, I swim on my back, I swim backwards, I spin around in there, a sort of agility to swim in that liquid fire . . . it's not at all unpleasant . . . I notice that my body is all black . . . It's a beautiful black body, very limber, stretched out, muscular . . . and now I decide to go down a bit deeper . . . so I take my submarine stroke, if you can call it that, and I go down head first all while kicking with my feet and stroking with my arms . . . I'm going down and I'm going down . . . now it looks like . . . it's . . . it's fire that's much clearer, that becomes white, luminous. . . . Now I'm surrounded by air or a liquid that's extremely dazzling . . . it's really beautiful . . . it's really beautiful . . . it's as if I was swimming in . . . swimming in . . . a sort of pool of diamonds . . . diamonds that sparkle

. . . I'm swimming in this dazzlement . . . dazzlement of luminous diamonds . . . they're not diamonds, but the fact that I'm passing through there makes the fire still more luminous . . . it's dazzling to swim in there . . . I'm moving ahead horizontally, and I'm trying to swim faster . . . it's as if instead of having air bubbles, there are bubbles . . . there are . . . there are diamond sparkles . . . it's really dazzling to swim in there . . . it's very beautiful . . . all I have to do is make a stirring up motion and before me I see very luminous things . . . it's very beautiful, and I'm swimming along in there . . . it's very beautiful . . . it's very pleasant . . . I'm swimming horizontally, and I decide to go down a bit farther . . . I go down a bit deeper there *it's as if it was pure light* . . . it's not as much fire as it is light . . . so I swim in the light . . . again it becomes . . . when I make motions, the splashes are of an extraordinary clearness . . . they're almost like crystals of light, coming about when I make motions in this sort of substance . . . it's not hot, no . . . it's rather nice . . . it's not at all unpleasant. . . . I get an inkling that it's the end of that because I'm beginning to see a sort of black hole . . . in fact there's less and less light . . . my body is less and less black, it took on its normal color, somewhat brownish, clearer . . . and I'm approaching this opening . . . it was between the rocks, and it's of the most absolute black, the most somber . . . and now I've passed from this layer of light which is now above me . . . again I've passed into a black abyss, into the bottomless pit . . . I'm diving into it now with more . . . with more courage, with more interest . . . I decide to fall into it head first . . . and I'm helping myself with swimming strokes to plung down as rapidly as possible . . . I'm moving along, I'm moving along head first at a vertiginous speed, extremely fast . . . I feel the air, if it's air, brushing against my body and whistling . . . I'm like a whistling meteor . . . I'm going down diagonally . . . I'm going down, I'm going down, I'm going down . . . it's not like a little while ago . . . a while ago I was letting myself sink, but now I'm directing myself downward . . . and now with all the energies that I have at my disposal, by movements of the arms, by movements of the feet, I go down, I go down . . . I'm aiming something, I'm aiming something . . . I'm aiming down below . . . I go down below, I put all my strength into it, and it goes down fast . . . I'm aiming . . . I don't see anything, but it's as if I was aiming something . . . I'm going to it in a direct line. . . ."

Similar to strategically interjected agreeable but preparatory phases which tend to occur during the central part of the abreactive period before particularly disturbing material is released are unusually peaceful, agreeable elaborations which may continue throughout an autogenic abreaction (e.g., 20-35 min.). When such prolonged processes of antithematic dynamics occur in the beginning of treatment with autogenic abreaction, they may be considered as an encouraging prelude for disagreeable and difficult material to come. To avoid the undue onset of unfavorable psychodynamic and psychophysiologic reactions which are related to the disturbing material to come, the interim period should be kept short (e.g., 2-4 days) and supportive medication prescribed (e.g., chlordiazepoxide, 10 mg., b.i.d.; meprobamate 400 mg., b.i.d.) for prophylactic reasons.

Apart from the recuperative, encouraging and presumably preparatory role of agreeable, positively loaded antithematic elaborations, thematic antitheses seem to fulfill other brain-designed functions.

Information obtained from pattern analyses indicate that psychophysiologically and psychodynamically oriented mono- or multidimensional antithematic changes tend to undergo a certain number of repetitions. During such repetitions progressively oriented mono- or multidimensional modifications ensue. Associated with such thematic and antithematic modifications is what may be called a "narrowing of the gap" of initially existing phenomena of antithematic contrast. In other words, antithematic elaborations appear to play a role in facilitating developments toward brain-desired functional readjustment, and as progress in this direction is made, the contrast effect of antithematic elaborations decreases and finally disappears. Occasionally these positively oriented reintegrative developments are accompanied by corresponding elaborations as, for example, a double image with synchronized presentation of the contrasting elements (Case 137, p.   ) which may fuse or melt into each other, or simply continue with the brain-preferred combinations of thematic elements by making the antithematic counterpart disappear (see Case 131).

*Case 133:* A 37-year-old technician (homosexuality, hypothyroidism, ecclesiogenic syndrome). During advanced phases of progressive neutralization of homosexual dynamics, the brain engages in thematic antitheses alternating between homosexual and heterosexual themes. In the following passage, a cinerama-type pattern with active self-participation focuses on confrontation, contact and exploration of female genitals. A thematic shift induces confrontations with the antithesis (masculine genitals) which elicits rejection, and is followed by a synchronized elaboration of antithematic elements in the form of an integration-promoting double image (female and male body). The masculine image disappears while the confrontation with the female body continues and is followed by a shift toward a brain-desired reality-related heterosexual development.

"I caress her legs with my hands and I find her skin very soft, and I move up to her thighs, and I stop just after having stroked the hairs of the vagina, and she doesn't seem offended by this gesture, but doesn't seem to appreciate it any more than that, then with the tip of my second finger, I penetrate the vagina to rub the clitoris, and suddenly I draw it out and briskly rub her hairs and I give her little pats on the vagina and the image remains fixed. . . . Now it's the image of a naked man instead of the woman . . . his penis is in erection and I believe that I'm angry at seeing it as such . . . and with the back of my hand I slap his penis . . . and I go on slapping his penis for a good while and I want him to disappear. . . . Now there are two images, a close-up of the one with the naked man arguing with the one of the naked woman . . . and it's the woman that stays on . . . and I observe her for a long time . . . and I find myself in a studio at Radio St. Laurent, and I see a woman announcer to whom I'm paying compliments for her beautifully tanned complexion. . . ."

Processes of brain-directed neutralization focussing on elements or combinations of elements which may be considered as belonging into the complex topics of "love and hate" may be subject to alternating patterns of antithematic nature during sufficiently advanced phases of neutralization of negatively loaded brain-disturbing material. With the exception of patterns which aim at neutralization of brain-disturbing material related to specific interpersonal situations (or periods) characterized by a relative or absolute affective and sexual deprivation by engaging in thematically relevant dynamics of love-making, the brain-designed sequence of thematic priorities emphasizes engagement in negatively interfering variables as, for example, thematically related anxiety or aggression. Antithematic elaborations (e.g., affection, love-making) only occur after brain-desired levels of neutralization of the negatively interfering variables has been achieved. A transitory occurrence of alternating sequences (e.g., aggression–affection–aggression–affection) indicates that the level of neutralization of, for example, aggressive material is still insufficient.

Of further interest are antithematic dynamics which involve a contrasting shift of the direction (or object) of the same thematic material (e.g., aggression against dead objects–aggression against other persons–aggression against oneself; masturbating animals–masturbating others–masturbating oneself). As different degrees of thematic dissociation (see p. 295 ff.) and variable forms of self-involvement (see Table 44, p. 296) tend to play a significant role in the specific monodimensional or synchronized multidimensional features of the antithematic directional shift, highly variable combinations of antithematic changes have been observed. In this connection, it is, however, important to remember that adequate levels of thematic neutralization are rarely reached in cases where brain-antagonizing forms of resistance do not permit *direct active self-participation* (see Table 44, p.    ), including the relevant dynamics of alternating antithematic directional shifts (e.g., killing oneself). Of particular therapeutic, positively oriented significance are brain-directed (not patient- or therapist-directed) antithematic shifts which imply a change from a passive dependent role (e.g., being tortured by devils, being eaten up by beasts) to an active independent mastering role (e.g., beating the devils, rendering the beasts inoffensive; see Case 121, p. 278).

# 25. Thematic Anticipation

Brain-designed programming of thematic neutralization also provides a mechanism which, foreseeing its own course of action, provides advance notice before relevant material or dynamics are released and assume more concrete forms. This brain-determined type of thematic forewarning permits an anticipatory response which is specifically related to the following somehow expected yet unknown thematic sequence of neutralization. When brain-designed elaborations of thematic anticipation are interjected during developments which are going to be potentially disturbing, patients may state: "I have the impression that this and this is going to happen." Thematic anticipation is considered a specific brain-designed maneuver which aims at reduction and elimination of brain-antagonizing surprise reactions, thereby providing a possibility of adjustment with increase of the patient's level of tolerance during subsequent tension-producing phases of thematic neutralization. In this manner the brain facilitates its own program-related course of self-curative action by actively supporting the patient's attitude of passive acceptance and reducing the possibility of producing forms of resistance.

Apart from anticipatory reactions which may occur before the beginning of an autogenic abreaction as, for example, during the *immediate preabreactive phase* (see p. 162), three types of thematic anticipation may be distinguished: (a) anticipatory reactions occurring during or directly after the induction phase, (b) anticipatory reactions in multiple choice situations occurring during processes of neutralization, and (c) specific anticipatory reactions which are interjected directly prior to relevant thematic elaborations.

When anticipatory reactions occur during the induction phase or during the latent period, they are associated with one particular or several apparently different themes which cross the patient's mind (e.g., the dream of two nights ago, certain themes of the last autogenic abreaction, friction in the office). During this period of preparatory thematic scanning, when the functions participating in desirable passive acceptance are still relatively unstable, anticipatory reactions may facilitate the subsequent engagement in certain topics; or the expectancy of certain thematic developments may block the brain-desired thematic neutralization to a variable extent and for variable periods of time (see p. 114, *anticipatory resistance*). When brain-antagonizing anticipatory resistance is activated, the brain usually attempts to present the same theme in a more camouflaged manner, in order to follow and maintain its priority-related program of thematic neutralization (see Case 134).

*Case 134:* A 40-year-old male patient (sexual deviation, psychophysiologic reaction, gastrointestinal system). After the induction phase, the patient's thoughts focussed repeatdly on homosexual themes which were put aside (anticipatory resistance). Then the brain presents as a facilitating maneuver the innocuous looking Fletcher's Field (a large park), which initially also elicits a negative anticipatory reaction and is only accepted after a period of indecision. It is assumed that the first negative anticipatory reaction facilitated the acceptance of the second thematic approach (Fletcher's Field) which appeared to be less clearly connected with homosexual material.

*"I was entertaining the idea . . . seeing what would happen by fooling around with males which whom I have social contact now . . . I put it aside . . . I have a vague image of Fletcher's Field . . . I'm undecided . . . I try Fletcher's Field . . . I vaguely have an image of myself at ten . . .* and this little boy returns from Fletcher's Field to an Orphan's Home . . . and he is in front of the basement toilet . . . and there is an older boy . . . I'm 7 or 8 and he is 11 or 12 . . . we are both in the W. C. . . ." (the subsequent part of this autogenic abreaction focusses on neutralization of homosexual material).

Similar to elaborations of thematic anticipation occurring before the actual beginning of engagement in thematic neutralization, anticipatory reactions can be observed during processes of neutralization, when the brain produces situations which leave the patient with the impression that he can choose the thematic nature of the developments to follow (see Case 134; Case 135). For example, the patient walks down a corridor and then comes to the end with the choice of turning left or right. Anticipatory reactions manifested by hesitancy and indecision at this junction may be related to the associated thematic significance of left (e.g., all sinners go left to hell) and right (e.g., to heaven). Since the brain will pursue its program-related course of thematic neutralization of disturbing material anyway (whether the patient turns right or left), the elaboration of such interjected multiple choice situations are considered to assume the functionally facilitating role of thematic anticipation by permitting thematically related adjustments through, for example, delay, hesitancy, and decision-making.

*Case 135:* A 40-year-old male patient (sexual deviation, psychophysiologic reaction, gastrointestinal system). The passages below reflect characteristics of thematic anticipation in association with brain-designed multiple-choice situations.

"I slit open the tip of the condom-shaped stomach and out drops an object . . . it has the same size of the thing which came out of the box . . . it looks like an enlarged chestnut . . . about one foot across by ten inches high . . . my stomach shrivels back to normal . . . *I have two notions: (A) I cut it open and out flies a genie, and (B) I stamp on the chestnut, once, and out flies a gray smoke . . . I wait* . . . I take a knife and slit the top of it . . . it is hollow . . . as I part the opening, a wisp of gray smoke swooshed out . . . it's conical-shaped, with the apex pointing toward the floor . . . this is a thriller . . . I could investigate the room, but I follow the smoke . . . it's hovering in front of me. . . ."

In other instances, during straight-forward developments of thematic neutralization, when the brain intends to release particularly disturbing thematic material with self-destructive involvement, there is no choice situation, but merely a brief and specific forewarning of the events to come. The anticipatory response elicited by such interjected thematically specific preparatory elaborations are usually favorable and produce a facilitating mental attitude of readiness for the anticipated developments (see Case 136; Case 137; Case 138).

*Case 136:* A 26-year-old female teacher (anxiety reaction, moderate depressive reaction). During neutralization of accident material, the elaboration of self-destructive dynamics is facilitated by brain-designed thematic anticipation.
"Suddenly I see myself come sliding back down on this diagonal path . . . sliding coming straight for me . . . a terrible look on my face . . . completely disfigured out of fright . . . whatever it is I don't know . . . surrounded with rays of yellow, yellow phases, everything in a kind of a yellow shade . . . *I'm just standing there and I'm not going to budge . . . it's coming right for me and I'm going to just let it . . . the anticipation seems to be building up . . . anticipation of knowing what is going to happen* . . . suddenly this just crashes into me . . . an explosion of light rays of all sorts . . . the other me seems to have come back and integrated with the other me just standing there calmly . . . all the light has dimmed . . . there's more of a very calm predusk tone all around . . . I look calm and quiet, perhaps too much so . . . I know I feel better. . . ."

*Case 137:* A 50-year-old priest (obsessive-compulsive reactions, multiple psychophysiologic reactions, ecclesiogenic syndrome). The following passages contain two phases of thematic anticipation which appear to facilitate the continuation toward brain-desired neutralization of dynamics of self-destruction.
"Now I am suspended by my two arms in this tower . . . *I'd have to leave go . . . I'm hesitating a bit . . . I might hurt myself on the walls* . . . will I let go? I let go and I start falling . . . I'm falling very fast, I'm falling very fast . . . every once in a while I feel the walls . . . I'm still falling, I'm still falling . . . *I'm afraid of falling on spikes* . . . in fact, I fall on spikes, pales . . . I'm impaled . . . it hurts me . . . they go in from the back and I feel them coming out of my throat . . . my throat feels caught because I'm impaled. . . I was really impaled . . . I'm immobilized . . . I'm impaled inside of there . . . I'm going to rot here. . . ."

*Case 138:* A 27-year-old research worker (anxiety reaction, obsessive-compulsive manifestations, habit disturbance, ecclesiogenic syndrome). A preparatory phase of thematic neutralization is interjected during thematic developments which aim at neutralization of anxiety related to his father's death. This is thematically associated with a very disturbing childhood episode (thematic analogy) and neutralization of inadequate identification.

"I see my father walking on the grass . . . his head is bending low . . . he looks so anguished . . . *and I have the impression he could fall and die . . .* and this is what happens . . . he falls down and seems to be dead . . . and I go up to him . . . and I see his glasses and his moustache . . . I try to lift him up . . . I let him drop, and he's inanimate, and I have the impression that he's dead . . . I find all of this very cold . . . I see him on the ground again, and it reminds me of something that happened during my childhood . . . I was five or six years old and one evening one of my friends came to get my father who wasn't there, and he told my mother that his father had fallen . . . and that he was having a heart attack . . . and he was in the other house . . . he was still lying there when I arrived in the other house . . . and it upset me quite a bit . . . and I'm still on the grass and Dad is still lying there. . . ."

# 26. Thematic Progression and Regression

During various types of autogenic abreactions (see p. 49), processes of neutralization progress from combinations of thematic elaborations which are less complex in the beginning to thematic combinations which become more complex as neutralization continues. As this trend of *functional progression* reaches a certain brain-determined point, the progressive development stops, a *functional regression* to less complex elaborations occurs, and another phase of functional progression follows. Such alternating phases of functional progression and regression may be repeated a variable number of times. Associated with the increasing number of repetitions of phases of functional progression and regression, a general trend toward increasingly more complex and more positively oriented thematic features can be noted (see Fig. 19). Such patterns may involve motor, vestibular, affective or visual elaborations of thematic elements. The particular phenomenon of brain-directed arrest of progression in association with a drastic cutback of thematic elaborations distinguishes this pattern from the other dynamics of thematic repetition.

Although it is evident that patterns of alternating functional progression and regression are progressively advancing in a brain-desired positively oriented direction and appear to serve a neutralization-facilitating purpose, no satisfactory hypothesis concerning the brain-directed alternation of functional progression and regression can be offered at this point. Since similar phenomena of functional regression can be observed after interference of brain-antagonizing forms of resistance, it was initially believed that the peculiar pattern of thematic progression and regression also resulted from brain-antagonizing forms of resistance. However, more detailed studies in this area did not support this assumption. Further investigations are required to elucidate the reasons why certain brain-mechanisms desire or need an end to functional progression and prefer an interjection of functional regression.

Patterns characterized by serial repetitions of alternating phases of functional progression and drastic regression tend to have a frustrating effect on patients who are inclined to think that they are doing something wrong. In such cases, after participation of brain-antagonizing forms of resistance (see Part I, Vol. VI) has been excluded, it is therapeutically important to encourage the patient to go along with these

318

brain-desired patterns and to maintain an attitude of passive acceptance. After variable periods, phenomena of drastic functional regression
tend to occur less frequently and appear to give way to functionally
and thematically more flexible dynamics of neutralization.

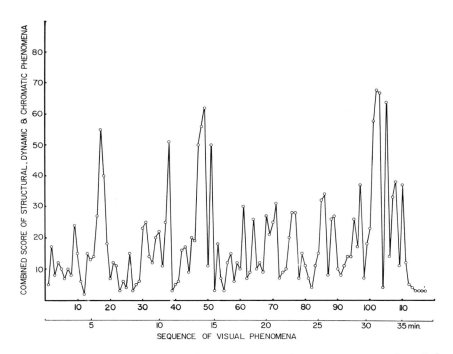

FIG. 19. Phases of functional progression and regression as reflected by
combined scores of structural, dynamic and chromatic components of 116
thematic sequence of consecutive visual elaborations (see also Fig. 8, p. 190;
Color Plate 4).

# 27. Thematic Resynchronization and Integration

It is assumed that a number of centrally coordinated brain functions participate in complex processes which aim at resynchronization and functional integration of thematic material which, for neutralization-facilitating purposes, have undergone thematic modifications (e.g., thematic disintegration, p. 292 ff.). This assumption is supported by ample evidence which is furnished by the brain itself as processes of autogenic neutralization are allowed to pursue their self-curative work of functional readjustment. Phenomena of thematic resynchronization and progressively advancing functional reintegration occur at different levels of psychodynamically or psychophysiologically oriented thematic dynamics as the brain-disturbing potency of certain thematic elements or an entire topic is reduced through processes of neutralization. Initially disintegrated, dissociated, thematically distorted, desynchronized, unrealistic and bizarre elaborations invariably show a progressive trend toward functional readjustment, brain-desired normalization and positively oriented reality. Whether this concerns brain-disturbing sexual deviations, depressive reactions, accident material or combinations of these and other brain-disturbing topics does not matter. The brain-desired progressive trend in self-normalizing direction is the same. This is reflected by gradual changes of the nature of brain-directed elaborations of thematic phases, of smaller sections, of larger parts, of entire autogenic abreactions and by the progressive orientation of longer series of autogenic abreactions. As initially prominent thematic elements lose their disturbing quality, they disappear from the brain-designed program of neutralization or they assume a more normal or adequate functional role in combination with other brain-desired thematic elements. Occasionally such developments are depicted by short sequences of double images (see Case 133, p. 312; Case 139, p. 320; see Vol. VI), double filmstrips (see Vol. VI), or series of simultaneously elaborated pictures as they may occur during phases of thematic verification (see Case 141, p. 322; Case 144, p. 327; Case 145, p. 327; Case 146, p. 328). Clinical improvements, gradual adjustment of disturbed behavior patterns, changes in attitude, increase of efficiency, productivity and creativity are considered as secondary manifestations of progressively oriented changes occurring during, and resulting from, autogenic abreactions (see Vol. VI).

*Case 139:* A 34-year-old housewife (anxiety reaction). After a series of thematically oriented preparatory autogenic abreactions, the patient's brain provides an integrative double image indicating that she basically had wished to marry Frank (which she had refused to admit), and that this was one of the reasons why her marriage with George did not work out.

"I think that is about the time mother had started the campaign: why don't you drop Frank . . . and I met George the following December, five or six months later. . . . I feel that gap is narrowing, it has to clinch together or that is where I will get an answer . . . and it was in the same spot, both incidents . . . symbolic gizmos . . . the hell with them . . . I feel the gap between that fall and the spring that I was engaged to George is very narrow, as if what? I am getting closer to the answer? . . . and I am afraid . . . it is stupid to be afraid to find out . . . are the two merging? I don't know . . . a very small part of me wants to stop it, I would say one-tenth . . . the rest . . . wants the answer . . . Damn it, what is it? . . . [crying] . . . why am I crying . . . why? It is still that room, it is still that semiobscurity or haziness or fuzziness . . . and that gap is closing more and more . . . *In a way, the two images are superimposed . . . one is as clear as the other, they are on the same level, they are of the same importance* . . . and *it is still not telling me anything . . . did I make it do it or did it happen* I don't know . . . George is sort of faded away and Frank took on importance . . . or became more predominant. . . ."

*Case 140:* A 33-year-old housewife (anxiety reaction, moderate depressive reaction, multiple phobias, ecclesiogenic syndrome). The following example (from AA 14) illustrates the pattern of neutralization characteristic for antithematic reversed (mother–son) Oedipus dynamics. After a period of violent aggression against her husband (see below), the brain shifted toward emphasis on affective and sexual dynamics involving her five-year-old son (Bobby).

"I push him into the furnace . . . I throw him into a stream, he crashes on the rocks . . . I throw garbage on him . . . Bobby and I, we drown him . . . we go with a lawn mower over him . . . and we take a scythe and cut him up with it . . . and push him into the water . . . I hide his books, so that he cannot find them, that he cannot read them anymore . . . I tear up his drawings . . . I cut all the bushes he planted around the house and I pull all the flowers out . . . Bobby and I, we eat what is reserved for him . . . now I understand why Bobby is so aggressive against his father, it's because he senses that I feel like that too, because he always tries to bother his father, taking things which belong to him, eating what was put aside for him . . . Bobby is taking more and more space in my heart . . . it seems that I transpose my erotic feelings onto Bobby . . . I caress Bobby, I embrace him affectionately, I make love to him. . . ."

*Remarks:* During her following appointment, two weeks later, the patient stated that after AA 14 she had noted a change in her attitude toward Bobby and his frequent desire to visit his aunt Mary. For the past two or three years, the patient never liked Bobby going to see his aunt whom he liked very much. She also knew that aunt Mary liked Bobby, and she felt quite jealous about this. Only recently she had told Bobby and Aunt Mary that such visits should be limited to one per month. The patient felt surprised that during the last two weeks she did not mind Bobby's visits any more and, on the contrary, she felt pleased about them and let him go whenever he wanted.

# 28. Thematic Verification

Brain-directed thematic verification may be considered as a specific type of thematic repetition which appears to be designed to verify whether various topics or sections of topics which were subjected to intensive processes of neutralization have been adequately neutralized or whether undesirable emotional or psychophysiologically oriented reactions are elicited and additional neutralization of certain thematic elements or phases is necessary (see Case 146, p. 328). Phases of thematic verification usually consist of thematically condensed versions of one or a number of disturbing themes in which cinerama-type autogenic abreactions are frequently presented in a pictorial telegram style, successively or in simultaneous presentation of thematically significant images which impress by a lack of dynamic features (see Case 141).

*Case 141:* A 49-year-old housewife (moderate depressive reaction, mild hypertension, overweight). During the initial phase of cinerama type neutralization of certain material which gave no indication for an impending shift toward a prolonged (10 min.) verification phase with postcard-like images covering central themes of about 25 AAs, the somewhat surprised patient gave the following out-of-context description.

"Now I see our cottage and our lake and everybody who was there last Sunday . . . I see all the pictures . . . everything . . . I see all the pictures like postcards . . . everything and I can't concentrate on one . . . all those pictures I always see . . . like postcards . . . and I see them all at once . . . the meadow, the fences, the horses . . . I just see all these pictures again . . . and our cottage . . . and myself swimming there, but I don't move, I am just in the lake . . ." (thematic shift).

In other instances thematically condensed filmstrips or a summarized version of earlier cinerama-type elaborations may be used (see Case 142, Case 143, Case 146, p. 328).

*Case 142:* A 30-year-old priest (sexual deviation, posttraumatic anxiety reaction, obsessive-compulsive reactions, multiple psychophysiologic reactions, ecclesiogenic syndrome). During AA 19 (cinerama with active self-participation), while talking to a brain-provided girl friend, a brief period of thematic verification involving three previously neutralized accidents is interjected. In contrast to earlier autogenic abreactions during which these accidents underwent neutralization in great detail with many repetitions and intensive emotional and psychophysiologic reactions, no further theme-related elaborations or disturbing reactions occurred during this period of thematic verification. After this, the original theme was taken up again and continued.

"For quite some time now I've felt the need to take off . . . and especially to not take any responsibility in face of life . . . *I see again many of the accidents*

*that I had . . . I see myself on the baseball field at school . . . hit on the face
with the bat . . . I see myself back home when I was five years old, the old
rattle-trap that runs over my body . . . enough to kill anybody . . . I see myself
on July 17, 1958 . . . getting knocked on the head when passing through a
door . . . I practically killed myself that time, I really hurt myself . . . that's
all. . . . Louise and I are still sitting on the bank of the river . . . she's
listening to me. . . ."*

*Case 143:* A 24-year-old student of theology (anxiety reaction, multiple
phobic and psychophysiologic reactions, ecclesiogenic syndrome). During AA
45, after an initial period of multithematic neutralization containing a number
of thematic elements which occurred many times before, the brain suddenly
interjected a verification phase. This consisted of a thematic sequence of
*static, photograph-like, superimposed* images which originally appeared in AA
2 and which at that time were associated with relatively strong emotional
reactions (e.g., apprehension, anxiety, restlessness, palpitations) and numerous
difficulties related to various forms of brain-antagonizing resistance. None of
these negatively loaded thematically related reactions occurred during the
verification phase (see the patient's comments, p. —). For direct comparison
relevant phases of AA 2 and AA 45 are given below.

*The patient's description of the initial part of AA 45:*
"I start out seeing a black disk within a yellow circle (the same one I saw
before during AA 41). This black disk transforms into a hole and this then
changes into hell . . . there I see black corpses . . . they are girls who are
burning me, especially my penis . . . then there is nothing. After this I am on
the ski slope where I was last Thursday . . . on the slope I fall and twist my
left leg and at that moment I experience pain in my left knee . . . after this
I change the skis and go downhill again and, because these skis are not as
good as the other ones, I cannot manage as well as with the others and I am
unable to stop . . . this is why I am afraid that I am going to crush against a
big rock . . . this rock changes into a hole and I find myself again in hell. . . .
There I see a number of naked girls lying on the floor . . . they are calcinated
by fire and look black like coal . . . among these girls I see Jack. . . . Then I
am on the beach of *N* . . . it is a nice summer morning . . . the sun is shining
and I let myself warm up by the sun . . . I see the tail of a fish which I throw
into the wood . . . then I am in a canoe on the same lake . . . after this I am
swimming across the *X* river . . . the water is nice and the river is very
beautiful . . . in the middle of the river I let myself drown, like it actually
happened about one year ago . . . after this I continue to swim across the
river. . . . Then I am again in hell and devils crush my head with a pick . . .
this is followed by a scene which I saw during AA 2 . . . this time, however, the
old images of AA 2 pass very fast and it appears to be only a sort of review of
those images which guided me to get out of the difficult situation . . . these
review images passed very rapidly *en bloc* and were rather of a dream-like
nature in the sense that *the images were superimposed instead of following in
sequence* as they developed originally during AA 2. For direct comparison I
continue the report of AA 45 with a parallel transcript of AA 2."

**Passages of the patient's description of AA 2**

"It is a desert and I ask Dr. *L.* to terminate . . . he suggests to go on . . . I get up and I can make a step, but the earth starts to give away There is only a thin layer of sand covering graves made of dry and rotten wood . . . with each step the boards come off and expose the coffins containing skeletons . . . I make another step and I crush another coffin, I sink into it and land with one foot on a skeleton which rises straight from its coffin and starts hitting my head with his head . . . as I want to look at him, he has disappeared . . . from there on it is the same thing all around me: skeletons and coffins which are ready to go at each of my steps . . . finally I succeed to get away from this area and manage to go up a small mound of grass . . . that is scarcely better, I discover that I am on an artificial mound of grass which surrounds a grave in a cemetery . . . on top of the grave there is a black coffin which opens by itself . . . the corpse is very ugly . . . he has a black-purplish-bluish face and is dressed in black . . . I did not know what to do at that point. Dr. L. suggested to give him water to drink . . . . He disappears at the moment I give him something to drink . . . I get up and walk around in the cemetery between two rows of corpses and south of the church toward the charnel house . . . I enter and I look around . . . there are coffins all around . . . I advance a bit . . . the door closes abruptly and I am a prisoner in a charnel house which seems to be made of lead all around . . . it is impossible for me to escape . . . in the center there is a coffin on black trestles . . . I approach, there is nobody in the coffin. . . . At that point Dr. L. asks me if I could try to lie down in the coffin. . . . I try, I walk around it and I walk around it again . . . without succeeding to get into the coffin . . . my knees are paralyzed when I try to get up and into it . . . suddenly one of the trestles gives away and the coffin falls down into a hole of its size, which is infinitely deep . . . the black coffin has now changed into a black pillar of the same size . . . I

"I am in the desert and I start walking . . . and. . . . I see boards giving away. . . . Exposing skeletons in the graves. . . .

Following this I am in a cemetery of *X* and I see a dark green lawn, but it is a lawn which surrounds a grave. . . .

Then I walk in the cemetery . . . toward the charnel house. . . .

And the door closes by itself. . . .

And I start hitting my head against the wall. . . .

**Passages of the patient's description of AA 2**

**Continued description of AA 45**

get closer and start hitting my head against it . . . the pillar is very soft and like a cork and my head sinks into it . . . I am caught and loose my breath a bit . . . then, the part in which my head got stuck falls down and I am in a small window and start breathing again . . . then I escape through the small window and get away from the charnel house by flying very high into the sky above the church . . . I loose my wings and I am about to fall exactly on the tip of the steeple of the church. . . . Dr. L. suggests a parachute and thus I can go down normally. . . . I end up on the road on the north side of the church and close to a house into which I intend to go . . . I go up the stairs and enter the house which is dark and humid . . . it is a house which has been abandoned for a long time . . . I make a step forward and the floor crushes and I find myself in a humid basement which is dirty and dark . . . there are black animals . . . I try to see and as I do that, the cellar becomes lighter . . . now it is a basement with cement walls, empty and absolutely clean . . . there is really nothing. . . . Dr. L. suggest I look into the corners, and there is a big corpse with a halloween pumpkin-like face . . . I crush it with one blow . . . then I see a coffin and I go over and open the lower part . . . I discover the lower part of a body . . . from the feet up to the lower part of the abdomen it appears to be transformed into a mass of tiny white worms . . . there is only the form of the body which seems to support the mass of mobile tiny worms. . . . At this point Dr. L. suggests to go and open the small window in the corner of the room. . . . I go there . . . the window is very badly located between the wall and a big cement pillar . . . as I am there the wall and the pillar move closer together and threaten to crush me . . . I look at the pillar, which then moves infinitely far away and, the window then becomes the end of a corridor-like room with daylight illumination . . . I want to walk in the corridor, but it changes abruptly into a steep slope which I fall down . . . I find myself at the bottom

Thus I make a little hole and leave by . . .

flying out. . . .
And I fall back on . . .

the road and . . . there is a house not far away . . .

where I fall down into a basement. . . .

And there I see a coffin in a corner . . . and in the coffin is a corpse . . . and the lower part of the body looks like a mass of tiny white worms. . . .

**Passages of the patient's description of AA 2**

of a sort of a well . . . it is very deep but the day-light is still visible above. . . . There is a ladder which I could use to get out of the humid and dark bottom of the well . . . I want to go up, but the bars are rotten and break and I fall back into the bottom of the well. . . . Dr. *L.* suggests to examine the bottom of the well very carefully because there might be something. . . . I look around and find behind me a rotten board which I can remove easily with my hands . . . I take it off and discover again a very ugly corpse which is lying there . . . he has a black-purplish-blue face and is dressed in black . . . it is myself . . I look at myself for quite a while and the corpse dis-appears . . . after this I want to go up and get out of the well . . . as I look up I see a big square block coming down right on my head . . . I fix the the cement block and it transforms into a car-ton which opens up at both ends . . . others fall on top and I am in a sort of long tube which is like a smaller version of the well . . . nothing happens and I am still in this tube made of cartons. . . . Dr. *L.* suggests I examine the carton . . . I scratch the carton and discover that the inner part is again filled with the same tiny white worms which I already saw in the coffin a little while ago. . . . An intervention of Dr. *L.* at this point seems to be of particular importance for the further development of this trip: [These tiny worms are they perhaps sperm?] . . . The answer is positive and the tube of carton boxes transforms into my penis . . . at this point the ejaculation starts . . . the well fills up to my knees and then empties by itself . . . and fills up again the same way . . . I taste the liquid . . . it has no taste . . . the well empties again and I try to go up . . . the opening of the well closes and I return . . . go down again and start over again . . . I drink the liquid and spit it out immediately . . . finally the well opens up and it is now clean . . . and has a cement wall . . . there is now an iron ladder, very solid and I can go up without difficulty. . . ."

These are sperm.

I succeed in getting out of this basement.

. . . by a prolonged ejacu-lation. . . ."

*The patient's comments:* "There seem to be some important differences between AA 2 and the review phenomenon in AA 45. The visual elaborations during AA 2 were very dynamic and various degrees of tension and anxiety accompanied the different phases. In AA 2 it was a process of a gradually developing discovery which went through various stages, multiple details and repetitions. The images were in sequence like a sort of cinerama and at that time I did not know what was going to happen next. The review during AA 45 was of a different nature. The phase of visual elaborations was comparatively short, up from a certain point I somehow knew what was going to happen, the images were *superimposed and static.* This reminds me of a fast review of an old story by looking at a series of old photographs. There was no tension and no anxiety during this period."

Phases of thematic verification have been seen during terminal elaborations at the end of highly differentiated and complex processes of neutralization of significantly disturbing material and at longer intervals covering a variable number of topics which underwent neutralization during series of autogenic abreaction. Both types of verification, the *immediate terminal verification* (see Case 144) and the *long-term verification* have many features in common. The elaborations which compose phases of terminal or long-term verification are of neutral or positively oriented nature. In contrast to their earlier versions they appear to be inoffensive. They are characterized by undistorted reality features and do not elicit any particular interest or any appreciable emotional or psychophysiologic reactions (e.g., crying, dizziness, palpitations, motor discharges, disgust, aggression, tension), and patients tend to express their now positively oriented feelings during or after such a thematic review (see Case 144). A particular feature of long-term verification phases is their unpredictable interjection into the mainstream of other processes of neutralization (see Case 141, p. 322; Case 143, p. 323; Case 145, Case 146, p. 328).

*Case 144:* A 49-year-old housewife (moderate depressive reaction, mild hypertension, overweight). After 64 minutes of cinerama-type reconfrontations with very disturbing material accumulated 25 years earlier, a terminal verification phase is elaborated.

"Now I see it all again, the sanatorium, the patients, the girls, the little house, and mother and myself sitting in the grass with Jack . . . it's like a stack of transparent postcards . . . I feel all right now . . . everything seems to be all right now . . . I feel very calm and relaxed. . . ." (termination).

*Case 145:* A 37-year-old housewife (anxiety reaction, multiple psychophysiologic reactions). In AA 46, during the central abreactive phase a brain-directed thematic shift interjected a reconfrontation with her childhood home. After briefly revisiting different rooms with some emphasis on her parents' bedroom which had appeared on many occasions during neutralization of brain-disturbing childhood material (e.g., sexual episode in mother's bed, father's death), the patient found herself suddenly outside and for the first time she pronounced a characteristic feeling of genuine disinterest in her childhood home.

"And again, there is something strange . . . I think it is that I felt as I did at that time (referring to childhood episode) . . . but I am not longing for it anymore . . . I just looked at the house . . . here is where I used to live . . . this is it . . . no desire to go in . . . there is not that longing anymore. . . ."

In case certain thematic components of material presented during a verification phase elicit undesirable emotional or psychophysiologic reactions, thus indicating that brain-desired levels of neutralization have not been attained in certain areas, the verification phase is followed by thematic re-engagement and relevant dynamics of neutralization (e.g., thematic repetitions; see Case 146).

*Case 146:* A 29-year-old housewife who was hit by a car (see Case 126, p. 294 ff.). During AA 28 after many difficult and disagreeable autogenic abreactions which were almost entirely devoted to neutralization of the accident material, a verification phase is presented in movie-like fashion. However, in this case, thematic neutralization is incomplete. For example, a thematically related transitory reaction (i.e., "My right ankle starts hurting") occurs, and one particular thematic section is filtered out to undergo additional neutralization (i.e., "The up-on-the-hood and falling-down phase") by thematic repetition.

"It is all like in a movie . . . I see myself walking there . . . but I am not there myself . . . I see myself limping in the movie . . . *and now my right ankle starts hurting, and there is a pain going down from my knee* . . . and there is the intersection, the East/West Street and the car and I am limping . . . but it is as if I dream all this . . . boring . . . it repeats itself again and again . . . in my unconscious it is as if I am fed up with all this, it is quite boring . . . always the same thing . . . it is as if I am sitting in a cinema and they play this movie . . . not interesting at all . . . it starts from the beginning, as I start walking across the East/West Street, and the car hits me . . . up on the hood . . . turning . . . falling down . . . lying on the pavement . . . limping to the snack bar . . . the snack bar . . . the ambulance, the hospital and then it starts over again and rather fast . . . this goes on and on, it is so boring I don't even bother to look at it, always the same thing . . . *now only a part of the film repeats itself, the up-on-the-hood and falling-down phase,* over and over again . . . and now it is not a movie anymore, it is as if I do it myself . . . up on the hood, turning and falling down . . . it slows down now and I am getting so tired . . . I perform this like a sort of gymnastic exercise . . . now I have to force myself to do it, I am so tired . . . now I remain lying on the pavement, I can't go on anymore, I am so tired . . . now I see the same thing again as in a movie. . . ."

# 29. Thematic Termination

Essential features of elaborations which are characteristic for dynamics of thematic termination as, for example, those occurring during terminal phases of autogenic abreactions have been presented in the chapter *Terminal Phase* (see p. 76 ff.). Other phenomena which are associated with the self-regulatory dynamics of thematic termination have been discussed in connection with thematic verification (see p. 322 ff.).

When processes of neutralization have reached a terminal phase after a relatively short period (e.g., 15 min. after the beginning of the abreactive period), it is advisable not to apply the standard termination procedure immediately, but to wait and see what is going to happen. In most instances, after a phase with relatively neutral or agreeable elaborations, the brain will engage in another topic of neutralization. When such a thematic shift does not occur and patterns characteristic for delayed termination (see p. 84 ff.) are elaborated or the patient falls asleep, it is appropriate to apply the standard termination procedure at a convenient point. When a Bright Light Phase (see Vol. VI) or phenomena of similar nature (see Case 27, p. 86) occur during the central abreactive phase, there is usually an indication that decisive progress in neutralization of particularly disturbing thematic elements has been achieved. However, such interjected Bright Light Phase (or similar elaborations) may be, but are not necessarily, a manifestation of thematic termination.

The termination of neutralization of minor elements or sections of thematically more complex material usually ensues in an uneventful manner by (a) simply disappearing from the brain-designed program of thematic neutralization or by (b) becoming a normalized integral part of more complex sections of the same topic. Only when larger portions of very complex material or when a number of interrelated areas of disturbing material have reached brain-desired levels of neutralization do characteristic terminal phase elaborations (see p. 78 ff., Table 17, p. 83) and brain-designed phenomena of thematic verification tend to occur.

Phases of thematic verification are assumed to be manifestations which, apart from performing a self-controlling screening function, indicate that brain-desired levels of neutralization and certain functional readjustments have been achieved for the time. This hypothesis implies that the originally existing pathofunctional potency of accumulated disturbing material has been reduced to levels which permit improved functions at more adequate levels of integration. Such developments are associated with improvements of the patient's psychodynamic and psychophysiologic reactivity. However, for now, it is not believed that even where previously existing psychodynamic and psychophysiologic deviations of reactivity have disappeared for prolonged periods (e.g., months, years) that processes of autogenic neutralization can erase the physiologic manifestations of recorded disturbing material. It is assumed that successively neutralized areas of disturbing material are not completely inactive but that they continue their interference-generating activities at a significantly lower level. This assumption is supported by observations which showed that relatively short and transitory processes of thematic reneutralization have occurred after longer intervals (e.g., months, years) of "thematic silence" of disturbing material which, according to phases of thematic verification and other evidence (e.g., thematic silence, clinical improvements), had reached brain-desired levels of neutralization. This seems to indicate that the brain needs to be given adequate opportunity to re-engage periodically in transitory and brief processes of thematic reneutralization of still existing records of disturbing material. Since sufficiently intelligent and technically experienced patients can do so whenever they want, periodic thematic reneutralization may be similar to the practice of autogenic exercises, considered as a benecial form of mental hygiene.

# Author Index

# Subject Index